Early Diagnosis and Interventional Therapy in Cerebral Palsy

PEDIATRIC HABILITATION

Series Editor

ALFRED L. SCHERZER
Cornell University Medical Center
New York, New York

ADDITIONAL VOLUMES IN PREPARATION

Early Diagnosis and Interventional Therapy in Cerebral Palsy

An Interdisciplinary Age-Focused Approach

Third Edition

edited by

Alfred L. Scherzer

Joan and Sanford I. Weill Medical College
Cornell University
New York, New York

MARCEL DEKKER, INC.   NEW YORK · BASEL

βS

The previous edition was published as *Early Diagnosis and Therapy in Cerebral Palsy: A Primer on Infant Developmental Problems, Second Edition, Revised and Expanded* by Alfred L. Scherzer and Ingrid Tscharnuter.

ISBN: 0-8247-6006-9

This book is printed on acid-free paper.

Headquarters
Marcel Dekker, Inc.
270 Madison Avenue, New York, NY 10016
tel: 212-696-9000; fax: 212-685-4540

Eastern Hemisphere Distribution
Marcel Dekker AG
Hutgasse 4, Postfach 812, CH-4001 Basel, Switzerland
tel: 41-61-261-8482; fax: 41-61-261-8896

World Wide Web
http://www.dekker.com

The publisher offers discounts on this book when ordered in bulk quantities. For more information, write to Special Sales/Professional Marketing at the headquarters address above.

Current printing (last digit):
10 9 8 7 6 5 4 3 2 1

PRINTED IN THE UNITED STATES OF AMERICA

3/22/05

Preface to the Third Edition

How surprising to recall that the first edition of *Early Diagnosis and Therapy in Cerebral Palsy* was published in 1982. With the tools then available, clinical focus on diagnosis of the very young child seems, in retrospect, more a hope than a serious endeavor. Yet the volume was well received and led to a second edition in 1990. The interim changes reflected more experience with the very young child, and a shift in focus, away from the older established schools of therapy toward more activist, invasive treatments.

Preparing the third edition has revealed truly remarkable changes. These changes are reflected in a slight revision of the title. Fundamental research at the molecular and cellular levels has advanced our understanding of mechanisms involved in etiology and epidemiology. Developmental neurology has extended our understanding of normal and abnormal behavior of the early preterm infant. Screening and assessment have become more sophisticated, with an exponential increase in the number of standardized instruments. The developmental screening and evaluation process has matured considerably, with the availability of very sensitive neuroradiologic tools. The accumulation of clinical experience with the very young child has enabled a more directed approach to infant differential diagnosis.

Interventional therapy has also moved forward in many new and different directions. Therapy has become oriented more toward a dynamical systems approach, emphasizing functional change, and maintaining physiological conditioning. Advances in the use of botulinum toxin, intrathecal baclofen, and selective dorsal rhizotomy to reduce spasticity have taken center stage, without uniform criteria for either individual or sequential application, or clear evidence of long-term effects. Cerebral palsy has increasingly found itself a prime target for alternative treatments during this era.

Perhaps the most startling innovation in the decade since the last edition has been advances in research. Outcomes research, including an indication of the strength of evidence, has emerged in this period, and has just begun to influence the field of cerebral palsy.

This third edition reflects these dramatic changes. We focus on the infant from birth to three years in order to highlight specific concerns about diagnosis and treatment in this group. This approach provides a model for dealing with older age group categories as well. It is apparent that an understanding of how to deal most effectively with the individual with cerebral palsy can best be approached through consideration of the options for the specific age group involved.

The authors comprise a truly interdisciplinary group that has worked to prepare this volume in much the same collaborative way that they would to treat an infant with cerebral palsy. We all feel it is a privilege to bring forward these important changes in the field at the start of a new century.

Alfred L. Scherzer

Preface to the Second Edition

The first edition of *Early Diagnosis and Therapy in Cerebral Palsy,* issued in 1982, sought to fill a major need for professionals in bringing together in one source comprehensive information regarding diagnosis and management of the very young child with cerebral palsy. At the same time, we hoped to demonstrate how this framework might serve equally in developing programs for other types of nonprogressive deficits with similar needs. That we succeeded in filling this gap is well illustrated by the wide use of this text over the years and its continued demand by a variety of professionals.

In the years since the original issue, there have been many new and exciting developments in the field. Among these of major interest are new approaches to early screening and identification, refinements in concepts and approaches to therapy, considerations of alternative surgical approaches to treatment, and an explosion in early intervention strategies increasingly based more on an educational than on a traditional medical model.

Clearly the time has come to incorporate these developments into this text which has found much favor with our colleagues. We therefore take pleasure in bringing forth this second edition with the hope that it will continue to fill the needs of those devoted to the care of the handicapped child in this ever-changing field.

Alfred L. Scherzer
Ingrid Tscharnuter

Preface to the First Edition

Until relatively recent years, cerebral palsy was primarily of professional interest to a limited number of specialists dealing with specific aspects of treatment, such as orthopedics and neurology. Indeed, these are the specialties which initially shaped its definition and scope, dating from the days of Little and Freud. Children came to attention late, when significant limitations in development and milestones were noted, or severe orthopedic deficits were apparent. Intervention was frequently concerned with static neurologic assessment, and treatment often exclusively focused upon orthopedic surgery or a form of limited individual muscle therapy. The approach was to deal with the specific functional deficits as they appeared.

A much broader concept has subsequently emerged with the awareness that cerebral palsy represents a major multidisciplinary developmental disorder in which timely intervention by a variety of specialties is essential, and a coordinated, directed approach is required. In addition, traditional therapy involving individual muscle training has given way—mostly through clinical work with cerebral palsy—to a more comprehensive and dynamic approach of movement education which emphasizes the sensorimotor duality and is therefore conducive to learning new motor skills. Clinical experience with cerebral palsy has also promoted an expansion in the understanding of sensorimotor development. Today, abnormal motor behavior typically associated with cerebral palsy is seen as the outcome of a long process of postural compensations to underlying deficits, such as abnormal postural tonus or poor integration of postural reflexes. While early and primary postural compensations consist of more subtle deviations from the norm, motor skills building on these deviant patterns become more and more abnormal.

Newer knowledge concerning infant development and recognition of early common findings among infants with nonprogressive central nervous system deficits has now placed cerebral palsy within the spectrum of major developmental disabilities. In fact, its early identification and management presently serve as a model for other types of multiply handicapping conditions.

Recent perinatal management and neonatal intensive care technologies have further influenced the outlook for the child with potential disability. Children are now surviving who until recently had an abysmal prognosis. Evidence indicates a reduction, as well, in degree of disability, although an increase in severity is suggested especially among those high-risk and low-birth-weight infants who formerly did not survive. It seems likely that chronic developmental disorders in children are destined to be a major and increasing concern for pediatrics of the future.

It is in this setting that the concepts of early diagnosis and intervention have taken root and a sizable literature has emerged. Current data are clinically supportive of early intervention and the notion is intuitively appealing on the basis of developmental theory. An explosive interest has been generated in this field, yet there is a paucity of sources available for comprehensive reference and documentation.

The present text attempts to fill this gap by putting into perspective the evolution of cerebral palsy from a narrow focus as an orthopedic disability to a broadly conceived developmental disorder. The emphasis is on the process of developmental diagnosis, and current clinical approaches to evaluation, management, and treatment are detailed. The need for continuous, systematic, and standardized re-evaluation is stressed. Suggestions are made for developing research methods which will ultimately lead to establishing the effectiveness of any given treatment approach.

It is hoped that the text will provide a useful guide for those who deal with a wide variety of developmental disabilities in young children. Considerable emphasis is placed on identifying early patterns of postural maladjustments so that they can be corrected as far as possible before leading to more severe abnormalities. Its focus is to provide a more uniform and standardized approach to diagnosis and treatment. Only in this way will it be possible to objectively evaluate and guide individual therapy activities. Ultimately, this will greatly aid in the much needed quest for research methodologies and firm data concerning the early intervention process.

Alfred L. Scherzer
Ingrid Tscharnuter

Contents

Contributors

Margaret J. Barry, P.T., M.S., P.C.S. Assistant Professor, Department of Physical Therapy, Youngstown State University, Youngstown, Ohio

Charlene Butler, Ed.D. Health and Special Education Consultant, Seattle, Washington

Judy M. Gardner, M.A., CCC-SLP Speech Pathologist, DuPage Easter Seals, Villa Park, Illinois

Gay L. Girolami, P.T., M.S. Executive Director, Pathways Center, Glenview, Illinois

Vidya Bhushan Gupta, M.D., M.P.H., F.A.A.P. Associate Professor of Clinical Pediatrics, Metropolitan Hospital Center, New York Medical College, New York, New York

Diane Fritts Ryan, OTR/L Occupational Therapist, DuPage Easter Seals, Villa Park, Illinois

Alfred L. Scherzer, Ed.D., M.D., F.A.A.P. Clinical Professor Emeritus of Pediatrics, Joan and Sanford I. Weill Medical College, Cornell University, New York, New York

1
History, Definition, and Classification of Cerebral Palsy

Alfred L. Scherzer
Joan and Sanford I. Weill Medical College, Cornell University, New York, New York

I. CEREBRAL PALSY IN HISTORICAL PERSPECTIVE

A. Ancient Egypt

As with most human phenomena, the earliest documentation of cerebral palsy goes back to the ancient Egyptians. A tablet in the Temple in Memphis dating from the fifth century BC memorializes its adult male caretaker who has characteristics consistent with spastic right hemiplegia (1) (Fig.1). Features suggestive of spastic diplegia during this period have also been uncovered by the French neurologist, Charcot (2) (Fig. 2).

B. Elizabethan Times

Evidence that the condition was well known and perhaps not an uncommon occurrence in Elizabethan times is found in the work of Shakespeare. In Richard III, Gloucester sets the stage for the tragedy by first identifying his feelings of anger and frustration at being born prematurely, and describing the stigmata of cerebral palsy (3):

> I that am curtailed of this fair proportion,
> Cheated of feature by dissembling Nature,
> Deform'd, unfinish'd, sent before my time
> Into this breathing world, scarce half made up,
> And that so lamely and unfashionable

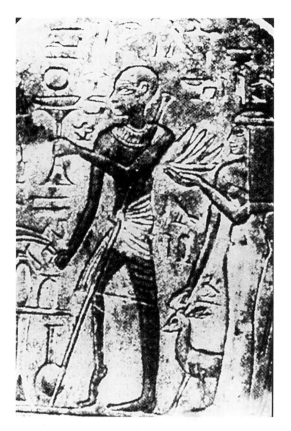

Figure 1 Caretaker of the Temple in Memphis (fifth century BC) with characteristics of spastic right hemiplegia. (From Ref. 1.)

> That dogs bark at me as I halt by them;
> Why, I, in this weak piping time of peace,
> Have no delight to pass away the time,
> Unless to spy my shadow in the sun
> And decant on mine own deformity;
> (Act I, Scene I, lines 18–27)

C. The Nineteenth Century

While the physician Cazauvielh was the first European to study cerebral paralysis scientifically (4), it was the French orthopedic surgeon, Delpech, who is credited with expressing the earliest professional interest in cerebral palsy. His influence

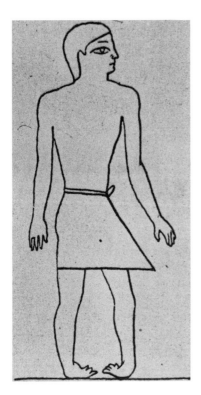

Figure 2 Cerebral palsy in ancient Egypt. A crippled individual with deformities of the feet and atrophy of the extremities suggestive of spastic diplegia. From an ancient Egyptian monument (Charcot and Richer, Les difformes et les malades dans l'art, 1889.)

later helped form the basis for modern treatment. Delpech was also concerned with the deformities resulting from poliomyelitis. His description of the tendo-achilles lengthening for equinus was the first published in the literature (5).

The procedure caught the interest of John Little, an English orthopedist, who as a child had contracted polio, which left a residual equinus deformity (Fig. 3). Little consulted Delpech about the operation, but was discouraged by the possibility of complicating infection. Instead, Little went to Germany, where the procedure was also being performed by George Stromeyer (Fig. 4), and under-went the operation. The successful correction of his lifelong deformity and the care he received from Stromeyer made a deep impression on Little. He subse-quently devoted himself to perfecting the procedure upon his return to England, and later even named his third son in honor of his German colleague and mentor (6).

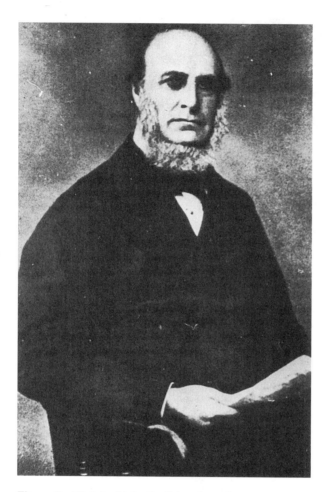

Figure 3 W. John Little, English orthopedist whose studies of cerebral palsy provided the first data on etiology.

As his practice developed (7), Little took an increasing interest in the correction of various deformities in children. He began to recognize many associated with paralysis, and particularly with generalized spasticity (8). His definitive work in 1861 (Fig. 5) drew upon 20 years of experience and documented possible correlations between abnormality of pregnancy, labor, delivery, and subsequent developmental deficit (Fig. 6) (9). Little reasoned that spasticity and deformity were primarily due to cerebral hemorrhage and anoxia secondary to trauma of

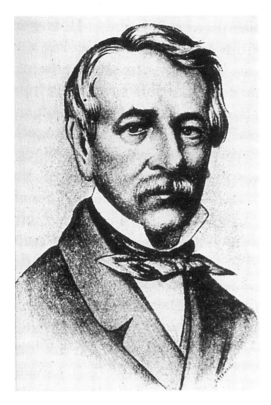

Figure 4   George Stromeyer (1804–1876) mentor and long-time colleague of W. John Little. (From Ref. 6.)

the birth process (Fig. 7). Thus the entity later to be known as Little's Disease became established.

It is of interest that neuropathological autopsy evidence from children with congenital hemiplegia appeared to be inconsistent at the time (10, 11), and clearly was a factor in professional resistance to Little's findings. Osler was eventually able to show a neuroanatomical correlation of structural brain pathology and spastic paralysis (12).

Interest in the condition spread to other medical disciplines. Gowers was among the earliest physicians to support Little's view that the etiology of cerebral palsy was trauma to the brain at or near term (13). Sigmund Freud, initially a practicing neurologist concerned with children, became greatly interested in the relationship between nonprogressive neurological deficits and prematurity

ON THE INFLUENCE OF ABNORMAL PARTURITION,

DIFFICULT LABOURS, PREMATURE BIRTH, AND ASPHYXIA NEONATORUM, ON THE MENTAL AND PHYSICAL CONDITION OF THE CHILD, ESPECIALLY IN RELATION TO DEFORMITIES*

W. J. LITTLE, M.D.

Senior Physician to the London Hospital; Founder of the Royal Orthopædic Hospital;
Visiting-Physician to Asylum for Idiots, Earlswood, etc.

(Communicated by DR. TYLER SMITH.)

Figure 5   Title page of Little's historic paper in 1861. (From Ref. 9.)

Abstract of Cases of Spastic Rigidity. Labour Abnormal or Premature, or Asphyxia at Birth.

Case No.	Initials and Date	Age (Yr.)	Description when First Seen	History obtained from Parents, etc.
I	Esther T. (78.)	4	Contraction of flexors and adductors of lower extremities slight; left particularly affected.	Mother confined at seventh month of gestation through over-fatigue. Strabismus convergens of left eye. (A later child subject to fits; another never rallied at birth.)
II	Frances Ann F. 1840 (80.)	7	Spastic rigidity of adductors and flexors of thighs, flexors of knees, and posterior muscles of legs; left most affected.	Mother's first pregnancy; at full period; labour tedious and difficult, but "straight". Mother suffered from fright 2 months before confinement; never felt movements of fœtus afterwards. Child stuporous, or alternately crying or convulsed, 4-5 days after birth. Unable to suck until 5 days old. Ran alone on toes at 4 years. Intellect unaffected. "Irritable nervous system." General appearance of irregular muscular action.
III	Lydia C. April 1844 (81.)	6	Spastic contraction of lower extremities; knees separable 1 foot. Gastrocnemii. especially left, much contracted. Left arm contracted, but extensible. Makes slight attempts to walk.	Mother had great anxiety during gestation; a fright 2 days before confinement: Child insensible 2 or 3 days after birth. "Fits" after birth. Strabismus. Constipated. Says "mamma" and "papa" only. Expresses aversion and pleasure. Idiotic. Died suddenly in convulsions a month after report. Had previous convulsions occasionally, apparently excited by loaded stomach.

Figure 6   Data from Little's paper. (From Ref. 9.)

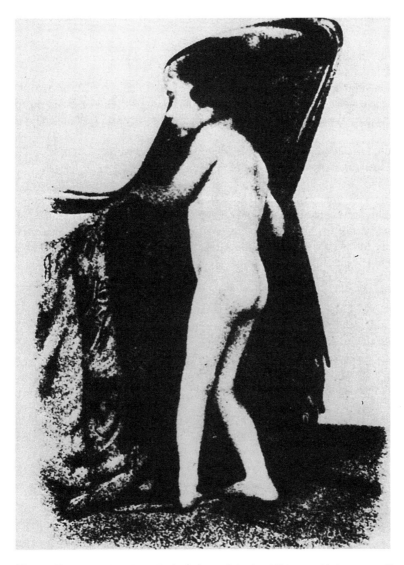

Figure 7 Little related paralysis and spasticity in children to birth trauma (from Ref. 9). Caption under original photo reads: Contraction of adductors and flexors of lower extremities. Left and weak. Both hands awkward. More paralytic than spastic. Born with navel-string around neck. Asphyxia neonatorum one hour. See Case XLII.

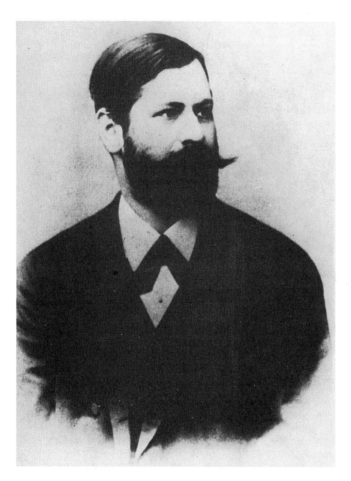

Figure 8   Sigmund Freud studied nonprogressive neurological deficits and prematurity in children.

(Fig. 8). He was well aware of Little's causal conceptualization of birth abnormality and spastic paralysis, but placed greater etiological emphasis on intrauterine developmental abnormality and less on birth trauma (14). To this day, Little's concern with birth trauma, and Freud's emphasis on abnormal intrauterine growth, remain as the two basic etiological pillars of *congenital* cerebral palsy (15).

Recognition of an association between infection and the development of permanent brain abnormality in previously normal children had also appeared about this time (16, 17). These studies provided the roots for a growing awareness of *acquired* cerebral palsy as a discrete entity.

D. Pre World War II

The interest in identification and etiology of spastic conditions initiated in the latter part of the nineteenth century maintained only limited momentum early into the twentieth century. Specific approaches to treatment were also slow in developing and had relatively little impact. Physical therapy made a start in the United States through the work of Jennie Colby at Children's Hospital in Boston (18). Colby was a gymnast with an interest in massage therapy, which she channeled into developing remedial exercises for a variety of paralytic conditions. Her work was purely empirical and was incorporated into the program of the newly emerging neurology clinic established by Crothers (19); new concepts in psychology and mental health were also contributed by Elizabeth Lord (20).

Orthopedic surgery to correct specific deformities gained greater popularity through the work of Stoffel, who early perfected neurectomy as a specific procedure for managing contractures (21). Surgery was viewed enthusiastically because of the easily measurable, immediate, and selected improvement. However, initial surgical benefit was often followed by disappointing long-term results.

As the psychological, developmental, neurological, and surgical considerations became more apparent, a broader approach was needed. The impetus began with Crothers and the interdisciplinary model in Boston. It was greatly expanded upon by Winthrop Phelps, an orthopedist who became devoted to finding ways to meet the needs of handicapped children, and who ultimately established a comprehensive community rehabilitation center in Maryland (22). Phelps developed the multispecialty approach in the period before World War II, when interest within the medical field was relatively scarce.

E. The Modern Era

The years immediately following World War II saw a merger of the extensive experience gained during the conflict with rehabilitation medicine, and rapid maturation in a variety of related medical specialties. Renewed interest in the handicapped child became apparent in a number of professional groups. Community demands for action began to stir. The National Society for Crippled Children and Adults (Easter Seal Society) established a Cerebral Palsy Division in 1946 with a National Advisory Medical Council. This group of professionals soon recognized the need for a forum for interdisciplinary information and exchange of ideas.

It was in this setting, in 1947 that the American Academy for Cerebral Palsy

(AACP) was born in Chicago (23). Conceived as a multispecialty professional organization to stimulate research and training in the field of the handicapped child, the AACP joined together the major medical disciplines with related therapeutic, educational, and psychological services. The founders, all of whom were in the original Easter Seal Group, had become convinced that only through a combined effort could there be any hope of having measurable impact (Fig. 9). The founders of the Academy included Phelps, who was the first president, Temple Fay (neurophysiologist), Bronson Crothers (neurologist), Meyer Perlstein (pediatrician), George Deaver (physiatrist), and Earl Carlson (internist). What started as a small forum for discussion and interprofessional education was the beginning of a midcentury resurgence of interest and effort on behalf of the handicapped child (24).

Demand for local services and facilities occurred simultaneously. A local cerebral palsy committee was established in New York in 1948 (25). It sponsored local hospital diagnostic services and provided treatment and educational pro-

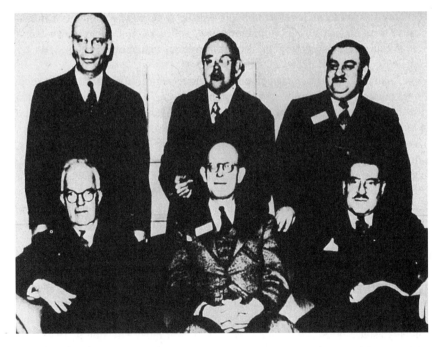

Figure 9 The founders of the American Academy for Cerebral Palsy, 1947. Standing (left to right). Dr. George Deaver (physiatrist), Dr. Earl Carlson (internist), Dr. Meyer Perlstein (pediatrician). Seated (left to right): Dr. Bronson Crothers (neurologist), Dr. Winthrop Phelps (orthopedist), Dr. Temple Fay (neurophysiologist).

grams based largely on the model developed in Maryland by Phelps in the 1930s. A New York State and, ultimately, a national United Cerebral Palsy Association followed, with chapters subsequently developing throughout the United States (26).

Of necessity, the emphasis of these programs was on diagnosis and treatment of the child with established deficits, frequently with severe deformity of a long-standing nature. Children were being seen with degrees of deformity comparable to Little's reports of the previous century. The difference lay in awareness that an approach much broader than orthopedics alone was needed. In addition to the medical specialties, psychological services, and therapies, serious effort was now made to provide appropriate special education, and supportive social services programs. Services have subsequently developed in a multitude of community clinics and agencies for children with all kinds of developmental problems, and identification of affected individuals has become more efficient. There has also been an increasing trend away from a rehabilitative to a "habilitative" approach. The aim is to employ whatever means are necessary to bring a child to a level of maximum potential in all areas of development, and particularly to ensure functional independence as an individual.

Technological developments in perinatal care starting from the late 1960s and early 1970s (27) have given further impetus to this concept. Improved obstetrical management of the high-risk mother is now widely available and complements a system of intensive neonatal care aimed at reducing mortality significantly and lower morbidity from neurological and developmental deficit. A significantly greater number of infants formerly classified as "at risk" are now surviving, and more effective methods of early identification of neurological abnormality enhance this trend. Although still imperfect in many respects, the present system of care in the western world has generally "caught up" with the late case of the untreated child having multiple deficits. In this respect, the goals of the 1950s to treat those with existing definitive handicaps are being met. As in the management of many medical conditions, the initial emphasis and interest lie with the most obvious and severe forms of the condition. As these become treated and greater understanding of cause is approached, emphasis will be placed on more subtle forms and, finally, on earlier diagnosis and treatment. So it is with cerebral palsy as we enter a new century.

Contributions from the areas of developmental psychology and neurology, and the experience of transdisciplinary methods with very young children, have also become particularly influential (28). A parallel and logical outcome is the development of early interventional treatment. The data on the effect of early intervention have been emerging since the 1970s (29) and infants are now increasingly being referred as a standard procedure of care.

In little more than 100 years there has been a virtual revolution in concept and thought concerning cerebral palsy. Conceived initially as an orthopedic deficit with a neurological basis, it has come to be recognized as a multihandicapping condition requiring the attention of many specialties and services. More importantly, cerebral palsy is currently seen as a major disorder in *development*, which emerges as the child grows, and requires very early identification and management. Thus, what had been approached initially and for many years largely from an orthopedic perspective has emerged as the prototype of nonprogressive developmental disability. This has facilitated a better understanding in management of the full range of infant developmental problems.

Recognition of this broader concept was given in 1977 when the AACP officially became the American Academy for Cerebral Palsy and Developmental Medicine (AACPDM) (30). Little's early concern with physical deformity alone has thus expanded, at last, to an appreciation of the full range of developmental disabilities in the affected child.

II. TOWARD A DEFINITION OF CEREBRAL PALSY

Confusion continues to exist concerning the term cerebral palsy and its generally accepted meaning. Cerebral palsy refers to a nonprogressive central nervous system deficit. The lesion may be in single or multiple locations of the brain, resulting in definite motor and some degree of sensory abnormality, as well as other associated disabilities. It occurs as a result of in utero factors or events at the time of labor and delivery (congenital cerebral palsy), or a variety of factors in the early developing years (acquired cerebral palsy). A well-established estimate of case distribution suggests 85% for the congenital form and 15% for the acquired type (31). Burgess was the first to make use of the term "cerebral palsy" in 1888 (32). Soon after it appeared in the English literature by Osler (12) and Sachs and Peterson (16); in France it was used by Brissaud (33), and in Germany by Rosenberg (34) and Freud (35). Phelps was the major popularizer of the term in the United States. In conjunction with Phelps' work in developing a comprehensive treatment program, cerebral palsy came to be known as the major nonprogressive motor deficit occurring in children (36).

The AACPDM and the United Cerebral Palsy Associations have both reinforced the neurodevelopmental aspects of the definition (37). Confusion of terms and overlap with other nonprogressive central nervous system (CNS) disorders may be present. The distinction in cerebral palsy is that it is a *static brain lesion* resulting in *motor* deficit with associated handicaps. The primary *motor* nature of the condition provides a clear distinction from other static encephalopathies such as mental retardation syndromes, organic brain deficits, attention deficit/hyperactivity disorders, and the pervasive developmental disorders.

That the motor features of cerebral palsy may change with development is a well-recognized phenomenon, and is reflected in the following definition proposed at the 1990 international meeting on epidemiology held in Brioni, Yugoslavia: "... an umbrella term covering a group of non-progressive, but often changing, motor impairment syndromes secondary to lesions or anomalies of the brain arising in the early stages of its development" (38).

III. CLASSIFICATION OF CEREBRAL PALSY

A. Motor Types

The type of motor deficit in cerebral palsy may take several forms. Neuroanatomical association with the clinical syndrome may be highly varied and differs with maturity of the fetus or infant at the time of insult (39). The *spastic* variety is most common and generally correlates with a fixed lesion in the motor portion of the cerebral cortex.

The *dystonic* form, commonly referred to as *athetoid* cerebral palsy, reflects involvement in the extrapyramidal system. Frequently there is intermittent tension of trunk or extremities and a variety of uninhibited movement patterns, which sometimes have been the basis for confusion in classification. The Dystonia Medical Research Foundation has attempted to clarify and standardize use of the term, but does not specifically deal with the movement disorder that has a developmental etiology (40).

Pathological correlation with nonprogressive *ataxia* relates variably to a cerebellar pathways lesion, but is often uncertain (41). Abnormalities of cerebellar function are frequently associated with other disturbances of the CNS (42).

Mixed types are now increasingly diagnosed. These may include combinations of spasticity with dystonia or ataxia. Indeed, the concept that a single and discrete focus of abnormality is found in most cases of cerebral palsy has been seriously questioned (43). Nevertheless, the generally accepted clinical practice is to identify the predominant type that is exhibited.

Rigidity is a form previously identified fairly commonly, but it may have been confused with a severe degree of tension dystonia. It may possibly represent a severe decerebrate lesion.

B. Distribution

The clinical neurological lesion has variable distribution. Table 1 lists descriptive terms relating to distribution in common use.

C. Severity

Severity must also be considered as a basis for description and a guide for prognosis and treatment. About one-third of patients have generally been considered to

Table 1 Distribution of Cerebral Palsy Types

Location	Description
Monoplegia	One extremity
Hemiplegia	Upper and lower extremity on one side
Paraplegia	Both lowers
Diplegia	Quadriplegia with mild upper involvement
Quadriplegia	Equal involvement of uppers and lowers

be equally distributed among the mild, moderate, and severely involved categories. A review of severity in relation to etiology is found in Chapter 2.

Clinical judgment of severity in the very young infant can be difficult, but the Gross Motor Function Classification System developed by Palisano et al. provides helpful guidelines for children under and above age 2 (44). A description of the levels involved in the classification system is given in the Appendix.

D. Approaches to Classification

Type, distribution, and severity are essential components of the cerebral palsy diagnosis. They give meaning and direction to treatment and management of the patient, and provide a more uniform understanding of the problem than simply referring to a static motor encephalopathy. They also provide some estimate of prognosis.

Classification and uniformity of diagnostic description has always been controversial (45). Rosenberg was the first to tackle the problem (34). He included categories of generalized rigidity, paraplegic rigidity, bilateral spastic hemiplegia, bilateral athetosis, chorioform diplegia, and atypical forms. Freud and Rie (35) made a slight refinement, giving more recognition to athetosis. Categories included spastic hemiplegia, generalized rigidity, paraplegic rigidity, paraplegic paralysis, double hemiplegia, generalized chorea, and bilateral athetosis. These were the only classifications available until the mid-twentieth century and were largely the basis for understanding and describing the lesions up to that time.

The modern era in classification dates from the work of Fay in 1950 (46), who attempted to correlate the clinical expression of the motor deficit with anatomical location and pathophysiology; adding his understanding of subtypes, served to encumber the system beyond practical use (Table 2).

Phelps greatly refined these categories into a simpler and more practical clinical scheme (47). He included, flaccid paralysis, spasticity, rigidity, tremor,

Table 2 Cerebral Palsy Classification of Fay (1950)

1. Spastic paralysis–cerebral: nonspastic paralysis; atonic type.
2. Athetosis–midbrain: Deafness, tension; nontension; hemiplegia; tremor; cerebral release, emotional release, head, neck, arm; shudder-type; rotary-type, dystonia-type,
   flail-type.
3. Tremors and rigidities–basal ganglia: Parkinsonism types; decerebrate types.
4. Ataxia: Cerebellar, kinesthetic.
5. High spinal: Spastic-medulla.
6. Mixed: Diffuse.

Source: Ref. 46.

athetosis, and ataxia. This system was much more workable and useful just at
the time of resurgence of interest and community activity in the field. Phelps'
approach was slightly expanded and further refined by Perlstein (48), while Balf
and Ingram emphasized body parts most involved (49). In their clasic study of
cerebral palsy, Crothers and Payne preferred to divide cases into spastic, "extrapyramidal," and mixed types. The extrapyramidal category included athetosis,
chorea, dystonia, and ballismus (50).

The influence of these investigators was strong in the subsequent classification prepared by Minear for the American Academy for Cerebral Palsy. Distribution and degree of involvement, extent of treatment required, as well as motor
types were also included for the first time (51) (Table 3).

Some ambiguity exists in several of the Minear motor types (e.g., the distinction between tremor athetosis and a separate tremor category). How does
tremor differ from ataxia? Is there a physiological equivalent of atonia or is this
part of a developmental stage from which one of the other types ultimately

Table 3 Cerebral Palsy Classification of Minear (1956)

Spasticity
Athetosis tension; nontension, dys-
   tonia, tremor
Rigidity
Ataxia
Tremor
Atonia (rare)
Mixed
Unclassified

Source: Ref. 51.

Table 4 Brioni Cerebral Palsy Classification (1990)

Spastic	Hemiplegia
	Tetraplegia
	Diplegia
Ataxic	Diplegia
	Congenital (simple)
Dyskinetic	Mainly choreoathetotic
	Mainly dystonic

Source: Ref. 38.

emerges? Are some motor patterns unclassifiable because they are transient developmental features that change to other forms or eventually disappear?

The relevancy of these questions becomes apparent when we consider that the Minear classification was developed at a time when cerebral palsy was diagnosed late and solely on the recognition of a fixed motor deficit type. The developmental characteristics of the condition, and especially the emerging nature of the neurological lesion, were not then well appreciated. Depending upon the age at which a child was initially seen, the motor features would be variably evident.

At the 1990 Brioni meeting, the classification in Table 4 was proposed for simplicity and to enable epidemiological reporting (38).

Classifications suggested previously by Badell-Ribera (52) and more recently by Yokochi (53) have emphasized both degree of motor impairment and ambulatory status, but likewise have not dealt with the developing expression of the motor lesion in cerebral palsy.

Identification and referral of the infant who is not developing normally now provides an opportunity for very early diagnosis and management. A modern classification of cerebral palsy must consider its early developing signs and recognition of the emerging motor type. Such a classification could help to dispel confusion regarding diagnosis and provide better communication among the various professionals dealing with the child. An attempt is made to develop a basis for such an approach in Chapter 3.

IV. ASSOCIATED CONDITIONS

While the motor deficit in cerebral palsy is predominant, a number of associated conditions are frequently present and must be considered in the overall developmental needs of the affected child. These include abnormalities of vision, hearing and speech, seizure disorders, learning disabilities among the vast majority, and frequent social, emotional, and interfamily problems (54). Mental retardation is not necessarily present with cerebral palsy, but is more likely to be associated with severe spasticity (see Chapter 2). In addition, a recent finding suggests the presence of unique growth patterns, with evidence of poor linear growth in this population that requires further investigation (55). In every sense, therefore, the term "cerebral palsy" conveys the concept of a broadly based, multiply handicapping condition.

V. STATIC ENCEPHALOPATHY AND DEVELOPMENTAL ABNORMALITY

At the outset, it is essential to put into perspective the diagnostic implications of the term "cerebral palsy." It clearly represents a *fixed*, primarily motor, condition within the brain with variable etiology that is a prior event rather than an ongoing phenomenon (see Chapter 2). This distinguishes cerebral palsy from other central nervous system conditions that are associated with a continuing or progressive pathology, with loss of milestones acquired previously (56), and identifies cerebral palsy as a *static encephalopathy*. Moreover, the predominant motor deficit

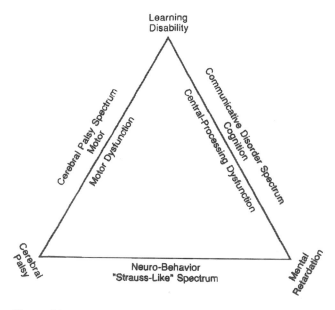

Figure 10   Cerebral palsy in the continuum of other static encephalopathies. (From Ref. 56.)

of cerebral palsy should be seen as part of a continuum within the spectrum of other nonprogressive developmental disabilities. These range from the cognitive mental retardation syndromes, behavioral attention deficit disorders and learning disabilities, through the mixed deficit pervasive developmental disorders.

Capute conceptualizes this spectrum as a "developmental triangle" linking and interconnecting each of these overlapping disorders (Fig. 10). In this view, the consequence of fixed central nervous system pathology (static encephalopathy) can give rise to a broad range of deficits in the motor, cognitive, and behavioral areas, either individually or in some combination. In the motor area, for example, abnormalities could range from the incoordination and clumsiness seen in attention deficit disorder to frank motor impairment in cerebral palsy. Therefore, anyone dealing specifically with diagnosis, management, and treatment of cerebral palsy, must keep in mind its predominant motor features and associated handicaps, yet be fully aware of and have the necessary clinical sophistication to deal with this entire range of nonprogressive developmental disabilities (57).

While the aberrant central nervous system in these conditions is the basis for delayed or abnormal developmental progress, it is essential to identify the primary impairment (cognitive, behavioral, or motor) that is outside the acceptable range and is the specific developmental abnormality characteristic of the child. These concepts are of great importance in understanding the developmental nature of the static encephalopathies such as cerebral palsy, and hence, their early identification (Chapter 3).

VI. CEREBRAL PALSY THROUGH THE LIFE SPAN

A. Birth to Three Years

The period from birth through 3 years is associated with rapid physical growth, neurological maturation, and social integration. This is a crucial time for clarifying the delays in development that have been experienced, beginning to deal with problems in daily management, and providing needed early interventional treatment. It is during these years that the discrete motor deficit in cerebral palsy makes its appearance and becomes a part of the growing child. But the extent and degree of motor deficit may still change with later growth, either becoming less pronounced or showing more permanent involvement. In order to avoid unnecessary or detrimental procedures, the range of applicable therapeutic approaches in this age group should therefore be conservative essentially and noninvasive while growth occurs.

B. Pre-School (Four to Six Years)

The preschooler will have a clearly recognizable motor deficit pattern whose degree and extent will be a major influence on development. Associated and concomitant problems in vision, hearing and speech, cognition and learning, behavior, and seizure status will become apparent. The need for mobility and social integration as well as the requirements associated with beginning formal schooling will all be demanding. The range of therapeutic choices that can be considered by professionals will also greatly broaden.

C. School Age

The child will be living with his unique motor problems and associated deficits while becoming integrated into the school situation. Family and social interaction will broaden, along with the beginnings of independence. Ongoing treatment will play an important part in prevention of further (secondary) deficits and maintaining attained levels of function.

D. Adolescence

Striving toward independence, and sexual maturity and the need for conformity and social acceptance are all variably experienced by the child with cerebral palsy during this period. Residual motor or other limitations will affect advancement in school and direction for later vocational development. Mental health needs may be a major requirement, while there is often simultaneous resistance to any suggested therapy modality. The transition to adulthood presents many special problems especially where there is limited agency contact (58), particularly for the young adult with cerebral palsy compared to those with other chronic conditions (59).

E. Adult

Attaining of adult status brings with it a wide range of levels of independence, from residential supervision (60) to complete integration into the adult community. The former may require treatment services to maintain function (61), while the latter may be able to manage with little or no additional therapy or services. Secondary effects of cerebral palsy may play an important role (62). General health maintenance issues, including appropriate fitness activities, employment, social and family status, and social acceptance will all be of increasing importance.

F. Senior Adult

Advancing age often brings with it accelerated motor deterioration in the person with cerebral palsy (63). Pathogenesis is not entirely clear and more data are needed on this now emerging population to better understand these changes.

Health-care issues and secondary effects of cerebral palsy become of increasing importance (64), particularly for women (65). Resumption of active therapy services in some form may be required in order to maintain/regain function. All of the social, emotional, and economic effects of reduction or loss of independence will come into play, possibly necessitating additional supportive and mental health services.

Cerebral palsy has specific implications in each of these life stages. It needs to be viewed specifically within each of them in order to focus on differing requirements for identification, care, and management. While cerebral palsy is a lifelong condition, the changes at a given age are crucial to understanding the unique age effects that will require professional assistance. In this sense, cerebral palsy should be considered as a grouping of age-related conditions, each with its own set of problems and challenges for management.

VII. THE CHALLENGE TO FOCUS ON THE INFANT

The child from birth to 3 years presents a unique combination of circumstances. On the one hand, the brain is in a rapid state of differentiation and maturation. Identification of specific abnormalities to account for the developmental delays may be elusive, and diagnosis becomes a major challenge. On the other hand, clinical experience indicates that very early initiation of assistance in daily management of the child and in providing a treatment regimen is crucial. Tailoring both management and treatment to the unique situation of an infant whose diagnosis may still be emerging presents another major challenge. These challenges offer opportunities to help the child to function and develop in better contact with the environment, to enhance the dynamics of intrafamily relationships, and perhaps to lessen or even prevent extensive deficits in the future. For these reasons, the special needs of the infant and young child from birth to 3 will be the focus of the chapters that follow.

VIII. CURRENT TRENDS

In contrast with Little's day, we are now fortunate enough to have available techniques for early identification and tools for early intervention of the infant with cerebral palsy. Even those with severe involvement may be expected to develop some independent function and eventually make their contribution to society. This progress has become possible as the traditional, primarily orthopedic approach in cerebral palsy has increasingly expanded to include multiple professionals who must deal with the array of needs of the child who has developmental disabilities. Concurrent early intervention special education programs up to age

3 have expanded both resources and the range of modalities that can now be offered. And extension to preschool and school services that now offer inclusion and mainstream programs enables increasing numbers of these children to become successful in finding a place within the community. For those who require continued supervision and assistance, opportunities are expanding for meaningful independence within a residential setting.

The advent of managed care within the United States health system has become pervasive, just as the interdisciplinary approach to the child with developmental disabilities is reaching universal acceptance. It remains to be seen whether the economics of providing health care under this system will work to the advantage of this coordinated model of management.

APPENDIX: GROSS MOTOR FUNCTION CLASSIFICATION SYSTEM [44]

Level I

Before 2nd birthday: Infants move in and out of sitting and floor sit with both hands free to manipulate objects. Infants crawl on hands and knees, pull to stand and take steps holding on to furniture. Infants walk between 18 months and 2 years of age without the need for any assistive mobility device.

From 2nd to 4th birthday: Children floor sit with both hands free to manipulate objects. Movements in and out of floor sitting and standing are performed without adult assistance. Children walk as the preferred method of mobility without the need for any assistive mobility device.

Level II

Before 2nd birthday: Infants maintain floor sitting but may need to use their hands for support to maintain balance. Infants creep on their stomach or crawl on hands and knees. Infants may pull to stand and take steps holding on to furniture.

From 2nd to 4th birthday: Children floor sit *but* may have difficulty with balance when both hands are free to manipulate objects. Movements in and out of sitting are performed with adult assistance. Children pull to stand on a stable surface. Children crawl on hands and knees with a reciprocal pattern, cruise holding on to furniture and walk using an assistive mobility device as preferred methods of mobility.

Level III

Before 2nd birthday: Infants maintain floor sitting when the low back is supported. Infants roll and creep forward on their stomachs.

From 2nd to 4th birthday: Children maintain floor sitting often by "W-sitting" (sitting between flexed and internally rotated hips and knees) and may require adult assistance to assume sitting. Children creep on their stomach or crawl on hands and knees (often without reciprocal leg movements) as their primary methods of self-mobility. Children may pull to stand on a table surface and cruise short distances. Children may walk short distances indoors using an assistive mobility device and adult assistance for steering and turning.

Level IV

Before 2nd birthday: Infants have head control but trunk support is required for floor sitting. Infants can roll to supine and may roll to prone.

From age 2nd to 4th birthday: Children floor sit when placed, but are unable to maintain alignment and balance without use of their hands for support. Children frequently require adaptive equipment for sitting and standing. Self-mobility for short distances (within a room) is achieved through rolling, creeping on stomach, or crawling on hands and knees without reciprocal leg movement.

Level V

Before 2nd birthday: Physical impairments limit voluntary control of movement. Infants are unable to maintain antigravity head and trunk postures in prone and sitting. Infants require adult assistance to roll.

From age 2: Physical impairments restrict voluntary control of movement and the ability to maintain antigravity head and trunk postures. All areas of motor function are limited. Functional limitations in sitting and standing are not fully compensated for through the use of adaptive equipment and assistive technology.

REFERENCES

1. Christensen E, Melchior J. Cerebral Palsy—A Clinical and Neuropathological Study. Clinics in Developmental Medicine No. 25. London: William Heinemann Medical Books, Ltd., 1967.
2. Charcot JM, Richer PMLP. Les deformes et les malades dans l'art. Paris: Lecrosnier et Babe, 1889.
3. Wolman B. Physical deformity of Richard III. Br Med J 1978; 1(6107):234.
4. Cazauvielh J. Recherches sur l'agenesie cerebral et la paralysie congeniale. Arch Gen Med 1827.
5. Delpech M. Tenotomie de tendon d'Achilles. In: Churgerie Clinique de Montpellier, Observations et Reflexions Tirees des Travaux de Chirurgie Clinique de Cette Ecole. Paris:Gabon, 1828:181.

6. Schleichkorn J. The Sometime Physician. New York: Jay Schleichkorn, Ph.D. (self-published) 1987: 39.
7. Little W. Course of lectures on deformation of the human frame. Lecture number VIII. Lancet 1843; i:18.
8. Little W. On the Nature and Treatment of the Deformities of the Human Frame. London: Longman, Brown, Green and Longman, 1853.
9. Little W. On the influence of abnormal parturition, difficult labours, premature birth, and asphyxia neonatorum on the mental and physical condition of the child, especially in relation to deformities. Trans Obstet Soc London 1861; 3:293.
10. Cruvelhier J. Traite d'Anatomie Pathologique Generale. Paris: Balliere, 1862.
11. Cotard J. Etude sur l'Atrophic Partielle de Cerveau. Paris: Lefrancois, 1868.
12. Osler W. The Cerebral Palsies of Children: A Clinical Study from the Infirmary for Nervous Diseases. Philadelphia: Blakiston, 1889.
13. Gowers W. On birth palsies. Lancet 1888; i:709.
14. Freud S. Die infantile cerebrallahmung. In: Nothnagel J. Specialle Pathologie und Therapie. Band IX, Th.III. Vienna: Holder, 1897.
15. Kuban KCK, Leviton L. Cerebral palsy. N Engl J Med 1994; 330:188–195.
16. Sachs B, Peterson F. A study of cerebral palsies in early life based upon an analysis of one hundred and forty cases. J Nerv Ment Dis 1890; 17:295.
17. Batten F. Ataxia in childhood. Brain 1905; 28:484.
18. Colby J. Massage and remedial exercises in the treatment of children's paralysis: their difficulties in use. Boston Med Surg J 1915; 173:696.
19. Crothers B. Clinical aspects of cerebral palsy: life history of the disease. Q Rev Ped 1951; 6:142.
20. Lord E. Children Handicapped by Cerebral Palsy. New York: Commonwealth Fund, 1937.
21. Stoffel A. The treatment of spastic contracture. Am J Orthoped Surg 1913; 10:611.
22. Phelps W. The treatment of cerebral palsies. J Bone Joint Surg 1940; 22:1004.
23. Wolf J. The Results of Treatment in Cerebral Palsy. Springfield, IL: Charles C Thomas, 1969:10–11.
24. Vining E, Accardo P, Rubenstein J, Farrell S, Roizen N. Cerebral palsy: a pediatric developmentalist's overview. Am J Dis Child 1976; 130:643–649.
25. Katz A. Parents of the Handicapped. Springfield, IL: Charles C Thomas, 1961:23.
26. United Cerebral Palsy. The Story of U.C.P. New York: United Cerebral Palsy, 1949.
27. Merkatz I, Johnson K. Regionalization of perinatal care for the United States. Clin Perinatol 1976; 3:271–276.
28. Haynes U. The First Three Years-Programming for Atypical Infants and Their Families. New York: United Cerebral Palsy Association, 1974.
29. Tjossem TD, ed. Intervention Strategies for the High Risk Infant. Baltimore: University Park Press, 1976.
30. Greenspan, L. The conception, growth, and development of the developmentalist. Presidential address. 31st Annual Meeting of the American Academy for Cerebral Palsy and Developmental Medicine, Atlanta, GA, Oct 5–9, 1977.
31. Perlstein M. Infantile cerebral palsy: classification and clinical observations. JAMA 1952; 149:30.
32. Burgess D. A case of cerebral birth palsy. Med Chron Manchester 1888; 9:471.

33. Brissaud E. Maladie de Little et tabes spasmodique. Sem Med 1894; 14:89.
34. Rosenberg L. Der cerebralen Kinderlahmungen. Kassowitz. Beitr. Kinderheilkd. Neue Folge IV, 1893.
35. Freud S, Rie C. Klinische Studien Uber Die Hoslbseitige Cerebral-Lahmung der Kinder. Vienna: Perles, 1891.
36. Phelps W. Let's define cerebral palsy. Crippled Child 1948; 16:4.
37. American Academy for Cerebral Palsy and Developmental Medicine. Membership Directory By-Laws. Rosemont, IL: AACPDM, 1998:113.
38. Mutch L, Alberman E, Hagberg B, Kodama K, Perat M. Cerebral palsy epidemiology: where are we now, and where are we going? Dev Med Child Neurol 1992; 34: 547–555.
39. Aicardi J, Bax M. Cerebral Palsy. In: Aicardi J. Diseases of the Nervous System in Childhood. 2nd ed. London: MacKeith Press, 1998:210.
40. Fahn S. Generalized dystonia: concept and treatment. Clin Neuropharmacol 1986; 9 (suppl 2):S37–S48.
41. Miller G, Calca LA. Ataxic cerebral palsy—clinico-pathological correlations. Neuropediatrics 1989; 20:84–89.
42. Friede RL. Developmental Neuropathology, 2nd ed. Berlin: Springer, 1989.
43. Brett EM. Pediatric Neurology. 3rd ed. Edinburgh: Churchill Livingstone, 1997.
44. Palisano R, Rosenbaum P, Walter S, Russell D, Wood E, Galuppi B. Development and reliability of a system to classify gross motor function in children with cerebral palsy. Dev Med Child Neurol 1997; 39:214–223.
45. Ingram T. A Historical Review of the Definition and Classification of the Cerebral Palsies. In: Stanley F, Alberman A, eds. The Epidemiology of the Cerebral Palsies. Philadelphia: Lippincott, 1984:1–11.
46. Fay T. Cerebral palsy: medical considerations and classification. Am J Psychiatry 1950; 107:180.
47. Phelps W. Etiology and diagnostic classification of cerebral palsy. In: Proceedings of the Cerebral Palsy Institute. New York: Association for the Aid of Crippled Children, 1950.
48. Perlstein M. Medical aspects of cerebral palsy. Nervous Child 1949; 8:128.
49. Balf CL, Ingram TTS. Problems in the classification of cerebral palsy in childhood. Br Med J 1955; 2:163–166.
50. Crothers B, Paine R. The Natural History of Cerebral Palsy. Cambridge: Harvard University Press, 1959.
51. Minear W. A classification of cerebral palsy. Pediatrics 1956; 18:841.
52. Badell-Ribera A. Cerebral palsy: postural-locomotor prognosis in spastic diplegia. Arch Phys Med Rehabil 1985; 66:614–619.
53. Yokochi K, Shimabukuro S, Kodama M, Hosoe A. Motor function of infants with athetoid cerebral palsy. Dev Med Child Neurol 1993; 35:909–916.
54. Amosun SL, Ikuesan BA, Oloyede IJ. Rehabilitation of the handicapped child— what about the care-giver? P N G Med J 1995; 38:208–214.
55. Samson-Fang L, Stevenson R. Linear growth velocity in children with cerebral palsy. Dev Med Child Neurol 1998; 40:689–692.
56. Nelson KB, Ellenberg J. Epidemiology of cerebral palsy. Adv Neurol 1978; 19:421– 435.

57. Capute A. The "Expanded" Strauss Syndrome: MBD Revisited. In: Accardo P, Blondis T, Whitman B, eds. Attention Deficit Disorders and Hyperactivity in Children. New York: Marcel Dekker, 1991:27–36.
58. Stevenson CJ, Pharoah PO, Stevenson R. Cerebral palsy—the transition from youth to adulthood. Dev Med Child Neurol 1997; 39:336–342.
59. Fiorentino L, Datta D, Gentle S, Hall DM, Harpin V, Phillips D, Walker A. Transition from school to adult life for physically disabled young children. Arch Dis Child 1998; 73:306–311.
60. Knishkowy BN, Gross M, Morris SL, Reeb, KG, Stewart DL. Independent living: caring for the adult with cerebral palsy. J Fam Pract 1986; 23: 21–23.
61. Bachrach S, Greenspun B. Care of the adult with cerebral palsy. Del Med J 1990; 62:1287–1290.
62. Granet KM, Balaghi M, Jaeger J. Adults with cerebral palsy. NJ Med J 1997; 94: 51–54.
63. Murphy KP, Molnar GE, Lankasky K. Medical and functional status of adults with cerebral palsy. Dev Med Child Neurol 1995; 37:1075–1084.
64. Lollar D. Preventing Secondary Conditions Associated with Spina Bifida or Cerebral Palsy Proceedungs of a Symposium. Washington, D.C.: Spina Bifida Association of America, 1994.
65. Turk M, Geremski CA, Rosenbaum PF, Weber RJ. The health status of women with cerebral palsy. Arch Phys Med Rehabil 1997; 78 (12 suppl 5):s10-s17.

2

Trends in Etiology and Epidemiology of Cerebral Palsy

Impact of Improved Survival of Very Low-Birth-Weight Infants

Vidya Bhushan Gupta
Metropolitan Hospital Center, New York Medical College, New York, New York

I. ETIOLOGY OF CEREBRAL PALSY

Although relatively less frequent than mental retardation and epilepsy, cerebral palsy (CP) occupies a preeminent position among developmental disabilities because of the debate that surrounds its causation. The complexity of factors etiologically associated with CP, and with its various motor types, was apparent even to Little. He recognized, for example, that spastic paraplegia or diplegia was generally associated with a preterm but normal delivery, whereas spastic quadriplegia was more often found after an abnormal term delivery (1). Much of the confusion about the etiology of CP is due to the fallacy of attributing CP to various antecedents and conditions discovered in a group of CP patients, without establishing causality (2). A condition should be considered causal only if it is found consistently more often in those who have CP than in those who do not, and if CP occurs consistently more often in those who are exposed to the condition than in those who are not. To be causal, an association should be strong and biologically plausible. Even if an association is strong, plausible, and consistent, it may only be a link in a chain of events. CP, like many other diseases, is often multifactorial in origin with various factors working in tandem or simultaneously to cause it. This preamble to the following discussion about the etiology of CP

is meant to caution clinicians against rushing to attribute CP to an adverse perinatal event, without examining the prenatal antecedents of the case.

A.   Congenital Cerebral Palsy

Congenital CP refers to cases in which the etiology is traced to intrauterine, natal,
or perinatal factors and was estimated by Perlstein to include some 85% of all
cases (3). The most important associations of congenital CP are discussed below.

1.   Prematurity

About 40% of children with CP are either born prematurely or have low birth
weight (<2500 g). The prevalence of CP among very low-birth weight (VLBW)
infants (<1500 g) is 40 to 100 times higher than in normal weight infants (4,
5), and VLBW infants, who constitute only 0.68% of newborn survivors, contribute up to 28% of children with CP (6).

   Among children with low birth weight, gestational age is more important
than growth retardation. It is not clear which factors increase the risk of CP among
preterm infants—factors that result in preterm birth or medical complications that
frequently occur in premature infants because of their increased vulnerability to
pathophysiological disturbances? The following pathogenetic mechanisms have
been suggested.

1.   Prenatal antecedents cause early brain damage, which, in turn, predis-
     poses to preterm delivery.
2.   Prenatal antecedents independently cause brain damage and preterm
     birth.
3.   Prenatal antecedents cause preterm birth, which, in turn, causes dis-
     abling sequelae.
4.   Prenatal antecedents cause preterm birth, which results in homeostatic
     disequilibrium at birth that results in brain damage, and which, in turn,
     causes disabling sequelae.

   The underlying basis of most neurodevelopmental sequelae in the preterm
infant is white matter damage, collectively called perinatal leukoencephalopathy
(7). This term encompasses germinal matrix hemorrhage (GMH), periventricular
hemorrhage (PVH), intraventricular hemorrhage (IVH), periventricular hemorrhagic infarction, and periventricular leukomalacia (PVL). Preterm infants are
prone to GMH, PVH, and IVH because their cerebral circulation is sensitive to
changes of blood pressure (pressure-passive) and they lack supporting glia in
their germinal matrix. Large GMH/IVH, in turn, causes obstruction of the termi-
nal veins, resulting in hemorrhagic infarction (8). Periventricular hemorrhagic

infarctions are asymmetric and generally occur on the same side as a large GMH/ IVH. Periventricular leukomalacia or multifocal necrosis in the periventricular white matter, on the other hand, occurs due to ischemic necrosis in the end and border zones of long penetrating arteries. Paneth et al. have reported that white matter damage in the preterm infant is not confined to the periventricular area but may extend more widely into the subcortex and beyond (9), and is characterized by loss of oligodendrocytes with an increase in hypertrophic astrocytes (10). Loss of oligodendrocytes affects nerve cell growth, which, in turn, impairs myelination. Conditions such as respiratory distress syndrome, apnea, hypotension, infection, and patent ductus arteriosus can disturb cerebral blood flow because of its pressure-passive nature in preterm infants, resulting in hypoxia, acidosis, and ischemic necrosis (10). Periventricular leukomalacia may be mediated by cytokines, tumor necrosis factor–alpha, interleukin-6, and free radicals that are released as a result of hypoxia and ischemia. A schematic diagram describing the pathogenesis of CP in the preterm infant is given in figure 1.

The principal diagnostic tool to diagnose periventricular and intraventricular lesions in the preterm infant is cranial ultrasound. Transient periventricular densities, called flares, are associated with an 8 to 10% risk of CP, while IVH with ventricular dilatation (grade III IVH) and IVH with periventricular hemorrhage (grade IV IVH) have a risk of 60 to 70% (11). Though echolucent areas (darker areas with few echoes) are less common, they are more ominous. Echolucent lesions detected by ultrasonography (Fig. 2) are associated with risk of CP estimated to be as high as 100% (12). The diffuse white matter damage mentioned above is usually undetected by cranial ultrasound during life, except as distortion of the contours of cerebral ventricles or ventriculomegaly.

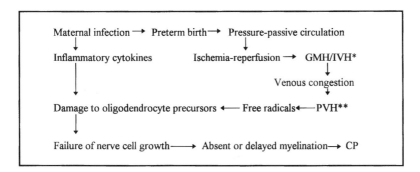

* Germinal matrix/intraventricular hemorrhage
** Periventricular hemorrhage

Figure 1   Events leading to cerebral palsy in preterm infant.

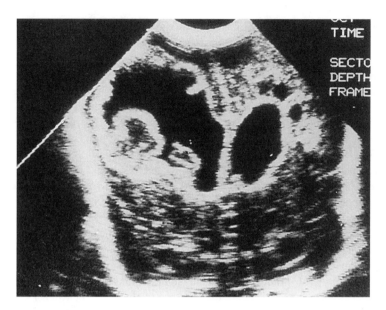

Figure 2 Ultrasound of a preterm infant with hypoxic-ischemic injury showing resolving IVH and porencephalic cyst on the right side and periventricular cystic leukomalacia on the left side. (Courtesy Syed Hossain, MD.)

Magnetic resonance imaging (MRI) is more sensitive in detecting white matter damage. In MRI, the child is placed in a magnetic field and changes in alignment of protons induced by the applied magnetic impulses are monitored and used to create images. The images are obtained under three conditions—T1, T2, and proton density (Fig. 3).

Although the pathophysiology of brain damage in preterm infants is better understood now, the causes of prematurity in preterm infants are still not fully understood. In multivariate analysis, the predictors of low birth weight are: low birth weight of the last infant born to the mother, fetal malformations, cigarette smoking, and placental inflammation or infection. Maternal and placental infection is related independently to preterm birth and to neurological damage leading to CP. Because of our poor understanding of the causes of prematurity, the incidence of preterm birth has not decreased despite advances in obstetric surveillance.

2. Birth Asphyxia

The relationship between asphyxia and developmental disabilities, especially CP, has intrigued the medical and lay communities since 1861, when William John

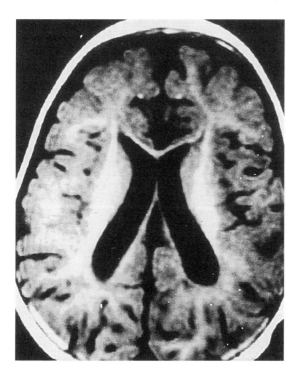

Figure 3   MRI (T1 weighted image) of a preterm infant at 14 months of age showing periventricular leukomalacia. (Courtesy Syed Hossain, MD.)

Little stated in his famous paper to the Royal Obstetrical Society of London "abnormal parturition, besides ending in death or recovery, not infrequently had a . . . third termination" in long-term disability (13). Birth asphyxia occurs when the organ of gas exchange (placenta or lungs), fails at the time of birth, resulting in oxygen deprivation (hypoxia), hypercarbia, and metabolic acidosis. Asphyxia leads to alterations in cerebral blood flow in a homeostatic attempt to maintain circulation to more vital areas. There is no damage if blood flow to the brain is maintained. If, on the other hand, blood flow is compromised (ischemia), depriving oxygen supply, cell death results due to release of free radicals and excitotoxic amino acids such as glutamate (Fig. 4).

If asphyxia is severe and total, an uncommon occurrence—involvement of the thalamus, brainstem and basal ganglia—occurs, with relative sparing of the cerebral cortex. If asphyxia is prolonged and partial, as is more common, bilateral parasagittal watershed injury occurs in term infants and bilateral periventricular end and border zone injury occurs in preterm infants. The neuoropathological

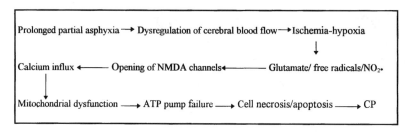

* Nitric oxide

Figure 4 Events leading to cerebral palsy in term infant.

picture of human asphyxia is similar to that seen in the rhesus monkey model of prolonged partial asphyxia (14), suggesting that most cases of human asphyxia have their onset in the prenatal period rather than being acute events triggered by labor and delivery. The asphyxial event has to be extreme and prolonged to result in neurological damage, and the neurological sequelae due to birth asphyxia are usually not limited to the motor system, but often include mental retardation and epilepsy as well.

It is difficult to estimate the exact incidence of birth asphyxia, because there is no universally accepted measure of this condition. It is estimated that the incidence of birth asphyxia ranges from about 1 to 2 per 1000, in full-term infants, to as much as 60% in extremely low-birth-weight infants. Between 10 to 60% of preterm neonates with asphyxia expire depending upon their gestation, while most full term infants survive (15, 16). Although survival after birth asphyxia is related to gestational age, the incidence of neurological impairment is similar in preterm and term infants (15). Based upon epidemiological data, about 12 to 20% of CP cases are related to intrapartum asphyxia (17, 18).

Despite evidence of a modest association between perinatal asphyxia and CP, it is difficult to establish that this association is causal in a particular child. Most cases of CP occur in infants who have no history of adverse perinatal events, and most infants who experience birth asphyxia recover without CP (19). Prediction is complicated by the absence of a universally accepted measure of birth asphyxia. Biochemical indices, such as low umbilical vein blood pH and buffer base, correlate poorly with Apgar scores (20, 21) and do not predict CP. Emergency cesarean sections, which are done solely because of abnormal biochemical indices, often deliver infants with no sign of birth asphyxia. Apgar scores are not a specific measure of birth asphyxia (22) because nonasphyxial conditions, such as maternal analgesia and anesthesia or infection, can also depress Apgar scores. Apgar scores have poor predictive validity and low sensitivity and specificity (23). In the National Collaborative Perinatal Project (NCPP), only about 12% of surviving children with Apgar scores of 0 to 3 developed CP (19). Fifty-five percent of cases of CP in the NCPP occurred in infants with 1-min Apgar scores of 7 or higher (19). Infants who suffer oxygen deprivation in the perinatal period show abnormal neurological signs within the first 12 h to the first week of birth. These signs, though not specific to asphyxial brain damage, are called hypoxic-ischemic encephalopathy (HIE) (24, 25) and are, by far, the best predictors of neurodevelopmental sequelae. Mild HIE, characterized by irritability, jitteriness, and increased tendon reflexes, carries little risk of subsequent handicap. Moderate to severe HIE, manifesting as seizures, altered state of consciousness, and abnormalities of posture, reflexes, and feeding and respiratory function, on the other hand, is associated with a 20 to 55% risk of long-term neurological sequelae (26). Hypoxic-ischemic encephalopathy is a better predictor of subsequent handicap than low Apgar scores or biochemical changes alone.

While individual indices of asphyxia are poor predictors of CP, infants with a constellation of factors, such as low Apgar scores for 20 min or more, moderate to severe HIE, HIE that persists for over 1 week, and severe acidosis, are more likely to have adverse neurological outcome. Neonatal seizures occurring in the context of prolonged depression are one of the strongest predictors of CP. Various neuroimaging techniques, such as ultrasound, CAT scan, and MRI, can be used to assess the extent of asphyxial brain damage and to predict CP. Radiological signs depend upon the maturity of brain, because asphyxial cerebrovascular disease affects the term and preterm infant differently (27). MRI appears to be the most sensitive technique to diagnose asphyxial brain damage in humans at present, with T2 prolongation (high signal) from edema occurring within 12 to 18 h of injury, and T1 shortening (high signal) and T2 shortening (low signal) appearing within 3 to 6 days of injury. While T2 prolongation is transient, T1 and T2 shortening predict permanent damage (28). The new techniques, such as diffusion and perfusion MRIs, MR spectroscopy, and near-infrared spectroscopy, hold more promise in detecting asphyxial brain damage in the infant (29).

The exact cause or causes of birth asphyxia are unknown. Freud, in 1875, had argued that Little had the causal sequence wrong—that babies may have had difficult birth because they were abnormal rather than the reverse (30). Many cases of birth asphyxia have prenatal antecedents that either directly damage the brain or make an infant more vulnerable to intrapartum stress leading to birth asphyxia, which in turn may cause CP. In the NCPP, of the 21% of children with CP, more than half had other characteristics, most often congenital malformations, that may have contributed to asphyxia, leading to CP. In a study by Hagberg, mothers of 42% of children who had birth asphyxia experienced bleeding during pregnancy, infarction of placenta, toxemia, or maternal diabetes. Most of these conditions limit supply of nutrients and oxygen to the fetus, a situation collectively called fetal deprivation of supply (31). In Hagberg's series, 62% of CP children who had history of fetal deprivation of supply had birth asphyxia (31).

Most cases of asphyxia and brain damage putatively caused by birth asphyxia are not preventable by intrapartum obstetric or neonatal interventions. Obstetricians use a number of techniques to prevent birth asphyxia and to detect fetal distress early, but most of the techniques have poor sensitivity and specificity. Intermittent auscultation to monitor fetal heart rate is a procedure of poor reliability (intraobserver agreement) and validity; thus it is of little use in preventing intrapartum stress. Continuous electronic monitoring does not show a major improvement over intermittent auscultation (32). Scalp vein pH is a very poor predictor of birth asphyxia. With an Apgar score of less than 7 at 1 min as the outcome measure, fetal heart rate monitoring plus fetal scalp sampling is 32% sensitive, and has a false positive and false negative rate of 43.6% and 19.9%, respectively (33). While the rates of electronic monitoring and cesarean sections have gone up significantly in recent years, the prevalence of CP has not declined. In a case-control study of the outcome in cases with and without adequate response to fetal distress, Niswander et al. found that 98% of the babies whose mothers received suboptimal care for fetal distress survived without CP (34).

The aim of treating a child who has suffered birth asphyxia is to limit brain damage. At present the treatment of birth asphyxia is not standardized and ranges from no therapy to sedation, anticonvulsants, fluid restriction, and osmotic diuresis. Though retrospective studies had suggested that magnesium sulfate administered to the mother for eclampsia during pregnancy was associated with decreased incidence of CP, prospective studies have failed to confirm this hypothesis (35). Hopefully, we shall have a rational approach to limit asphyxial brain damage in the future because studies are underway in animals to prevent formation and elimination of free radicals and excitatory amino acids.

While birth asphyxia has become less common as a cause of CP in developed countries, it continues to be an important cause of perinatal mortality and neurodevelopmental sequelae in developing countries, where it is often prolonged and severe due to suboptimal obstetric care; many cases are preventable (36). A community-based study in Zimbabwe found that a preventable factor was present in 76% of cases of perinatal asphyxia (37).

3. Other Perinatal Factors

Hyperbilirubinemia of the newborn due to Rh factor, ABO, or other blood group incompatibility, was formerly a major factor in the development of kernicterus, milder forms of athetosis, or mixed forms of cerebral palsy. Its impact has been greatly reduced by improved methods of early identification, exchange transfusions, and, above all, the preventive use of anti-Rh (D) immune globulin to immunize the mother immediately after her first pregnancy (38). Neonatal jaundice due to sepsis or physiological immaturity of the liver may still require careful attention.

Infection during the perinatal period may be significant, particularly if it leads to sepsis or meningitis. Herpes simplex encephalitis in the perinatal period can cause devastating brain damage resulting in cerebral palsy as well as mental retardation.

4. Prenatal Factors

Prenatal factors that have the potential of causing CP are present in a significant number of children with CP. As many as 70% of term infants with CP have a history of one or more adverse prenatal factors. In 30% of these cases, CP is causally associated with these prenatal factors, giving credence to Freud's view that difficulties at birth and the subsequent neurological syndrome of CP is the cart and not the horse in the causal sequence. Enamel hypoplasia has been noted to occur more often in children with CP, suggesting a prenatal cause for CP during the first trimester when enamel is formed (39). Foremost among the prenatal factors are maternal disorders that result in "fetal deprivation of supply," such as bleeding during pregnancy, placental infarction, toxemia, and twinning. According to Hagberg, about 30% of CP occurs in infants whose mothers had history of fetal deprivation of supply (31). Williams et al. reported a seven time higher relative risk of CP in twins as compared to their singleton counterparts, even when controlled for low birth weight and prematurity (40). Regardless of gestational age or birth weight, maternal prenatal conditions such as the general health status of the mother, untreated medical conditions, use of recreational drugs, alcohol, tobacco, and exposure to radiation are all known to have some effect on fetal development, but the exact relation to cerebral palsy is not established. Exposure to environmental toxins during pregnancy may be responsible for a few cases of CP, as occurred during the epidemics of methylmercury and fungicide poisoning in Japan and Iraq, respectively.

Certain endocrine problems during pregnancy have been reported to be associated with a higher risk of cerebral palsy; for example, hyperthyroidism or administration of thyroid hormones and estrogens during pregnancy (16). The role of the thyroid is especially intriguing because transient hypothyroxinemia of prematurity is a marker for neurodevelopmental problems, though its causal role has not been established, and it is not clear if thyroxine treatment in the neonatal period can prevent adverse outcome (41).

Maternal infections remain a major source of fetal central nervous system pathology. The primary conditions of concern are congenital rubella, toxoplasmosis, cytomegalovirus, and herpes. Each may be without serious or even noticeable clinical manifestations during gestation. While congenital rubella has been controlled in the United States, it continues to be a problem in developing countries. The latest on the list of possible congenital infections is the acquired immune deficiency syndrome (AIDS). It is well established that vertical transmission of HIV-1 virus frequently results in severe developmental disorders, including primary CNS motor conditions. Motor disorder in AIDS may progress so slowly that it appears consistent with cerebral palsy (42). Maternal fever and chorioamnionitis are also associated with significantly higher risk of disabling CP in the offspring (43). Maternal urinary tract infection has been linked to white matter damage in the offspring (44). Grether at al. have hypothesized that brain injury due to maternal infections is perhaps mediated by complement-induced injury to oligodendria and neurons, with alteration of blood-brain barrier and coagulation disorders that may result in clots, emboli, and bleeds. They reported significantly higher levels of α-, β-, and γ-interferons and other biochemical indicators of inflammation in 14 of 31 term infants with spastic diplegia (45).

Vascular factors have been implicated in the etiology of CP. Both arterial and venous infarctions are known to cause cerebral palsy. Strokes can occur in prenatal, natal, and postnatal periods and are associated with polycythemia, neurocutaneous syndromes such as Sturge-Weber syndrome and neurofibromatosis, maternal cocaine abuse, congenital cyanotic heart disease, and coagulopathies, dehydration, and meningitis (46). Factor V Leiden mutation may be an important cause of in utero cerebrovascular disease and hemiplegic cerebral palsy (47). If a vascular lesion occurs early during gestation, dysgenesis occurs with destruction and a cavity lined with dysplastic gray matter results. These cavities are called dysgenetic porencephaly or schizencephaly. If the lesion occurs late during gestation, a well-formed cavity with minimal glial reaction, called porencephaly, is formed. After 30 weeks of gestation, cavities with internal septation due to glial response result, a process called encephalomalacia (46).

CNS malformations, such as hydrocephalus and encephalocele, can result in permanent motor sequelae, depending on whether or not they are surgically corrected at the right time or not. Congenital brain malformations, such as absence of corpus callosum, isolated lissenencephaly, Miller-Dieker syndrome, polymicrogyria, schizencephaly, and cerebellar malformations, may be associated with cerebral palsy, but children with these congenital malformations often have seizures and intellectual deficits as well (46). Cerebral palsy associated with Sturge-Weber syndrome, neurofibromatosis, and other phakomatoses may be due to brain malformations or due to vascular accidents. The distinction between a brain malformation and brain damage is not clear cut because the same insult can result in brain malformation if it occurs earlier during morphogenesis and damage if it occurs late.

In view of the importance of prenatal factors in the etiology of CP one should not rush to blame events surrounding birth for CP. In most cases, it may be more prudent simply to state the factors elicited in history without stating that they, indeed, caused CP. Even if prenatal factors are causally associated with CP, in most cases these factors are not preventable.

5. Genetic Cerebral Palsy

Examples of multiple cases within a family and a higher incidence of cerebral palsy in offspring of consanguineous marriage suggest that there maybe a hereditary basis for cerebral palsy in a few cases (48). Genetically determined cases of spastic paraplegia, generalized athetosis, and ataxia are well documented (49). Glutaric acidemia, type 1, is an is important genetic cause of cerebral palsy in the Amish population of Pennsylvania, presenting as static encephalopathy once the children are past their infantile period of vulnerability to metabolic toxins (50). Metabolic conditions, such as ketoadipic aciduria, unclassified mitochondrial disease, and milder or later onset variants of classical lysosomal disorders and peroxisomal disorders, though strictly not CP, should also be considered in differential diagnosis of CP because these conditions may progress so slowly that they appear static (51).

6. Preconceptional Factors

In epidemiological studies, long intervals between menses, an unusually short or long interval since the previous pregnancy, and history of fetal wastage have been reported to be associated with higher risk of cerebral palsy (52).

B. Acquired Cerebral Palsy

Cerebral palsy is thought to be caused by a defect or lesion of the developing brain (53), but the period during which the brain continues to develop after birth is uncertain. Therefore, there is no consensus about the age until which CP can be acquired. While those interested in identifying antenatal and perinatal causes of CP consider only cases occurring between conception and the first month of life as CP, others also include as CP cases that occur in children who were apparently normal at birth but sustained brain damage during the first 2 years of life. Infective and traumatic factors are important causes of brain damage during this period. Among the infective cases, meningitis and encephalitis are the most important, with herpes simplex infection prevalent in the developed countries, and bacterial meningitis, tubercular meningitis, viral encephalitis, especially measles encephalitis, and cerebral malaria common in the developing countries. Trauma is particularly common once the child begins to walk and develops independence in the preschool period. Accidental causes include motor vehicle accidents, near drowning, accidental choking, and acute life-threatening events. Unfortunately, inflicted trauma in the form of shaken baby syndrome has become a frequent cause in the United States. Other conditions that may cause permanent motor sequelae include late-onset or inadequately treated hydrocephalus, neoplastic intracranial lesions that occur in the early developing years (54), intracranial hemorrhage due to an arteriovenous malformation, and cerebral infarction secondary to an embolus from a cardiac lesion or thrombosis in sickle-cell anemia.

Data regarding the incidence of static intracranial lesions with permanent residue that develop beyond the perinatal period are limited. Records of Perlstein's cases suggest that approximately 15% of CP cases are acquired postnatally (3). A report from Finland identified postnatal causes in 13 (19%) of 69 cases (55). While most cases of congenital CP are not preventable, many of the postnatal cases of CP are.

II. EPIDEMIOLOGY OF CEREBRAL PALSY

Because of the probable role of perinatal factors in its causation (56), the frequency of CP is measured as a rate per thousand live births and not per thousand population alive at the time of diagnosis. This rate is called prevalence, not incidence. It is difficult to compute incidence in CP because there is a considerable gap of time between the onset of CP and its diagnosis, and a considerable number of cases that die or are lost to follow-up before diagnosis are not counted.

Prevalence of cerebral palsy in the industrialized countries of the world ranges from 2 to 2.5/1000 live births (Table 1).

Prevalence of CP in developing countries is believed to be higher than in developed countries because of a higher incidence of severe birth asphyxia (65, 66) and higher incidence of low birth weight, but no population-based studies are available to ascertain the true prevalence of cerebral palsy in developing countries.

Table 1 Prevalance of Cerebral Palsy in Population-Based Studies in Developed Countries

Country	Study (Ref.)	Prevalence/1000 live births
Australia	Stanley (57)	2.3
Canada	Robertson et al. (58)	2.6
Ireland	Dowding (59)	2.0
Finland	Rikonen (60)	2.5
Norway	Meberg (61)	2.1
Sweden	Hagberg et al. (62)	2.4
UK	Evans (63)	2.0
US	Yeargin Allsop (64)	2.1

Cerebral palsy has been found to occur in all countries of the world and in all ethnic groups (65, 66). The prevalence of CP is not related to ethnicity per se, but is mediated by the prevalence of low birth weight, maternal and obstetric factors, and consanguinity in an ethnic group. Although, in the United States, the incidence of low birth weight among blacks is double that among whites, no clear pattern of CP excess has been seen among blacks. Murphy et al. reported higher prevalence of CP among blacks in Metropolitan Atlanta (67), but no differences were reported by Haerer et al. from Mississippi (68). Similarly, no differences between blacks and whites were reported by Emond et al. from Britain (4).

The prevalence of cerebral palsy is higher among ethnic groups in whom consanguineous marriage is common, such as Pakistani immigrants in England and Saudi Arabians (65, 69).

Many studies report an excess of males among cases of cerebral palsy. Males tend to be more severely affected and have more dysmorphic features, but no explanation has been found for these findings, and, in fact, male predominance in CP maybe diminishing (70).

A.   Secular Trends in the Prevalence of Cerebral Palsy

Despite advances in obstetric and neonatal care, prevalence of cerebral palsy has been rising in the industrialized countries since the mid-1970s. (6,59,60,71). Hagberg et al. (62) reported rising prevalence of CP in western Sweden until the late 1980s when the overall CP prevalence fell, but CP among preterm infants increased. Although no change in the overall CP rates has been observed in Australia, a significant upward trend in CP rates among VLBW infants has been noted (57, 72). Similarly, in the counties of Merseyside and Cheshire in the United Kingdom, there has been a threefold increase in the CP rate in VLBW infant survivors in the 1980s, with most of the increase occurring in infants less than 1000 g (6).

B.   Cerebral Palsy and the Very Low Birth-Weight Infant

The increasing prevalence of CP in the developed countries seems to be due to improved survival of VLBW infants in whom the prevalence of CP is very high (73). Prior to intensive care, very few VLBW infants survived. Neonatal survival for singleton white infants in the United States increased by 7100 %, from 6.5 to 461.2 per 1000 live births for those weighing 500 to 999 g, and 200%, from 422.6 to 845.9 per 1000 live births, for those weighing 1000 to 1499 g between 1960 and 1983 (74). These changes in mortality translate into more than a twofold increase from 1960 to 1986 in the number of VLBW infants surviving the neonatal period. With continuing advances in neonatal care, the gestational age of viability is getting lower, and more extremely low birth weight (birthweight <1000 g) and extremely extremely (also called micro) low-birth-weight infants (<750 g) are surviving. At one perinatal center in the United States, the survival of infants with birth weights of 500 to 750 g increased from 23% during the period from 1982 to 1988 to 43% during the period from 1990 to 1992. While none of the children born at the gestation of 23 weeks survived in the 1982 to 1988 cohort, 7% of children with gestation of 23 weeks survived in 1990 to 1992 cohort, and the survival of infants with gestation of 24 weeks went up from 16% to 40% during the same period (75). In view of the above trends in newborn survival, the National Institute of Child Health and Human Development concluded, after a multicenter study, that obstetricians should be willing to perform cesarean sections at above 800 g or 26 weeks gestational age for fetal indications (76).

The improved survival of extremely low-birth-weight infants has not been accompanied by an increase in medical and neurodevelopmental sequelae in the survivors. Escobar et al. reported little variation in prevalence of CP in VLBW survivors since 1960 (77). At Rainbow Babies Hospital in Cleveland, outcomes among surviving extemely low birth weight infants at 20 months of age did not change appreciably from the 1982 to 1988 period to the 1990 to 1992 period, despite a twofold increase in survival (75). Lorenz et al. reviewed the English language studies published since 1970, reporting on mortality and disability in infants born at or before 26 weeks gestation, with birth weights less than 800 g, and concluded that the prevalence of major neurodevelopmental disabilities has not changed among survivors over time (78).

Despite the stable incidence of disability in VLBW infants, their improved survival alone is likely to increase CP prevalence, because the prevalence of CP in infants below 1500 g is 77/1000 live births, 60 times the prevalence in infants more than 2500 g (1.3/1000) and 9 times the prevalence in infants 1501 to 2500 g (8.5/1000) (57, 79). That this is indeed happening is supported by the ''changing panorama of CP.'' The relative proportion of low-birth-weight infants among CP has increased; low-birth-weight infants now contribute 40 to 50 % of patients with CP (6, 57) as compared to 30 to 35% in the past (6, 80).

With an increasing proportion of CP occurring among very low birth weight infants, there has been a change in the clinical type of CP as well. Diplegic CP is becoming more common because of improving survival of VLBW infants, while the dyskinetic type of CP is decreasing due to decreased incidence of bilirubin encephalopathy. In Sweden, diplegia and hemiplegia constitute 45 and 34% of all cases, respectively, with quadriplegia ranking a distant third (9% of cases) (62); in England, quadriplegia, hemiplegia, and diplegia constitute 36%, 32%, and 22% of cases, respectively (6). Dyskinetic CP which includes dystonic, athetoid, choreiform, and ataxic types of CP, accounts for about 13% to 16% of cases. About 20% of cases have mixed features of choreathetosis and spasticity. Spasticity is the most frequent motor finding, occurring in about 60% of children.

The hypotonic form of CP, not accepted by some to be CP at all (81), is the least common, occurring in about 1% of cases.

C.   Cerebral Palsy and Associated Abnormalities

Cerebral palsy is often associated with various other disabling conditions, a few of which are described below.

1.   Mental Retardation (MR)

Even though 25 to 30% of CP cases have severe intellectual impairment defined as IQ less than 50 (82, 83), as many as 50% of children with CP have normal intelligence. The rest have mild MR (IQ $\geq$ 50–70). No recent studies of the prevalence of MR in children with CP are available, but it is unlikely that the prevalence of MR in CP has increased. Intelligence is often spared in spastic diplegia, the form of CP whose prevalence has increased with increasing survival of VLBW infants.

2.   Epilepsy

From 25 to 45% of children with CP have epilepsy (84, 85). Epilepsy is most common in spastic hemiplegia, followed closely by spastic quadriplegia, and least commonly in spastic diplegia. Children with MR and spastic quadriplegia are more likely to have seizures than other children with CP. Partial epilepsy is the most frequently seen form of epilepsy in spastic hemiplegia, while major motor epilepsy and West syndrome are common in spastic quadriplegia. Seizures tend to occur earlier in spastic quadriplegia, at a median age of 6 months (85), than in spastic hemiplegia, in which they occur at a median age of 4 years (85). Epilepsy in patients with CP is more difficult to control because of associated brain lesions (86). For example, infantile hydrocephalus occurred in 26% of preterm children with CP in a population-based study in Sweden (62).

3.   Sensory Impairments

CP is often associated with visual and hearing impairments. Eighteen percent of preterm and 14% of full-term infants with CP had various degrees of visual impairment in a Swedish cohort (62). The association of hearing impairment with cerebral palsy is much less common and is mediated by prematurity (87) and to a much lesser extent by perinatal asphyxia (88). Of 547 preterm infants of 34 weeks gestational age or less, born between 1987 and 1991 in Lausanne, Switzerland, 1.46% developed bilateral sensorineural hearing loss (89). In a register of hearing-impaired children born in a region of the United Kingdom between 1984 and 1988, low-birth-weight infants were found to be at a significantly increased risk for hearing impairment, with an odds ratio of 4.5 rising to 9.6 for birth-weight less than 1500 g (87).

4. Behavior Problems

Behavior problems are common in children with CP. Using the National Health Interview Survey, Child Health Supplement for 1981 and 1988, McDermott et al. reported that parent-reported behavior problems were five times more likely in children with CP (25.5%) compared with children having no known health problems (5.4%). These problems included dependency, oppositional behavior, and hyperactivity (90).

III. SUMMARY

Cerebral palsy rose to prominence during this century as a metaphor for abnormal labor and delivery, and a ticket to colossal jury awards for damages, because of its putative association with birth asphyxia. However, many well-done studies, such as the NCPP, have established that birth asphyxia makes a minor contribution to the causation of CP, and many children with birth asphyxia have prenatal antecedents that cannot be prevented. Of the potentially asphyxiating perinatal conditions, such as abruptio placentae, placenta previa, prolapsed cord, cord compression, and tight nuchal cord, only tight nuchal cord was found to be significantly associated with CP in term infants (91). Failure of the advances in obstetric care and the ever escalating rate of cesarean section to decrease the prevalence of CP is a further testimony to the lack of a strong causal association between CP and birth asphyxia. While the advances in obstetric and neonatal care have failed to decrease the prevalence of CP due to birth asphyxia, there has been an amazing improvement in the survival of very low- and extremely low-birth-weight infants. As a corollary to the improved survival of VLBW infants in whom the prevalence of CP is higher than in full-term infants, the absolute number of low-birth-weight infants with CP has increased. This trend is likely to continue until we understand the mechanism of brain injury in the preterm infant and are able to devise interventions to address these processes. Until such time, we will have to contend with a higher prevalence of cerebral palsy, preterm survivors with spastic diplegia forming the majority of them.

REFERENCES

1. Little WJ. On the influence of abnormal parturition, difficult labours, premature birth, and asphyxia neonatorum on the mental and physical condition of the child, especially in relation to deformities. Trans Obstet Soc London 1861; 3:293.

2. Susser M, Hauser WA, Kiely JL, Paneth N, Stein Z. Quantitative estimates of prenatal and perinatal risk factors for perinatal mortality, cerebral palsy, mental retardation and epilepsy. In: Freeman JM, ed. Prenatal and Perinatal Factors Associated with Brain Disorders. Bethesda: U.S. Department of Health and Human Services, 1985:359–439.

3. Perlstein M. Infantile cerebral palsy: classification and clinical observations. JAMA 1952; 149:30.

4. Emond A, Golding J, Peckham C. Cerebral palsy in two national cohort studies. Arch Dis Child 1989; 64:848–852.

5. Hagberg B, Hagberg G, Zetterstrom R. Decreasing perinatal mortality—increase in cerebral palsy morbidity. Acta Paediatr Scand 1989; 78:664–670.

6. Pharoah PO, Platt MJ, Cooke T. The changing epidemiology of cerebral palsy. Arch Dis Child Fetal Neonatal Ed 1996; 75:F169–73.

7. Leviton A, Gilles FH. Acquired perinatal leukoencephalopathy. Ann Neurol 1984; 16:1–8.

8. Volpe, JJ. Brain Injury in the premature infant: neuropathology, clinical aspects, and pathogenesis. MRDD Res Rev 1997; 3:3–12.

9. Paneth N, Rudelli R, Monte W, Rodriguez E, Pinto J, Kairam R, Kazam E. White matter necrosis in very low birth weight infants: Neuropathologic and ultrasonographic findings in infants surviving six days or longer. J Pediatr 1990; 116:975–984.

10. Bendersky M, Lewis M. Effects of intraventricular hemorrhage and other medical and environmental risks on multiple outcomes at age three years. J Dev Behav Pediatr 1995; 16:89–96.

11. Cooke RWL. Early and late cranial US appearances and outcomes in VLBW infants. Arch Dis Child 1987; 62:931–937.

12. De Vries LS, Dubowitz LM, Dubowitz V, Kaiser A, Lary S, Silverman M, Whitelaw A, Wigglesworth JS. Predictive value of cranial ultrasound: a reappraisal. Lancet 1985; 2(8447):137–140.

13. Accardo P. William John Little and cerebral palsy in the nineteenth century. J Hist Med Allied Sci 1989; 44:56–71.

14. Myers RE. Four patterns of perinatal brain damage and their conditions of occurrence in primates. Adv Neurol 1975;10:223–234.

15. MacDonald HM, Mulligan JC, Allen AC, Taylor PM. Neonatal asphyxia: I. Relationship to obstetric and neonatal complications to neonatal mortality in 38,405 consecutive deliveries. J Pediatr 1980; 96:898–902.

16. Mulligan JC, Painter MJ, O'Donoughue PA, Allan AC, Taylor. Neonatal asphyxia: II. Neonatal mortality and long-term sequelae. J Pediatr 1980; 96:903–907.

17. Nelson KB, Ellenberg JH. Antecedents of cerebral palsy: multivariate analysis of risk. N Engl J Med 1986; 315:81–86.

18. Freeman JM, Nelson KB. Intrapartum asphyxia and cerebral palsy. Pediatrics 1988; 82:240–249.

19. Nelson KB, Ellenberg J. Apgar scores as predictors of chronic neurologic disability. Pediatrics 1981;68:36–44.

20. DeSouza SW, Richards B. Neurological sequelae in newborn babies after perinatal asphyxia. Arch Dis Child 1978; 53:564–569.

21. Lauener PA, Calame A, Janecek P, Bossart H, and Monod JF. Systematic pH measurements in the umbilical artery: causes and predictive value of neonatal acidosis. J Perinatal Med 1983; 11:278–282.

22. Sykes GS, Molloy PM, Johnson P, Gu W, Ashworth F, Stirrat GM, Turnbull AC. Do Apgar scores indicate asphyxia? Lancet 1982; 1(8270):494–6.

23. Low JA. Fetal asphyxia in the antepartum and intrapartum period. Perinatal Asphyxia, Its Role in Developmental Deficits in Children. Proceedings of a symposium held in Toronto, Ontario, 1988.

24. Sarnat HB, Sarnat MS. Neonatal encephalopathy following fetal distress: a clinical and encephalographic study. Arch Neurol 1976; 33:696–705.

25. Robertson C, Finer N. Term infants with hypoxic/ischemic encephalopathy: outcome at 3.5 years. Dev Med Child Neurol 1985; 27:473–484.

26. Sarnat HB, Sarnat MS. Neonatal encephalopathy following fetal distress—a clinical and electroencephalographic study. Arch Neurol 1976; 33:695–706.

27. Allan WA, Riviello JJ. Perinatal cerebrovascular disease in the neonate. Pediatr Clin North Am 1992; 39:621–650.

28. Barkovich AJ, Hallam D. Neuroimaging in perinatal hypoxic-ischemic injury. MRDD Res Rev 1997; 3:28–41.

29. Wyatt JS. Magnetic resonance spectroscopy and near-infrared spectroscopy in the assessment of the asphyxiated term infant. MRDD Res Rev 1997; 3:42–48.

30. Freud S. Infantile Cerebral Paralysis. Coral Gables, FL: University of Miami Press, 1968:257.

31. Hagberg G, Hagberg B, and Olow I. The changing panorama of cerebral palsy in Sweden 1954–1970. III. The importance of fetal deprivation of supply. Acta Pediatr Scand 1976; 65:403–408.

32. Thacker SB. The efficacy of intrapartum electronic fetal monitoring. Am J Obstet Gynecol 1987; 156:24–30.

33. Banta HD, Thaker SB. Assessing the costs and benefits of electronic fetal monitoring. Obstet Gynecol Surv 1979; 34:627–642.

34. Niswander KR. Asphyxia in the fetus and CP. In: Pitkin RM, Zlatnik FJ, eds. The Yearbook of Obstetrics and Gynecology. Chicago: Yearbook Publishers, 1983: 9.

35. Paneth N, Jetton J, Pinto-Martin J, Susser M. Magnesium sulphate in labor and risk of brain lesions and cerebral palsy in low birth weight infants. Pediatrics 1997; 99(5). URL: http://www.pediatrics.org/cgi/content/full/99/5/e1.

36. Kumari S, Sharma M, Yadav M, Saraf A, Kabra M, Mehra M. Trends in neonatal outcome with low Apgar scores. Indian J Pediatr 1993; 60: 415–422.

37. De-Muylder X. Perinatal mortality audit in a Zimbabwean district. Paediatr Perinat Epidemiol 1989; 3:284–293.

38. Spellacy W. Management of the High Risk Pregnancy. Baltimore: University Park Press, 1976.

39. Paneth N. The etiology of cerebral palsy. Ped Ann 1986; 15:191–201.

40. Williams K, Hennessy E, Alberman E. Cerebral palsy: effects of twinning, birthweight, and gestational age. Arch Dis Child Fetal Neonatal Ed 1996; 75:F178–182.

41. Paneth N. Does transient hypothyroxinemia cause abnormal neurodevelopment in premature infants? Clin Perinatol 1998; 25:627–43.

42. Belman AL. Acquired immunodeficiency syndrome and the child's central nervous system. Pediatr Clin North Am 1992; 39:691–714.

43. Grethers JK, Nelson KB, Emery ES III, Cummins SK. Prenatal and perinatal factors and cerebral palsy in the very low birth weight infant. J Pediatr 1996; 128:407–414.

44. Leviton A, Gilles F, Neff R, Yaney P. Multivariate analysis of risk of perinatal telencephalic leucoencephalopathy. Am J Epidemiol 1976; 104:621–626.

45. Grethers JK, Nelson KB, Dambrosia JM, Phillips TM. Interferons and cerebral palsy. J Pediatr 1999; 134:324–332.

46. Grant PE, Barkovich AJ. Neuroimaging in CP: issues in pathogenesis and diagnosis. MRDD Res Rev 1997; 3:118–128.

47. Thorarensen O, Ryan S, Hunter J, Younkin DP. Factor V Leiden mutation: an unrecognized cause of hemiplegic cerebral palsy, neonatal stroke, and placental thrombosis. Ann Neurol 1997; 42:372–375.

48. Hughes I, Newton R. Genetic aspects of cerebral palsy. Dev Med Child Neurol 1992; 34:80–86.

49. Silver JR. Familial spastic paraplegia with amyotrophy of hands. Ann Hum Genet 1966; 30:69–75.

50. Ploch E, Christensen E, Colombo JP, Weiss-Wichert P, Wenger E. Macrocephaly and dystonic cerebral palsy in a child with type I glutaric aciduria. Am J Hum Gent 1991; 48:1214.

51. Cohn RM, Roth KS. Metabolic Disease: A Guide to Early Recognition. Philadelphia: Saunders, 1983.

52. Kuban KCK, Leviton A. Cerebral palsy. N Engl J Med. 1994; 330:188–195.

53. Bax M. Terminology and classification of cerebral palsy. Dev Med Child Neurol. 1964; 6:295–297.

54. Phelps W. Etiology and diagnostic classification of cerebral palsy. In: Proceedings of the Cerebral Palsy Institute. New York: Association for the Aid of the Crippled Children, 1950.

55. Rantakallio P, von Wendt L. A prospective comparative study of the etiology of CP and epilepsy in a one-year birth cohort from Northern Finland. Acta Paediatr Scand 1986; 75:586–592.

56. Kiely JL, Paneth N, Stein S, Susser M. Cerebral palsy and newborn care. I: Secular trends in cerebral palsy. Dev Med Child Neurol 1981; 23:533–538.

57. Stanley FJ, Watson L. The cerebral palsies in Western Australia: Trends, 1968 to 1981. Am J Obstet Gynecol 1988; 158:89–93.

58. Robertson CM, Svenson LW, Joffres MR. Prevalence of cerebral palsy in Alberta. Can J Neurol Sci 1988, 25:117–122.

59. Dowding VM, Berry C. Cerebral palsy: Changing patterns of birthweight and gestational age (1976/81). Irish Med J 1988; 81:25–29.

60. Riikonen R, Raumavirta S, Sinivuori E, Seppala T. Changing Pattern of Cerebral Palsy in the Southwest Region of Finland. Acta Paediatr Scand 1989; 78:581–587.

61. Meberg A. Declining incidence of low birth weight—impact on perinatal mortality and incidence of cerebral palsy. J Perinat Med 1990; 18:195–200.

62. Hagberg B, Hagberg G, Olow I, Wendt Lv. The changing panorama of cerebral palsy in Sweden. VII. Prevalence and origin in the birth year period 1987–1990. Acta Paediatr Scand 1996; 85:954–960.

63. Evans P, Elliot M, Alberman E. Evans E Prevalence and disabilities in 4 to 8 year olds with cerebral palsy. Arch Dis Child 1985; 60:940–945.

64. Yeargin-Allsopp M, Murphy CC, Oakley GP, Keith Sikes R. A multiple-source method for studying the prevalence of developmental disabilities in children: The Metropolitan Atlanta Developmental Disabilities Study. Pediatrics 1992; 89:624–630.1.

65. Al-Rajeh, Bademosi O, Awada A, Ismail H, Al-Shammasi S, Dawodu A. Cerebral palsy in Saudi Arabia: a case-control study of risk factors. Dev Med Child Neurol 1991; 33:1048–1052.

66. Srivastava VK, Laisram N, Srivastava RK. Cerebral palsy. Indian Pediatr 1992; 29: 993–996.

67. Murphy CC, Yeargin-Allsopp M, Decoufle P, Drews CD. Prevalence of cerebral palsy among ten-year-old children in metropolitan Atlanta, 1985 through 1987. J Pediatr 1993;123:S13–20

68. Haerer AF, Anderson DW, Schoenberg BS. Prevalence of cerebral palsy in the biracial population of Copiah county, Mississippi. Dev Med Child Neurol 1984; 26: 195–199.

69. Sinha G, Corry P, Subesinghe D, Wild J, Levene MI. Prevalence and type of cerebral palsy in a British ethnic community: the role of consanguinity. Dev Med Child Neurol 1997; 39:259–262.

70. Blair E, Stanley FJ. Issues in the classification and epidemiology of cerebral palsy. MRDD Res Rev 1997; 3:184–193.

71. Takeshita K, Ando Y, Ohtani K, Takashima S. Cerebral palsy in Tottori, Japan. Neuroepidemiology 1989; 8:184–192.

72. Stanley FJ. Survival and cerebral palsy in low birthweight infants: implications for perinatal care. Pediatr Perinatal Epidemiol 1992; 6:298–310.

73. Bhushan V, Paneth N, Kiely J. Impact of improved survival of very low birth weight infants on recent secular trends in the prevalence of cerebral palsy. Pediatrics 1993; 91:1094–1100.

74. Kleinman JC, Fowler MG, Kessel SS. Comparison of infant mortality among twin and singletons. United States 1960 and 1983. Am J Epidemiol 1991; 133:133–143.

75. Hack M, Friedman H, Fanaroff AA. Outcomes of extremely low birth weight infants. Pediatrics 1996; 98:931–937.

76. Bottoms SF, Paul RH, Iams JD, Mercer BM, Thom EA, Roberts JM, Caritis SN, Moawad AH, Van Dorsten JP, Hauth JC, Thurnau GR, Miodovnik M, Meis PM, McNellis D. Obstetric determinants of neonatal survival: influence of willingness to perform cesarean delivery on survival of extremely low-birth-weight infants. National Institute of Child Health and Human Development, Network of Maternal-Fetal Medicine Units, Bethesda, Maryland, USA. Am J Obstet Gynecol 1997; 176: 960–966.

77. Escobar GJ, Littenberg B, Petitti DB. Outcome among surviving very low birthweight infants: a meta-analysis. Arch Dis Child 1991; 66:204–211.

78. Lorenz JM, Wooliever DE, Jetton JR, Paneth N. A quantitative review of mortality and developmental disability in extremely premature infants. Arch Pediatr Adolesc Med 1998; 152:425–435.

79. Pharoah POD, Cooke T, Cooke RWI, Rosenbloom I. Birthweight specific trends in cerebral palsy. Arch Dis Child 1990; 65:602–606.
80. Hagberg B, Hagberg G, Zetterstrom R. Decreasing perinatal mortality—increase in cerebral palsy morbidity. Acta Paediatr 1989; 78:664–670.
81. Grethers JK, Cummins SK, Nelson KB. The California cerebral palsy project 339. Paediatr Perinatal Epidemiol 1992; 6:339–351.
82. Cockburn JM. Psychological and educational aspects. In: Henderson, JL ed. Cerebral Palsy in Childhood and Adolescence. Edinburgh: E&S Livingstone, 1961.
83. National Institute of Health on causes of mental retardation and cerebral palsy: task force on joint assessment of prenatal and perinatal factors associated with brain disorders. Pediatrics 1985; 76:457–458.
84. Aicardi J. Epilepsy in Children, 2nd ed. New York: Raven Press, 1994.
85. Hadjipanayis A, Hadjichristodoulou C, Youroukos S. Epilepsy in patients with cerebral palsy. Dev Med Child Neurol 1997; 39:659–663.
86. Aksu E. Nature and prognosis of seizures in patients with cerebral palsy. Dev Med Child Neurol 1990; 32:661–668.
87. Sutton GJ, Rowe SJ. Risk factors for childhood sensorineural hearing loss in the Oxford region. Br J Audiol 1997; 31:39–54.
88. Borg E. Perinatal asphyxia, hypoxia, ischemia and hearing loss: an overview. Scand Audiol 1997; 26:77–91.
89. Borradori C, Fawer CL, Buclin T, Calame A. Risk factors of sensorineural hearing loss in preterm infants. Biol Neonate 1997; 71:1–10.
90. McDermott S, Coker AL, Mani S, Krishnaswami S, Nagle RJ, Barnett-Queen LL, Wuori DF. A population-based analysis of behavior problems in children with cerebral palsy. J Pediatr Psychol 1996; 21:447–63.
91. Nelson KB, Grethers JK. Potentially asphyxiating conditions and spastic cerebral palsy in infants of normal birth weight. Am J Obset Gynecol 1998; 179:507–513.

3
Diagnostic Approach to the Infant

Alfred L. Scherzer
*Joan and Sanford I. Weill Medical College, Cornell University,
New York, New York*

I. THE CONCEPT OF NORMAL NEUROLOGICAL MATURATION

The work of Gesell and others firmly established both uniformity and the concept of variation in the normal developmental sequence of children (1–3). Acquaintance with this basic framework is essential to a working understanding of the growth process. More importantly, it is the cornerstone upon which identification of abnormal development rests. Underlying this framework is an orderly maturational sequence of the entire central nervous system (CNS).

Review of current data regarding structural neurological differentiation is helpful in understanding the complex process at work in earliest development. There is an extremely active and ongoing sequence of neurological maturation following birth that is continuous with in utero development (4). Massive development of neurons, axons, and dendrites takes place during this period, as the neurochemicals increasingly enable electrical transmission of signals between synapses (5). By age 2, the number of synapses is said to reach adult levels; by age 3, the brain has twice the number of adult synapses. This number remains high through age 10, then gradually becomes reduced to adult levels in adolescence (6). Myelination, or development of the nerve insulation sheath, is also an active, continuous process that takes up to at least the first two years of life before completion (7). Neuromaturation thus has enormous potential for growth throughout the preadult years.

Initially, growth of nerve pathways, interconnections, and cell fibers proceeds actively to the trunk and extremities, while brain stem connections affecting tone and earliest spontaneous motor patterns remain predominant (8). Maturation proceeds toward "higher" centers, ultimately reaching the cortex with independence in full voluntary control. However, some degree of voluntary movement is present even in the neonate. Newborn spontaneous patterns of motor behavior, previously considered to be infant reflexes, are viewed by Prechtl to occur endogenously through central pattern generators, rather than being reflex in nature (9). As growth proceeds, the infantile primitive motor patterns give way to more complex postural motor patterns and to mature voluntary behavior. Initial mass behavior activity on an involuntary basis is replaced by individual responses under voluntary control, and integration proceeds at the various levels of CNS activity. Postural tone, or the maintenance of the body in space, becomes integrated simultaneously as part of the developmental process.

Complex general movements (GMs) that involve the head, trunk, arms, and legs have been identified by 9 to 10 weeks of fetal life through the use of video studies (10), and are said to persist up to 3 to 4 months post-term (11, 12). Earliest preterm general movements are fluent, changing with age in range, variation, and speed. The preterm GMs give rise to writhing GMs near term, with less trunk involvement (13, 14). These give way to irregular fidgety GMs involving the entire body by 2 months post-term, prior to their normal disappearance (15).

Motor maturation has traditionally been thought to be hierarchical in development, proceeding in a predetermined cephalocaudal direction, with motor control of the head, neck, and trunk preceding extension of the trunk, ultimate weight bearing, and walking. More recent data from longitudinal studies of infant kicking (16), and postural control during reaching (17), among others, demonstrate that infants are not preprogrammed for motor coordination and activity. Instead of the predetermined concepts of the past, a dynamic systems approach is now generally accepted in which there is individual self-organization of movement with interaction between tasks and environment over time. However, there is a need for further evidence to support the theory.

Maturation of the normal central nervous system occurs simultaneously at many different levels. Although there is an orderly sequence in development, considerable variation is seen within individual children in achieving stages of motor and intellectual achievement. Thus, a child's intelligence may be considerably ahead of his or her locomotion ability, yet ultimately development may reach average levels. There is also a range of variation that exists among infants in reaching established levels of neuromaturation (18).

Motor development should be seen as a succession of integrated milestones leading to more complex and independent function (19). Each stage is interdependent and relates closely to progressive control of higher centers of the nervous system and reduced influence of involuntary motor behavior patterns (20). Many stages will develop simultaneously. Each milestone, therefore, is not necessarily perfected before going on to the next (21). Also, a "competition of motor patterns'' is suggested in which a child naturally practices new activities, with temporary suppression of others, until learning is complete. Older and more established activities may then be resumed and added (22).

Finally, the dynamic systems theory now emphasizes the influence of the child's tasks and the environment as factors beyond the nervous system that influence motor development (23). Obviously, any evaluation or assessment of the infant must take account of these variables and their interaction. In turn, the concept opens new approaches to influencing maturation through changing tasks offered to the child as well as altering the environment (24).

Thus the infant is initially dominated by tone and early motor patterns mediated through the brain stem, and by mass responses as physical and biochemical growth of the nervous system proceeds. The orderly process simultaneously leads to maturation of tone, gradual inhibition of earliest primitive motor patterns, emergence of postural motor patterns, progression of developmental milestones, and an increasing degree of voluntary behavior. Environmental influences will have a profound effect on this process throughout (25, 26).

The challenge for those dealing with developmental problems in very young children is to accurately assess and comprehend the significance of delay that falls outside the limits of typical variability. Is it normal or pathological? Knowledge of the normal orderly sequence of developmental achievement, and patterns of integration of behavior, is the basis upon which possibly significant deviation in maturation can be gauged. Appendix A includes a comprehensive outline of developmental stages and normal motor milestones from birth to 3 years for detailed reference (27).

II. OVERVIEW OF ABNORMAL INFANT NEUROLOGICAL DEVELOPMENT

Although the theme of development is one of a continuum with many variations constantly under environmental influence (24), its physiological basis is exceedingly complex. Any aberration of the central nervous system does not necessarily coincide initially with distinct and observable focal motor dysfunction in the developing infant. Instead, evidence of malformation or insult will generally be apparent only in abnormalities of general movements, tone, patterns of motor behavior, and developmental milestones.

General movements have been classified into "mildly abnormal" and "definitely abnormal" with the use of video and EMG recording (28). Mildly abnormal GMs are said to lack fluency, while definitely abnormal GMs lack all fluency, complexity, and variation (14). Strong correlation and specificity of abnormal GMs and neurological abnormality increases by the third month postterm (15).

Tone is often altered, with either excessive or diminished quality. This is mediated through brain stem pathways and may well be an early indication of brain stem malfunction (29). In particular, one may see a discrepancy between proximal and distal tone, that is, between the trunk and extremities.

Alteration in appearance, intensity, or expression of *primitive motor patterns* will occur (30). The normal course of early disappearance of primitive motor patterns through inhibitive pathways will be affected, with either delay or failure in the development of later *postural motor patterns* (31).

Developmental milestones will be delayed in progression, with prolonged fixation at a given stage. The extent of abnormality will relate to the degree of delay in brain stem and nerve pathway maturation. The nature of the total central nervous system fixed pathology would directly affect both.

Motor abnormality appears relatively late in infant development, as nerve pathways become more functional. This is a natural outcome of the selective nerve growth process. Differential rates or order of appearance of motor deficit are manifest. The abnormal motor features emerge as the damaged nervous system matures. In cerebral palsy, for example, evidence of spasticity may be first noted only at 7 to 9 months of age. Dystonia will not generally be apparent before 18 months and may be delayed beyond 2 years. Ataxia is frequently not manifest before 30 months to 3 years. Identification of mixed motor features may be further delayed while nervous system development progresses and relative dominance of one motor form interchanges with another. Immature initial CNS development may result in poor overall organizational ability of the infant, affecting irritability, feeding, and sleeping, for example. These findings will ultimately need to be distinguished from true specific sensory and motor deficits. In fact, transient neurological deficits are common in such infants, and a long-term perspective on progression in development is essential to achieve an accurate picture of developmental status.

III.   PREDICTION OF DEVELOPMENTAL ABNORMALITY

A.   Physiological Screening

1.   Biochemical

From time immemorial there have been concerns about ultimate development of the newborn with signs of distress. Prediction of outcome based on clinical experience alone finally gave way in the 1950s to the Apgar score, which has also been used as a guide for resuscitation and as a statistical tool (32). The scoring system was based on observations of color, respiratory effort, heart rate, tone, and reflex activity (33). However, lack of correlation has been found with this group of factors and later chronic neurological deficits (34, 35). Similarly, each of the variables in the score has been shown to be a poor predictor of later outcome (36).

The use of blood acidemia and base deficits in the newborn as markers of asphyxia with later neurological sequelae have also shown poor correlation (37, 38). Predictability is improved with the addition of a low 5-min Apgar score and the need for intubation at term (39). Various newborn spinal fluid components have been shown to be effective markers of hypoxic-ischemic encephalopathy (40). However, they would not ordinarily be obtained without evidence of obvious neurological abnormality.

Predictive effects of newborn urine products have also been considered since asphyxia results in injury to the kidney. Paucity of urine flow (oliguria) and elevated β_2-microglobulin at 36 h have been found to correlate with later neurological deficits (41). A more recent finding has shown a high correlation between the ratio of urinary lactate to creatinine within the first 6-h of birth in those infants who are likely to develop hypoxic-ischemic encephalopathy (42). It should be kept in mind that even if these or other biochemical markers of hypoxic-ischemia stand the test of time and experience, they deal only with asphyxia and ischemic injury to the brain, which represent but one etiological basis among many for static encephalopathy (see Chapter 2).

2. Prenatal

Prenatal screening has also had extensive development, including amniocentesis, chorionic villus sampling, and the use of ultrasound. These tools are used to monitor the pregnancy and to identify specific abnormalities that may include developmental disabilities such as Down syndrome (43).

3. Neuroimaging

Cranial ultrasonography, cranial tomography, and magnetic resonance imaging (MRI) now have considerable capability of documenting peri and intraventricular lesions, as well as demonstrating hypoxic-ischemic encephalopathy in premature and high-risk infants (44). Moreover, definite image patterns have been found to be associated with the clinical course of the infant (45,46). And, most recently, proton magnetic resonance spectroscopy (MRS) is being used to observe abnormal intracellular cerebral metabolites within hours of birth, which correlates well with later neurological deficit (47). Nevertheless, all of these techniques deal with only one possible etiology of developmental disabilities.

B. Developmental Screening

Recognizing that early development is a dynamic and changing process has led to extensive efforts to anticipate and predict developmental abnormality in very young children. A large variety of rating/screening instruments have burgeoned within recent years, with varying degrees of accuracy for prediction of (1) developmental delay; (2) definite developmental abnormality; and (3) specific developmental diagnoses. Among those most commonly used at the present time are the following.

1. Developmental Scales

Amiel-Tison (48)
Bayley (49)
Brazelton (50)
Dubowitz (51, 52, revised)
Haataja et al. (53)
Peabody (54)
Prechtl (21)

2. Developmental Screening Tests

Denver Developmental Screening Test (Denver II) (most commonly used) (55)
Batelle Screening Test (56)
Clinical Adaptive Test (CAT)/Clinical Linguistic and Auditory Milestone Scale (CLAMS) (57)
Knobloch Revised Screening Inventory (58)
General Movements (GMs) Assessment (30, 59, 60)

3. Motor Assessment Instruments

Alberta Infant Motor Scale (AIMS) (61)
Early Motor Pattern Profile (EMPP) (62)
Gross Motor Function Measure (GMFM) (63)
Movement Assessment Inventory (MAI) (64)
Test of Infant Motor Performance (TIMP) (65)

Clearly, reliability, sensitivity, and validity of any of these instruments vary greatly, while predictive power increases with the age of the child (66). At present none are well-standardized (67). Moreover, none of them deal effectively with early differential diagnosis for the infant less than 12 months.

In addition to the use of, or findings from, various existing scales, it is essential to have the perspective of a dynamic evaluative approach that: (1) identifies factors relating to significant risk for disability; and (2) utilizes variables that can be followed to make an early determination of specific developmental abnormality.

The scales currently in use have limitations in both these areas. However, they can provide an important *screening function* as a basis of referral for full evaluation. Alternatively, specific screening tests, such as the Denver, the CAT/ CLAMS, or the Bayley, can provide important information about the functioning level of the infant, and may provide a baseline for change over time.

With these considerations in mind, we offer in the following sections a broad developmental evaluation approach to identification of the infant from birth to 3 years based upon clinical experience and long-term follow-up.

IV. DEVELOPMENTAL EVALUATION APPROACH TO DIAGNOSIS

The complex developmental nature of the condition with its late emerging motor signs makes early identification of cerebral palsy a diagnostic challenge. There is obviously no early pathognomonic sign, x-ray, or laboratory test that, in itself, is confirmatory. Evidence to substantiate a diagnosis must be gathered in an orderly and consistent sequential way, with full knowledge of the total maturation process, rather than fixation on any given focal neurological sign or physical deficit. This is the basis of the developmental approach to diagnosis.

One must start with concern about risk and an index of suspicion. The beginning point is often the pediatrician, family practitioner, or other health professional who is consulted by a concerned parent whose child is not making typical progress in motor milestones or speech. Too often the matter may not be given serious consideration if a specific motor abnormality is not found. The parent may be reassured that the child "will grow out of it," and told to return if no progress is forthcoming, in the hope that delayed development will ultimately speed up and reach a typical pattern. A similar situation may occur, as well, even in a highly sophisticated neonatal intensive care unit. For example, an infant is discharged following treatment for respiratory distress syndrome. Subsequent difficulty in feeding and ordinary infant management, when brought to the attention of medical staff on follow-up clinic visits, may be attributed to immaturity, poor organization at home, or emotional upset within the family environment. In fact, each of these situations may represent a child with significant developmental delays due to a fixed brain lesion that ultimately will appear as one of the major motor forms of cerebral palsy. Parental concern may well be appropriate while the professional response is dilatory or insensitive.

Professional awareness is the starting point in early diagnosis and must be based upon sensitivity to possible neurological deficit in any infant with developmental delay or behavior problems. The obvious first priority is to utilize history, physical examination, and appropriate laboratory studies to rule out the possibility of a progressive CNS disorder. With the assurance that progressive CNS pathology is not present, the basis of parental concern must be probed further, rather than merely looking for a discrete structural or neurological abnormality. Knowledge of the developmental process needs to be incorporated by the professional and used appropriately as with any other diagnostic tool. Only in this way will it be possible to develop a realistic and appropriate sense of whether a child is, in fact, at risk of cerebral palsy or other developmental disability. The index of suspicion should then generate initiation of a full process of developmental evaluation, and not simply a physical examination. This should be recorded using an outline such as that illustrated in Appendix B.

It is essential to follow a systematic and uniform multifactor developmental evaluation approach in order to identify the specific diagnosis (if possible) in children who clearly have a nonprogressive developmental disability (68). Table 1 provides an outline of the developmental evaluation procedure that is detailed in the following sections.

A. Developmental History

1. Chief Complaint

The chief complaint or concern of the parent presents the initial focus. Often, this is diffuse and sometimes disorganized, with confusion about the actual problem. ''Advice'' from friends and relatives, and poorly understood information gleaned from the media, may greatly color the real issues. The time-consuming procedure of directing and putting into order these concerns may discourage even the most patient examiner. Skillful and well-directed interviewing, however, will channel unrelated or even diffuse information into a pattern that can be integrated into the history (69). The examiner should elicit not only the area of most concern, but also the age and circumstances at which the problem was first noted. This will be helpful in guiding discussion about the needs of the family.

An accurate and complete history is the first step in the process of developmental evaluation. Adequate records must be obtained where possible. However, birth and hospital records may not be sufficiently detailed or accurate, particularly if obstetrical or neonatal events have been complex or traumatic. On the other hand, reliability and possible bias of the parent or guardian should be weighed in assessing the information given. It is important to obtain information using a well-organized, logical sequence of questions, so that gaps or omissions will be minimal. Factors that may be of significance are discussed below.

2. Family and Genetic History

Parental and sibling health should be reviewed, particularly as it relates to the prepregnancy period. Endocrine and metabolic disorders such as thyroid, pituitary

Table 1 Developmental Evaluation Procedure

A. Developmental History
    1. Chief complaint
    2. Family and genetic history
       a. Pregnancy
       b. Labor/delivery
       c. Perinatal/neonatal
    3. Developmental milestones
    4. Other developmental features
    5. Reviews of systems
    4. Other developmental features
    5. Reviews of systems
    6. Past medical history
B. Developmental Physical Examination
C. Developmental Neurological Examination
    1. General observation
    2. Quality of general movements
    3. Tone
    4. Patterns of motor behavior
       a. Primitive
       b. Postural
    5. Sensation
    6. Cranial nerves
    7. Cerebellar function
    8. Dystonia
    9. Motor signs
       a. Upper motor
       b. Lower motor
    10. Neurological soft signs.
D. Developmental Screening Instruments
E. Laboratory Evaluation

abnormality, or diabetes may be relevant. History of seizures and other CNS problems should be detailed, including any evidence of mental retardation, learning disorders, attention deficits, cerebral palsy, seizures, emotional disorders, congenital malformations, or multiple handicapping conditions among any family members. Evidence for any genetic disease should be elicited, particularly possible patterns of genetic developmental transmission, including conditions such as Down's syndrome, Sturge-Weber syndrome and related disorders, genetic forms of cerebral palsy, and evidence for familial organic learning disorders or varieties of mental retardation.

(a) Pregnancy.   Experiences during the pregnancy are important and relate to feelings of well being or anxiety, presence of bleeding, health problems,
and fetal movements. Each of these experiences may give an indication of pertinent abnormality. Persistent bleeding may indicate intrauterine developmental
abnormality, especially if it occurred early in the pregnancy. Infection, toxemia,
and use of medications, such as diuretics, anticonvulsants, and various types of
antibiotics, may be of importance. The use or abuse of tobacco, alcohol, and drugs
should be questioned. Late-onset or diminished fetal movement may indicate a
poorly developing fetus. History of possible trauma or stress should be carefully
evaluated.

Length of gestation and the presence of prematurity may be crucial. It is
often difficult to obtain an accurate history of pregnancy length due to conflicting
dates and various obstetrical calculation methods. Every effort should be made
to document possible premature gestation to better assess the relation to birth
weight and the extent of developmental risk.

(b) Labor and Delivery.   Details of labor should include extent of labor
before delivery and rate of progression. Evidence for dystocia or prolonged labor
should be considered as well as precipitate or rapid labor. Either may be of considerable significance. A prolonged period between membrane rupture and delivery could be a basis for fetal infection. Obstetrical features of the delivery must
include use of anesthesia, mechanical events such as version, abnormal presenta-
tions, use of instrumentation, and rationale for caesarian section if performed.
The place of delivery may be relevant, especially if at home, en route to the
hospital, or under unusual circumstances.

(c) Perinatal and Neonatal Events.   Assessment of the child's condition
at birth requires information about birth weight, presence of a nuchal cord, respiratory status, the need for prolonged oxygen treatment, continuous apnea, cyano-
sis, or resuscitative procedures. History of possible sepsis, meningitis, neonatal
seizures, and the presence of any type of congenital malformation is important.
Jaundice shortly after birth due to possible blood group incompatibility should
be distinguished from subsequent hyperbilirubinemia in the neonatal period, possibly related to breast-feeding, galactosemia, infection, such as hepatitis, or structural abnormality of the liver. Reports of an abnormally small or large head circumference should be given appropriate consideration for microcephaly or
hydrocephaly.

History of progress up to the first month should be selectively examined
for an overview of the entire neonatal period. Particular attention should be given
to evidence of poor extrauterine adjustment of the infant. This could include
marked irritability, hyperactivity, limited or negative environmental contact, or
inability to develop a reasonable feeding and sleeping schedule. Adjustment to
feeding, in particular, may be crucial, especially if the child sucks or swallows

poorly and is thought to have "colic." Colic may be one of the earliest signs of central nervous system malfunction and represents one of a number of problems in infant organization and adaptation referred to as "behavioral soft signs," discussed later in this chapter.

3. Developmental Milestones

The gross motor developmental milestones present an orderly sequence through which the child is expected to progress normally and are a major indicator of developmental progress (70). The range of normal compared with late and abnormal appearance is given in Table 2. Note the wide range of normal appearance in each modality and the marked delay observed in a group with cerebral palsy. An arrest or delay at any given stage is usually the basis for initial parental referral. This is the reference point from which the examiner must go back and bring into focus the chief complaint as a first step in the developmental evaluation process. The fundamental requirement is to make a distinction between the delayed developmental progress of a possible static encephalopathy, in contrast to the child with a history of regression from previously achieved function who may have a progressive or degenerative condition (71).

Table 2 Normal Development Compared with Average Development of 100 Cerebral Palsy Children

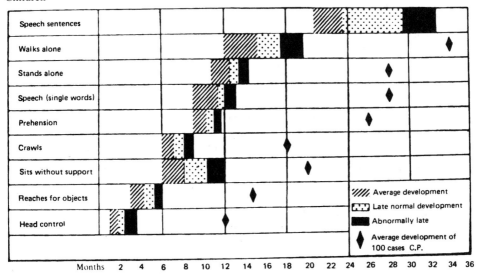

Source: Courtesy of Crippled Children and Adults of Rhode Island, Inc., Providence, Rhode Island.

It is useful to elicit information about developmental milestones in the following order, specifically inquiring about when each of the modalities was achieved: (1) smiling; (2) head control in prone position; (3) grasping; (4) transferring objects from hand to hand; (5) sitting; (6) crawling, including quality of motion; and (7) independent walking with quality of movement and evidence of any deficits.

Oral development should be carefully reviewed for any difficulties in sucking, chewing, tongue thrusting, and drooling, problems in tooth eruption, enamelization, jaw structure, and dental development. Onset of speech should be noted, including intelligibility and quality of sounds, with a description of progression to phrases and sentences, or any evidence of regression. Verbal behavior is most important, bearing in mind verbosity, repetitive speech, and early evidence of echolalia. Information should also be obtained about hearing acuity and discrimination, visual development, and the onset of and response to environmental stimuli.

Patterns of sleep should be noted, with attention to getting to sleep and wakefulness. Also levels of ability in taking off clothes, dressing, and early self-care should be considered.

It is essential to emphasize that the developmental milestones present the major clinical parameter of progressive central nervous system growth and integration. Delay or arrest beyond the normally acceptable range may provide the most significant index of suspicion for developmental disability, particularly when considered in conjunction with abnormality in developmental history, including family background, pregnancy, labor, or delivery. No one factor alone will necessarily be definitive, but all taken together can form a framework to establish the diagnosis.

4. Other Developmental Features

Social and emotional variables give an insight into personality integration. Attention should be given to temper tantrums, breath holding, hyperactivity, limited attention span, and ability to separate from family and adjust in new situations. Play interests are important and should be age appropriate. These interests will closely correlate with any obvious physical deficits or limitations. Reaction to and participation in group activities, such as nursery classes, gives an insight into demands for attention, supervision, and ability to react both physically and socially. This may also provide an early indication of behavioral problems, learning disabilities, or fine motor function, and should be noted. Independence in self-care activities should be assessed, including feeding, dressing, and toileting. Problems with the latter may have both neurological and emotional aspects that should be carefully weighed.

5. Review of Systems

Particular consideration should be given to general medical or health problems and previous hospitalizations either associated with or related to possible neurological deficit. Examples would include any evidence of headaches, tics, seizure activity, unexplained vomiting, lethargy, personality change, or loss of previously achieved function. Any of these symptoms could be related to hydrocephalus, an intracranial vascular lesion, or neoplasm. Details of any seizure activity should include association with fever, frequency, duration, and character of the movements.

6. Past Medical History

Apart from seizure history, information should include data from any previous neurological evaluation with description of electroencephalogram, CAT or MRI scans, and other findings. Results of psychological and developmental evaluations should be obtained. Documentation of medications in use should include rationale and effect. Previous treatment including occupational, physical, and speech therapies should be noted, with details of associated changes and the child's response. Similar data are needed about bracing or assistive devices used, and types of surgery performed.

At the conclusion of the developmental history, the examiner should indicate an impression of parental interest, attitude, and ability to deal with the child. During the course of the interview, it is generally possible to arrive at some awareness of these interpersonal factors that can later provide a basis for needed supportive services.

B. The Developmental Physical Examination

The setting of the examination is important and should provide a relaxed, unhurried atmosphere for parent and child. Obtained measurements of height, weight, and head circumference should be plotted on appropriate standards and analyzed.

Observation of the child gives the first indication of environmental response, social interaction, and relation to parent. Much of this observation can be done while obtaining the developmental history. Evidence should be noted for possible visual or hearing deficits and the quality of verbal response or speech. Level and appropriateness of activity and behavior can also be gauged. Structural abnormalities must be detailed in an orderly manner through examination of skin, head and neck, trunk, abdomen, back, spine, and extremities. Obvious malformations could immediately identify conditions such as Down's syndrome, Sturge-Weber syndrome, neurofibromatosis, tuberous sclerosis, hydrocephalus, meningomyelocele, encephalocele, hemiplegia, and brachial plexus paralysis (72).

Many other minor structural deviations may also be apparent early. Some may be part of a syndrome complex, such as abnormal facial features in fetal alcohol syndrome. Others more frequently will not form part of a specific classification, but their presence may suggest associated central nervous system malformation.

Examination of the head requires careful measurement of head size with accurate recording on a standardized instrument (73). Simultaneous check of size and shape of fontanelles should lead to immediate referral if there is any evidence of hydrocephalus or premature suture closure. Also, failure of head growth over a period of months, particularly in a girl, may be an indication of a progressive disorder, such as Rett Syndrome (74). Possible microcephaly should be noted, as well as cleft palate or lip, structural problems of tongue, mouth, nose, and jaw, and abnormal set or configuration of the ears. These structural anomalies are not unusual in children with severe developmental deficits.

Examination of the eyes is not as difficult in small children as might be anticipated if the parent assists. The procedure may be most rewarding. Readily obtainable peripheral eye findings may include strabismus, hypertelorism, epicanthus, cataracts, congenital glaucoma, heterochromia, corneal ring (Wilson's disease), depigmented iris of albinism, blue sclerae of osteogenesis imperfecta, scleral pigmentary deposits with ochronosis, or a cloudy cornea noted in mucopolysaccharidosis.

The fundi must be carefully examined for evidence of retinal inflammation as in rubella, toxoplasmosis, or cytomegalovirus infections. Retinal degeneration may indicate a nonspecific degenerative condition, or retinitis pigmentosa, while macular degeneration is specific for Tay-Sachs disease, Nieman-Pick disease, and Gaucher's disease. Also to be noted are retinal changes indicative of intracranial pressure due to hydrocephalus or tumor, and evidence of possible vascular lesions or malformation.

Neck examination should consider signs of webbing and shortening associated with Klippel-Feil syndrome, platybasia and basilar impression, or possible Turner's syndrome. Congenital torticollis is seen in conjunction with other anomalies, and enlarged thyroid is of major concern. Also, a check should be made for bruits, both in the neck and head, for vascular malformations. Chest evaluation should consider anomalies of the bony thorax such as pectus excavatum and carinium, absent ribs, or aplasia of the pectoralis muscles. Lungs and heart should be assessed for normal functioning.

Abdominal fullness or asymmetry may suggest hydronephrosis associated with renal anomalies, Wilms' tumor, or neuroblastoma. Enlarged liver or spleen would give rise to many diagnostic considerations relating to developmental abnormality including biliary atresia, galactosemia, or Wilson's disease, hemoglobinopathy such as in sickle cell anemia or thalassemia, or congenital red cell abnormality in spherocytosis. Hernia is a common finding, often seen in connection with other malformations.

Genitalia should be noted for ambiguity, abnormality in size or shape, testicular descent, presence of hypo or epispadius. Testicular enlargement may be associated with fragile X syndrome. Extremities should be examined for syndactyly, abnormal palmar creases seen in Down syndrome, shortening or asymmetry present in hemiplegia or hemihypertrophy. The hips must be carefully assessed for possible dislocation.

Observation of the back should check for lumbosacral hemangioma, anomalous hair, dermal sinus, or raised lesion consistent with meningomyelocele. Spinal deviation including fixed scoliosis, kyphosis, or excessive lordosis needs further review.

C. Developmental Neurological Examination

1. General Observation

The child's activity in relating to the environment should be carefully noted during the physical examination, with special emphasis given to awareness, interest in the environment and examiner, irritability, attention span, and evidence for hyperactivity. Observation of gross motor function and posture can be done simultaneously, including head, neck, and trunk control, sitting, crawling, standing, walking, and hand use. Attention to patterns of movement may indicate the presence of asymmetry consistent with hemiplegia or evidence of dystonia. Character of the cry, voice, and sounds should also be readily apparent.

2. Quality of General Movements

Whether or not video and EMG recording capability is available, it is important to be aware of the writhing character of GMs in the normal term infant, which change to a fidgety, irregular pattern by 2 months. Quality of GMs should be assessed when the infant is awake, active, and not crying (75). There is significant correlation of the quality of these GMs with normal and abnormal neurological development, especially in preterm and immediate post-term ages (76).

3. Tone

Tone should be assessed early in the examination when the child is most relaxed. A useful method is to pull the arms forward to sitting and standing positions with the child supine and observe ability to maintain head and neck upright and stabilize the trunk. Obvious hypotonicity will be apparent with lag of the head and trunk (Fig.1). On the other hand, maintenance of a hyperextended trunk and rigid standing with support in the very young infant may be the earliest indication of pathological hypertonus (Fig.2). Distinction should be made between tone of extremities and trunk and any disparity noted. A pattern of hypertonic extremities

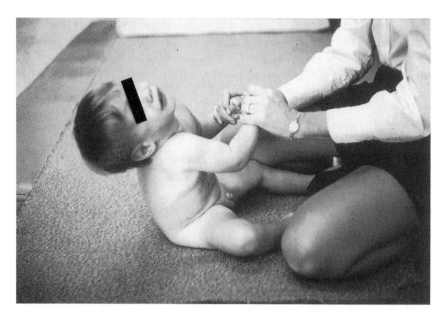

Figure 1 Hypotonia of head and trunk when child is brought to sitting.

with hypotonicity of the trunk may be an indication of underlying athetosis. The ability of a newborn to dorsiflex the foot completely onto the shin is considered normal and any restriction may suggest abnormal tone (77) (Fig. 3). Degree of head lag has been quantitated as a standardized reference for comparison with the norm (78).

The floppy child seems to have relatively little control over one joint upon another. Such a finding raises the possibility of a wide differential diagnosis including mental retardation, cerebral palsy, and varieties of myopathies. Generally, children who have a cerebral palsy diagnosis and are extremely hypertonic early may eventually have the athetoid form, while those with initial hypotonia may later become spastic (79).

4. Patterns of Motor Behavior

Assessment of earliest behavior provides a major insight into brain stem function and CNS developmental integration. It may provide the earliest indication of fixed motor deficit consistent with cerebral palsy long before any discrete motor signs are present. Two major categories function dynamically as the nervous system develops toward maturation of higher centers. The first is a group of primitive motor patterns present at birth and without which the infant would not

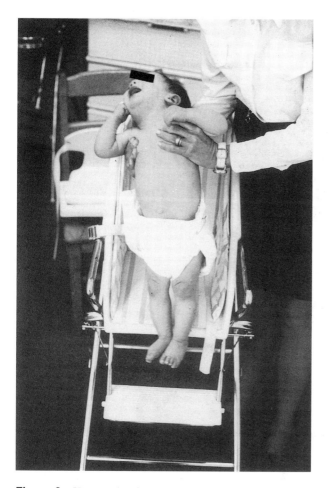

Figure 2 Hypertonia of entire body using under arm support.

be viable. Most of this motor behavior typically disappears by 4 to 6 months with maturation (80), as the postural motor patterns become manifest and remain throughout life. The latter are closely associated with and underlie rolling, sitting, crawling, and, eventually walking.

   (a)   Primitive Motor Patterns.   The major primitive motor patterns that have been described include startle, Moro, palmar and plantar grasp, rooting, sucking, placing, truncal incurvation, asymmetrical tonic neck, crossed extension, tonic labyrinthine, and others. Since a large number of primitive motor patterns

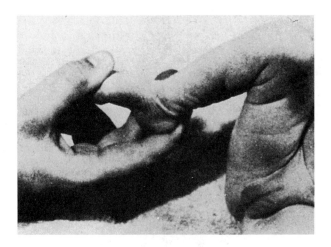

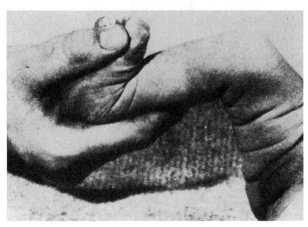

Figure 3 A normal newborn can dorsiflex the foot right onto the shin. (From Ref. 4, © 1966.)

are present, and some authors make no distinction between primitive and postural behaviors, there is controversy concerning which have the greatest clinical meaning and predictive significance. Dagarssies places relatively little importance upon truncal incurvation, but considers crossed extension to be critical in maturation (30). Capute et al., on the other hand, include truncal incurvation among the major predictive motor patterns (reflexes) being intensely evaluated in an extensive long-range study (81). The revised Dubowitz scale utilizes the following: tendon, suck, gag, palmar grasp, plantar grasp, Moro, and placing (52). Gupta favors rooting, Moro, crossed extension, plantar, positive support, placing, asymmetyrical and symmetrical, palmar, tonic labyrinthine, and Landau (82). Haataja et al. focus on tendon reflexes, arm protection, vertical suspension, lateral tilting, and forward parachute in their optimality score for the infant between 2 and 24 months of age (53).

Our own clinical experience has led to use of the following primitive motor patterns in the diagnostic evaluation: Moro, palmar grasp, asymmetric tonic neck, rooting, and sucking (Fig. 4a–e). Weak expression such as poor rooting, sucking, or limited Moro response, would be consistent with abnormality, particularly if there is associated asymmetry. Any persistence of these motor patterns beyond 4 to 6 months would provide a strong index of suspicion for significant fixed motor brain deficit, particularly in association with an abnormal developmental history. An obligatory asymmetric tonic neck (ATN) is always abnormal, especially if the child cries in this position. A strong and persistent ATN is frequently later associated with dystonic cerebral palsy (83).

(b) Postural Motor Patterns. A number of postural motor patterns are also identified whose diagnostic relevance is variously recognized (84). Among those we have found to be clinically relevant are neck righting, parachute or protective extension, and the Landau (Fig. 5a–c).

An overview of these developmental patterns of motor behavior is shown in Table 3, indicating the sequential disappearance of the primitive motor patterns and appearance of postural motor patterns. Each of these should be tested during the diagnostic evaluation and considered in relation to timing, strength of expression, and symmetry. Use of abnormal patterns of motor behavior in infant differential diagnosis will be discussed in detail later in the chapter. In general, it should be noted that both delayed disappearance of primitive motor patterns and delayed appearance of posturals is consistent with cerebral palsy. Normal primitive disappearance and delayed posturals is more characteristic of mental retardation (85).

5. Sensation

Sensory modality evaluation should include response to touch and pain. Where indicated, specific responses at various dermatome levels should be obtained to rule out possible lower motor lesions.

6. Cranial Nerves

Cranial nerve function may be difficult to evaluate in small children. An accurate observation of III, IV, and VI can be obtained for evidence of strabismus; V for

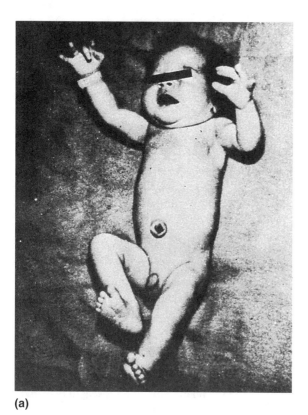

(a)

Figure 4 Primitive motor patterns that persist beyond 4 to 6 months and may indicate fixed motor brain deficiency: (a) Moro; (b) palmar grasp (from Ref. 4, © 1966); (c) strong, persistent asymmetric tonic neck; (d) abnormally delayed rooting; and (e) abnormally delayed sucking.

mandibular function; VII for corneal reflex and facial asymmetry; IX and XI for swallowing and gag reflex. Function of XII may be possible to estimate, especially if there is tongue deviation.

7. Cerebellar Function

Cerebellar dysfunction may be equally difficult to recognize in the infant and very small child. Exaggerated opticokinetic nystagmus should be elicited using response to horizontal movements. Ataxia may be indicated through observation

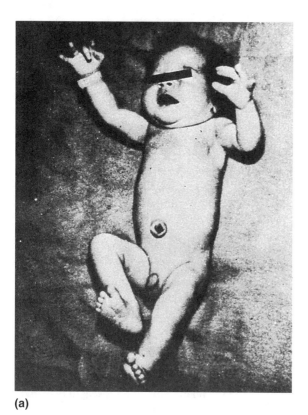

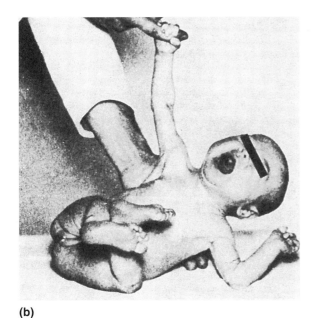

(b)

of balance of head, neck, and trunk, and demonstration of hand use with small objects.

8. Dystonia

Disparity of tone between trunk and extremities may be the first suggestive sign of dystonia, particularly if there is significant hypotonicity of the trunk. This may quickly alternate to truncal hypertonicity. Stiffness and hyperextension of the entire body, but particularly of the face, head, and upper limbs, may dramatically change. Apparent limitation in range of motion in the extremities may give way to full movement and no restriction if the child can be relaxed. In the slightly older patient, facial movements and grimacing may be observed together with movements of the upper limbs and an overpronated position of arms and hands. Variable tone remains a cardinal feature that may involve trunk and extremities. Depending upon the state of the child, these features may vary from time to time, especially in early developmental stages. Actual dystonic movement is likely to appear very late, often well beyond 18 months. The early stiffness noted before the child is fully relaxed may often be misdiagnosed as spasticity. Variability in findings related to dystonia has also played a part in the past confusion of cerebral palsy classification (see Chapter 1) particularly relating to types of "athetosis,"

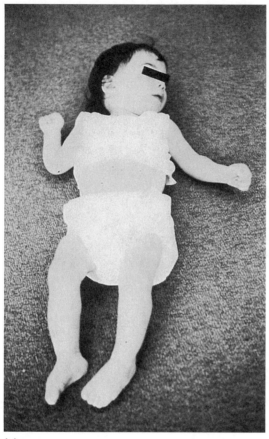

(c)

Figure 4 Continued.

and the relation to tremor, atonia, rigidity, and even ataxia. The clinical distinction between these can be most difficult in a very small child.

9. Motor Signs

(a) Upper Motor. Upper motor neuron signs can generally be elicited without difficulty, particularly if there is asymmetry. Markedly exaggerated deep tendon reflexes can be judged accurately indicating evidence for spasticity. Babinski sign may be variable and often cannot be definitely evaluated (86). Its significance even in newborns is also questioned since it may not be found at all

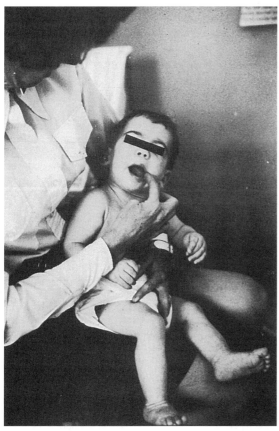

(d)

(87). Frequently, clonus can best be demonstrated by placing the child in the prone position and gently dorsiflexing the great toe or anterior part of the foot. This maneuver tends to displace voluntary motor activity away from the feet so that the reflex is not dampened.

 (b) Lower Motor. Lower motor signs should be considered when there is evidence of impaired sensation at segmental levels. Testing of strength should be attempted using estimates of muscle/joint resistance, and observing paucity of discrete extremity movements.

10. Neurological Soft Signs

Soft signs refer to a group of functional neurological findings that are general and not focal, often subtle, and may relate to faulty integration in early develop-

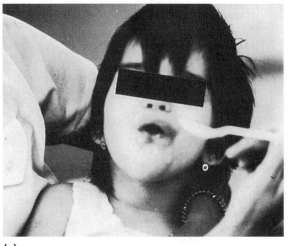

(e)

Figure 4 Continued.

ment (88). They give clues to underlying poor organization and possible central nervous system deficit. Early on they are manifest as ''behavioral'' soft signs and later may be identified as discrete neurological abnormalities in fine motor and integrative functioning. One of the earliest may affect sucking, swallowing, and feeding, and has already been mentioned previously in connection with neonatal ''colic.'' Persistent irritability, demanding behavior, continuous gross movement activity, markedly limited attention span, delayed speech with poor or repetitive expression, withdrawn and isolated behavior, and irregular sleep habits may all suggest underlying deficit in the infant.

For the older child, a systematic approach to observing other of these features is indicated if the subject is capable of some cooperation. This assessment would include visual tracking without moving the head, blowing out the cheeks, lateralizing the tongue, and demonstrating fine finger/ rapid succession movements.

The soft signs add another dimension to early differential diagnosis by either helping to confirm a diagnosis of cerebral palsy when used in conjunction with other positive motor findings or suggesting areas other than gross motor as the basis of developmental deficit. These might include mental retardation syndromes, attention deficit/hyperactive disorder, or the pervasive developmental disorders. More specific and directed diagnostic assessments could then be undertaken.

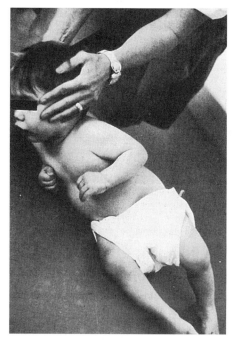

(a)

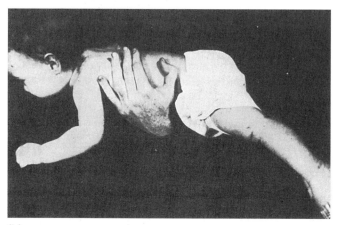

(b)

Figure 5 Postural motor patterns of diagnostic and prognostic significance: (a) neck righting; (b) protective extension (parachute) (Ref 84a); and (c) full extension in the Landau position.

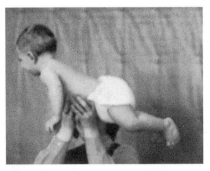

(c)

Figure 5 Continued.

D. Developmental Screening Instruments

The developmental neurological evaluation can be enhanced by the additional use of appropriate screening instruments noted previously to assess levels of function. The Denver Developmental Screening Test, for example, can be administered in a short time by the physician or other professional, and provides a visually descriptive index of functioning in fine and gross motor, language, and social skills (55). It has the added advantage of being easily updated and provides a visual impression of functional change.

The Clinical Adaptive Test (CAT) assesses problem-solving skills, while the Clinical Linguistic and Auditory Milestone Scale (CLAMS) screens language development from birth to age 3. Both are administered as an office procedure (57).

Table 3 Patterns of Motor Behavior and Age (Month) Normally Demonstrated

Months	1	2	3	4	6	9	12	15	18	24
Primitive										
Moro	+	+	±	±	0	0	0	0	0	0
Palmar	+	+	±	±	0	0	0	0	0	0
ATN	+	+	±	±	0	0	0	0	0	0
Rooting/suck	+	+	+	±	±	0	0	0	0	0
Postural										
Neck right	0	0	0	±	±	+	+	+	+	+
Parachute	0	0	0	0	±	+	+	+	+	+
Landau	0	0	0	0	0	0	+	+	+	±

Cognitive functioning of the infant can also be effectively evaluated in the office setting with the Bayley Infant Developmental Screener (49). Alternatively, referral could be made for formal psychological testing.

Other instruments, such as the WeeFIM, may be used equally to assess function initially, and changes in function with subsequent reevaluations (89). The interests, special concerns, and experience of the examiner with a particular test would determine selection.

E.　The Scope of Laboratory Evaluation

The extent to which laboratory procedures are needed to aid in diagnosis will depend upon the findings of the physical and neurological examinations in relation to the developmental history. For example, the child with a history of prematurity and neonatal anoxia, who is markedly delayed in milestones and has signs of generalized spasticity, will need few laboratory data to support a diagnosis of cerebral palsy. However, a patient who has a normal birth history and marked progressive developmental delay with a paucity of findings would require a very extensive work-up that might even include hospitalization. Considerable variation generally exists in the more typical situation between these two examples. A major benefit of an organized, sequential system of developmental evaluation is that it provides a focus and direction in the usual office or clinic setting that will help to determine the extent to which more detailed workup will be indicated. The child with a developmental delay must not be the subject of a shotgun approach using laboratory findings to determine whether a lesion exists. Rather, the dynamic and changing nature of the central nervous system, especially one in which there is some deficit, has to be viewed in its entirety.

Depending upon clinical indications, initial laboratory tests that may be useful include any or all of the following: complete blood count and urinalysis, serum lead level, TORCH titer, thyroid function studies, CPK, and urinary amino acid scan. Fragile X testing must be considered, as well as a more extensive genetics workup where indicated. Any evidence of micro- or macrocephaly *requires* either brain CAT scan or MRI, depending on clinical judgment.

The electroencephalogram (EEG) is much abused and frequently misused. However, it is mandatory where there is a definite seizure history, and a sleep EEG should be considered if subclinical seizures are suspected as in pervasive developmental disorder (90, 91). Where there is a behavior disorder or hyperactivity, the EEG generally has little to add. As a routine procedure, it has no place and should be discouraged. Unfortunately, many teachers and others who deal professionally with children have come to regard it as a major developmental diagnostic tool. They often need guidance and direction to discourage this approach.

V. FORMULATING THE DIAGNOSIS

A. Developmental Delay

It is not always practical nor desirable to place a diagnostic label on an infant. When dealing with the very young nervous system, it is often not completely clear at the time whether the evidence from developmental history, and physical, and neurological evaluations is compatible with cerebral palsy or other specific diagnoses. However, definite and significant developmental delay may be present and should be identified (92). The judgment and clinical maturity of the examiner will then determine how this is communicated and the subsequent course of action.

The professional is sometimes hesitant to inform parents of possible non-specific deficit because:

1. The index of suspicion is not high.
2. There is uncertainty about the diagnosis.
3. There is concern about unduly alarming parents.
4. There is lack of knowledge about available treatment and where to refer the child.
5. The professional is unconvinced of treatment effectiveness.

However, when significant deficits are evident and confirmation of an exact diagnosis such as cerebral palsy cannot be made with certainty, it is best to inform parents that the child shows definite developmental delay without using a more specific label. This preliminary diagnosis sets the stage for future action. It may confirm what the parents already know and help return balance and stability to the family. A threefold plan of action should then be recommended: (1) appropriate further diagnostic and laboratory testing; (2) referral for some form of early intervention program; and (3) a clear commitment to continuing reevaluation for specific diagnosis and assessment of functional change. This keeps open the possibilities for future interventional strategies and demands that the child be seen at regular periodic intervals to monitor change. Continuity of follow-up by the same professional group over a period of time is essential, if at all practical, to fully assess diagnosis, needs, and progress. Only in this way will it be possible to provide adequate communication and support for parents and plan appropriately for the future. The need for continuous reevaluation does not cease even when a specific diagnosis can be made.

The recognition of significant developmental deficit in the young child will lead to planning an appropriate program (see Chapter 4). The first concern is to develop specific *management* techniques and procedures to assist in caring for the child. These procedures are necessary because deficits may severely limit and alter the usual daily child- care regime. Second, simultaneous *treatment* or therapy is instituted to guide and stimulate a more normal pattern of neurological development and growth. Both management and treatment constitute the basis for the approach to the infant with a nonspecific developmental deficit diagnosis, as well as the young child with specifically identified cerebral palsy. The procedures should be continuous and flexible enough to deal with the neurological lesion as it becomes increasingly apparent and discrete.

B. Cerebral Palsy

It must be emphasized that the traditional motor forms of cerebral palsy are generally not present in the infant less than 1 year of age (93). These forms gradually emerge during the first year and beyond as the abnormal nervous system matures. The condition in very young children may appear merely as a nonspecific form of developmental delay. There will initially be ''definite abnormality'' in the quality of general movements within the first 3 to 4 months, with complete absence of fidgety movements (14, 60, 94). Tone will be aberrant, and there will be persistence of primitive motor patterns, with delay in disappearance, and late, often incomplete, emergence of postural motor patterns. Abnormal developmental history is crucial in diagnosis. Paucity of laboratory findings is to be expected. Where the developmental history is strongly positive and signs of abnormal quality of GMs, tone, and earliest motor behavior patterns are present, a probable diagnosis of cerebral palsy may be appropriate long before the definitive motor manifestations are apparent. Utilizing this sequential developmental evaluation procedure can provide a systematic basis for considering a presumptive or specific diagnosis within the first few months of life.

Consequences of the fixed motor lesion in cerebral palsy must be seen as emerging and concomitant with growth of the central nervous system itself. This is a dynamic, active process, at least from the initial moment of postnatal life and probably earlier. However, cerebral palsy is not to be conceived as merely one or more types of motor disturbance, but an array of developmental disorders that may affect the most primitive functions, as well as sophisticated voluntary actions, and often both.

In the older child, generally beyond 1 year, a diagnosis of cerebral palsy can often be made indicating a specific motor type. This diagnosis may change as the child grows and the definitive motor defect becomes more apparent (95). Motor signs may also disappear early in very mild cases (96, 97). Also, the identification of a particular type of cerebral palsy frequently coincides with the age at which a specific motor task is expected to be present. For example, inability to perform pincer grasp may be a first indication of upper extremity abnormality in hemiplegia (98).

As the child grows, one should formulate and update specifics of cerebral palsy type and distribution, as well as extent and degree of involvement, using a standard such as that of Palisano (99). For example, the diagnosis of cerebral palsy should be identified as spastic quadriplegia, level III. Where possible, it is useful to include these features in the diagnosis so that some prognostic outlook is available.

Understanding the broad developmental scope of the condition forms the basis for both identification and intervention for cerebral palsy. It is no longer acceptable to wait for emergence of the spastic foot, the dystonic posture, or the ataxic gait in deciding upon diagnosis or initiating treatment. Consideration must be given as early as possible to recognition of the global developmental abnormality that exists so that appropriate means can be directed to remediate the spectrum of deficit of the entire nervous system.

It is essential to keep in mind that cerebral palsy is always a presumptive diagnosis, since confirmatory evidence is indirect and is based upon behavior and development at a given time. One must always be on guard for any changes that may be consistent with progressive disease, however subtle or slow in nature. This is particularly true of cerebellar and mixed cerebral palsy types.

VI. DIFFERENTIAL DIAGNOSTIC CONSIDERATIONS

A. The Infant Developmental Evaluation Profile of Static Encepahalopathies

Very early differential diagnosis of nonprogressive infant developmental disorders (static encephalopathies) can be systematically approached utilizing a profile of information from the developmental evaluation procedure (Table 1). This profile (Table 4) will assist in heightening the index of suspicion of a given diagnosis

Table 4 Developmental Evaluation Profile

 I. History
   A. Behavioral soft signs
   B. Developmental milestones
 II. Physical Examination
III. Neurological Evaluation
   A. Quality of general movements
   B. Tone
   C. Reflex behavior
      1. Primitive
      2. Postural
   D. Focal signs

and, when the variables are considered together, can offer a specific recognizable pattern consistent with characteristics of the emerging disorder.

Table 5 compares early diagnostic features frequently seen in the developmental evaluation profiles of cerebral palsy, mental retardation, attention deficit/ hyperactivity disorder, and pervasive developmental disorders.

1. Congenital Cerebral Palsy

(a) History. There may be a positive history of abnormality in pregnancy, labor, or delivery, such as prematurity, respiratory distress, or other significant difficulty in the neonatal period.

(b) Behavioral Soft Signs. These are frequently found in the neonatal period. They may include colicky behavior with significant irritability, frequent problems in feeding, and failure to develop regular sleep patterns. Clinical experience indicates that the combination of a significant pregnancy or birth history, with colic-like behavior or sleep disturbance, are often preexisting factors when the developmental delay is indeed cerebral palsy (100).

(c) Developmental Milestones. It is important to recognize the well-established sequential nature of motor developmental milestones as well as the broad range of their emergence (Table 2). The child with cerebral palsy will be significantly delayed in reaching milestones, which is usually the basis of referral for evaluation. The degree of delay must be assessed and considered in relation to any abnormalities in the history and the possible presence of soft signs. Taken together, this will heighten the index of suspicion for a diagnosis of cerebral palsy.

(d) Physical Examination. In the infant with cerebral palsy the physical examination generally will not yield specific findings. The exception is the situation in which there is motor asymmetry. Frequently there have been delays both in growth and physical development with evidence of failure to thrive.

(e) Neurological Examination. "Definitely abnormal" GMs would be expected, which would show a lack of fluency (cramped) in the term infant and the expected fidgety quality in the child up to 3 to 4 months of age (60, 94). Movements are symmetrical up to 3 months and then become asymmetrical in the infant with hemiplegia (9).

Of major concern are abnormalities of tone. Infants with cerebral palsy may be excessively hypotonic with floppiness and poor control of head, neck, and trunk, and are often brought to attention of the health professional because of inability to sit. On the other hand, they may show marked hypertonia with stiffness and rigidity. Sometimes the child can be brought to a rigid standing

Table 5 Developmental Evaluation Profiles with Early Differential Diagnostic Features Frequently Seen

	Cerebral palsy	Mental retardation	Pervasive development disorders	Attention deficit hyperactivity disorder
I. History	often positive	gen. negative	possible family	possible family; often males
A. Behavior Soft Signs	colic, irritable, sleep problems	"easy baby"	colic, irritable, dificult management	colic, active, demanding, sleep problems
B. Milestones				
1. Motor	delayed	delayed	delayed	advanced
2. Speech	delayed	delayed	beginning onset, then regression	possible delayed appearance
II. Physical exam	not specific; delayed growth	not specific or syndrome	not specific; poor social response	not specific
III. Neurological Evaluation				
A. General Movements	"definitely abnormal"	?abnormal	?"mildly abnormal"	"mildly abnormal"
B. Tone	increased or decreased	hypotonia	hypotonia	normal
C. Motor Behavior Patterns				
1. Primitive	persists beyond normal	normal disappear	persists beyond normal	normal disappear
2. Postural	delayed appear	delayed appear	delayed appear	early appear
D. Focal Signs	appear late	absent	absent	absent

position at a very early age and considered to have advanced development by the parent.

(f) *Patterns of Motor Behavior.* Early motor patterns represent a powerful predictive feature in the diagnosis of cerebral palsy. (Table 3) (101). Primitive motor patterns will be delayed in disappearance (85). There may also be abnormalities in their expression, depending upon the degree of severity, such as an inadequate or incomplete Moro, rooting, or poor sucking. A very strong or obligatory asymmetric tonic neck is almost pathognomonic of emerging dystonia.

Equally important is the delay in appearance or incomplete expression of postural motor patterns (102). This combination of delay in disappearance of the primitives, with variable expression, and delay in the appearance of posturals is a significant predictor of cerebral palsy. This is especially true when viewed in relation to the totality of abnormalities in tone, delays in achieving milestones, the presence of soft signs, and an abnormal history.

(g) *Focal Signs.* It is essential to bear in mind that the specific motor forms of cerebral palsy appear late as the abnormal central nervous system matures. Focal neurological signs other than asymmetry are not generally seen in the infant. Instead, one must rely on more indirect indicators and multiple variables, such as the features included in the infant developmental evaluation profile.

2. Acquired Cerebral Palsy

Following an acute brain insult, cerebral palsy will be identified by specific or mixed motor type in a child who had previously been typical in development. Preceding features of tone, primitive or postural behavior patterns, and milestones all would have been appropriate.

3. Genetic Cerebral Palsy

Genetically based cases of cerebral palsy are reported, particularly where there is consanguinity (103, 104). Among the several motor forms, clear distinction must be made between hereditary spastic paraplegia and cerebral palsy as a true developmental disorder (105). Ataxia is most likely to have a genetic basis or to be slowly progressive and mistaken for cerebral palsy (106). Few data about parameters of early development are available concerning the relatively rare cases of genetic cerebral palsy that meet the criteria for static encephalopathy.

4. Mental Retardation

In contrast to cerebral palsy, Table 5 shows that the infant with emerging mental retardation generally has a negative history. The child is often "too easy" to deal with and does not have feeding problems or sleep disturbances. Significant delay in milestones is present. The physical examination is unremarkable other than for poor responsiveness to surroundings, unless specific morphological features are present. Definitive abnormalities of GMs have not been reported for the post-term infant, but have been observed in the fetus with Down syndrome (9). Significant hypotonia is the usual finding. Finally, a major differential point is the normal disappearance of primitive motor patterns, but significant delay in the appearance of the postural motor patterns (107). No focal neurological signs are present.

5. Pervasive Developmental Disorders

The term "pervasive developmental disorders" refers to a heterogeneous grouping of generalized developmental deficits in a child including social, behavioral, cognitive, learning, speech, and motor. Some of these children develop with persistence in abnormality in several or all of these areas. Others eventually separate out with all the features of autistic disorder. The ultimate course will not be apparent in the infant, but rather there will be evidence of delayed and aberrant development. A family history of some developmental abnormality may be found, but is not common. Abnormal behavioral soft signs are likely, especially with marked irritability, and difficulty in management. Limited responsiveness to the environment would be expected. There would be definite delay in motor milestones and often clumsiness. However, a pattern of normal or near normal initiation of recognizable words, with subsequent complete regression of speech, is regularly reported (108, 109). This regression may be an important early diagnostic marker in identifying pervasive developmental disorder (110). However, Landau-Kleffner syndrome should also be considered where onset of speech abnormality follows initial normal development (111).

The physical examination would be unremarkable, except for evidence of excessive activity or poor social responsiveness. The neurological evaluation may well show "mildly abnormal" quality of GMs (94). Hypotonia may be present, with delays in both disappearance of primitive and in appearance of postural motor patterns. Focal signs would not be expected.

6. Attention Deficit/Hyperactivity Disorder

For the infant with attention deficit/hyperactivity disorder, a positive family history of hyperactivity or learning disabilities may be noted, especially in the father or siblings. There may be some evidence of colic or sleep problems, and the child is often very active and demanding in behavior. Motor milestones may be significantly advanced. However, there is frequently a noticeable delay in developing speech patterns. The physical examination is not significant. "Mildly abnormal'' quality of GMs is reported (94). Tone is normal. Motor behavior patterns show normal disappearance of the primitives, but there is frequently early appearance of the posturals. No focal neurological signs are present.

B. Progressive CNS Disease

Progressive CNS disease must be given serious consideration when there are delays in development, the pregnancy and birth history is normal, no abnormalities are found on physical or neurological examination, yet there is marked abnormality or delay in early motor patterns of behavior or milestones. This would be particularly true if earlier milestones had been normal and subsequent development is aberrant. Hydrocephalus with persistent increased intracranial pressure should be seriously considered in children with full, open fontanelles and a markedly enlarged cranial circumference. Neoplasia or vascular malformations must also be ruled out in this situation.

The progressive lipoidoses would be evident by the cherry red macula in Tay-Sachs and Niemann-Pick diseases, and hyperpigmented yellow retinal lesions in Gaucher's disease. Cloudy cornea may be seen in mucopolysaccharidoses, and corneal ring in Wilson's disease.

Lesch-Nyhan syndrome occurs in boys in association with high uric acid levels and a specific enzyme defect (112). Positive family history is frequently noted. Unexplained high fevers are present and severe self-mutilation develops early. Without restraint, self-amputation of fingers will occur. At 12 to 18 months, typical severe generalized athetosis appears and has been frequently diagnosed as the congenital variety. Contrary to many reports, it is not invariably associated with mental retardation (113). Unfortunately, the condition is progressive and the prognosis grave.

Other nonspecific progressive disorders of gray or white matter should be considered where the initial history is normal in association with marked subsequent developmental delay. Pelizaeus-Merzbacher disease and a variety of leukodystrophies will be arrived at by exclusion. Alexander's disease is identified by progressive macrocephaly without increased intracranial pressure.

Patterns of primitive and postural motor behavior have not been well studied in these cases, but would vary considerably with age at onset, pathology, and degree of involvement.

1. Neuropathies

These are rare in young children and generally would not be a differential consideration. An infectious polyneuritis with significant functional residue could be considered when onset is acute and infection can be documented. Anterior horn cell infection as in poliomyelitis is generally identifiable without difficulty. Degeneration of the anterior horn cell as in Werdnig-Hoffmann disease or variants would be extremely rare, but should be considered.

2. Myopathies

A spectrum of benign intrinsic muscle disease is now recognized which may be seen in association with the "floppy child" and delayed milestones. These include nemaline myopathy, central core disease, and others (114). The outcome is generally favorable.

The muscular dystrophies might be a serious consideration where there is evidence of marked hypotonia, weakness, or possibly lower extremity contractures in the case of the newborn (115). Many different forms are now identified, including those with brain involvement, which show generalized delays (116). Particular attention should be given when there are delays in milestones, especially in a child not ambulating by 18 months, and to boys beyond the toddler stage who show increased delay in progression, or actual regression in gross motor development (117). Abnormality in previous patterns of motor behavior or tone would not be expected.

Myasthenia gravis with severe hypotonia may be seen transiently in newborns in association with maternal disease or may be present as a primary disease (118). The life-threatening nature of the condition should lead to prompt and extensive evaluation.

VII. PERSPECTIVE ON DEVELOPMENTAL EVALUATION

We have seen that cerebral palsy is a nonprogressive brain disorder of varying etiologies, with late-appearing focal neurological signs. Early diagnosis of the infant must first rule out the possibility of progressive disease. A comprehensive, multivariable procedure should then be used in search of often-seen characteristics that may form a distinctive profile. Awareness of early profiles of other static encephalopathies can be helpful in differential diagnosis. When a distinct diagnostic entity cannot be delineated, the term "developmental delay" should be used to indicate significant concerns about development. This will enable early referral on the often-long road to assistance with management and treatment. Regardless of the degree of diagnostic certainty, it is essential that the child be reevaluated at regular intervals to rule out the possibility of progressive disease, observe changes in motor signs and development, and allow for appropriate management and treatment.

APPENDIX A: NORMAL EMERGING DEVELOPMENT—
BIRTH TO 36 MONTHS

Neonatal Period (First 4 Wk)

Prone:	Lies in flexed attitude; turns head from side to side; head sags on ventral suspension
Supine:	Generally flexed and a little stiff
Visual:	May fixate face or light in line of vision; "doll's eye" movement of eyes on turning of the body
Reflex:	Moro response active; stepping and placing reflexes; grasp reflex active
Social:	Visual preference for human face

At 4 Wk

Prone:	Legs more extended; holds chip up; turns head; head lifted momentarily to plane of body on ventral suspension
Supine:	Tonic neck posture predominates; supple and relaxed; head lags on pull to sitting position
Visual:	Watches person; follows moving object
Social:	Body movements in cadence with voice of other in social contact; beginning to smile

At 8 Wk

Prone:	Raises head slightly farther; head sustained in plane of body on ventral suspension
Supine:	Tonic neck posture predominates; head lags on pull to sitting position
Visual:	Follows moving object 180 degrees
Social:	Smiles on social contact; listens to voice and coos

At 12 Wk

Prone:	Lifts head and chest, arms extended; head above plane of body on ventral suspension
Supine:	Tonic neck posture predominates; reaches toward and misses objects; waves at toy
Sitting:	Head lag partially compensated on pull to sitting position; early head control with bobbing motion; back rounded
Reflex:	Typical Moro response has not persisted; makes defensive movements or selective withdrawal reactions
Social:	Sustained social contact; listens to music; says "aah, ngah"

At 16 Wk

Prone:	Lifts head and chest, head in approximately vertical axis; legs extended
Supine:	Symmetric posture predominates, hands in midline; reaches and grasps objects and brings them to mouth
Sitting:	No head lag on pull to sitting position; head steady, tipped forward; enjoys sitting with full truncal support
Standing:	When held erect, pushes with feet

Adaptive: Sees pellet, but makes no move to it
Social: Laughs out loud; may show displeasure if social contact is broken; excited at sight of food

At 28 Wk
Prone: Rolls over; pivots; crawls or creep-crawls (Knobloch)
Supine: Lifts head; rolls over; squirming movements
Sitting: Sits briefly, with support of pelvis; leans forward on hands; back rounded
Standing: May support most of weight; bounces actively
Adaptive: Reaches out for and grasps large object; transfers objects from hand to hand; grasp uses radial palm; rakes at pellet
Language: Polysyllabic vowel sound formed
Social: Prefers mother; babbles; enjoys mirror; responds to changes in emotional content of social contact

At 40 Wk
Sitting: Sits up alone and indefinitely without support, back straight
Standing: Pulls to standing position; "cruises" or walks holding on to furniture
Motor: Creeps or crawls
Adaptive: Grasps objects with thumb and forefinger; pokes at things with forefinger; picks up pellet with assisted pincer movement; uncovers hidden toy; attempts to retrieve dropped object; releases object grasped by other person
Language: Repetitive consonant sound (mama, dada)
Social: Responds to sound of name; plays peek-a-boo or pat-a-cake; waves bye-bye

At 52 Wk (1 Yr)
Motor: Walks with one hand held (48 wk); rises independently, takes several steps (Knobloch)
Adaptive: Picks up pellet with unassisted pincer movement of forefinger and thumb; releases object to other person on request or gesture
Language: A few words besides mama, dada
Social: Plays simple ball game; makes postural adjustment to dressing

15 Mo
Motor: Walks alone; crawls up stairs
Adaptive: Makes tower of 3 cubes; makes a line with crayon; inserts pellet in bottle
Language: Jargon; follow simple commands; may name a familiar object (ball)
Social: Indicates some desires or needs by pointing; hugs parents

18 Mo
Motor: Runs stiffly; sits on small chair; walks up stairs with one hand held; explores drawers and waste baskets
Adaptive: Makes a tower of 4 cubes; imitates scribbling; imitates vertical stroke; dumps pellet from bottle

Language: 10 words (average); names pictures; identifies one or more parts of the body
Social: Feeds self; seeks help when in trouble; may complain when wet or soiled; kisses parent with pucker

24 Mo

Motor: Runs well; walks up and down stairs, one step at a time; opens doors; climbs on furniture; jumps
Adaptive: Tower of 7 cubes (6 at 21 mo); circular scribbling; imitates horizontal stroke; fold paper once imitatively
Language: Puts 3 words together (subject, verb, object)
Social: Handles spoon well; often tells immediate experiences; helps to undress; listens to stories with pictures

30 Mo

Motor: Goes up stairs alternating feet
Adaptive: Tower of 9 cubes; makes vertical and horizontal strokes, but generally will not join them to make a cross; imitates cicular stroke, forming closed figure
Language: Refers to self by pronoun "I"; knows full name
Social: Helps put things away; pretends in play

36 Mo

Motor: Rides tricycle; stands momentarily on one foot
Adaptive: Tower of 10 cubes; imitates construction of "bridge" of 3 cubes; copies a circle; imitates a cross
Language: Knows age and sex; counts 3 objects correctly; repeats 3 numbers or a sentence of syllables
Social: Plays simple games (in "parallel" with other children); helps in dressing (unbuttons clothing and puts on shoes); washes hands

Source: Ref. 27.

APPENDIX B: INITIAL DEVELOPMENTAL EVALUATION FORM

Date completed: Informant:
Reason for referral:
  Age problem recognized and symptoms recognized
A. History
  1. Family and genetic history
  2. Pregnancy history
  3. Labor and delivery
  4. Perinatal and neonatal events
    a. condition at birth
    b. neonatal history

5. Developmental milestones
   a. head balance and control
   b. smiling
   c. grasping
   d. transferring
   e. rolling
   f. sitting
   g. crawling
   h. walking
6. Oral development
   a. feeding and sucking
   b. tongue and mouth problems
   c. speech onset development
   d. dental development
7. Hand preference
8. Other developmental features
   a. hearing
   b. vision
   c. sleep
   d. self-care
9. Social/emotional/behaviorial characteristics
10. School experience
11. Review of systems
12. Past medical history/previous evaluations
B. Physical/developmental evaluation
C. Diagnostic Formulation
D. Plan for Management/Treatment

REFERENCES

1. Gesell A, Amatruda C. Developmental Diagnosis, Normal and Abnormal Child Development, Clinical Methods and Pediatric Applications. New York: Hoeber, 1947.
2. Pascal G, Jenkins W. Systemic Observations of Gross Human Behavior. New York: Grune and Stratton, 1961.
3. Bayley N. Value and limitations of infant testing. Children 1958; 5:129.
4. Illingworth R. The Development of the Infant and Young Child—Normal and Abnormal. Baltimore: Williams & Wilkins, 1966.
5. Shore R. Rethinking the Brain: New Insights into Early Development. New York: Families and Work Institute, 1997.
6. Huttenlocher P. Synapse elimination and plasticity in developing human cerebral cortex. Am J Ment Deficiency 1984; 88 488–496.

7. Clarke E, O'Malley C. The Human Brain and Spinal Cord. Berkeley: University of California Press, 1968.
8. Sherrington C. The Integrative Action of the Nervous System. New Haven: Yale University Press, 1961.
9. Prechtl HFR. Developmental neurology as a new method for early prediction of cerebral palsy. 53rd Annual Meeting of the American Academy for Cerebral Palsy and Developmental Medicine, Washington, D.C., Sept. 15–18, 1999.
10. DeVries JIP, Visser GHA, Prechtl HFR. The emergence of fetal behavior. I. Qualitative aspects. Early Hum Devel 1982; 7:301–322.
11. Hopkins B, Prechtl HFR. A qualitative approach to the development of movements during early infancy. In: Prechtl HFR, ed. Continuity of Neural Functions from Prenatal to Postnatal Life. London: Spastics International Medical Publications, 1984:179–197.
12. Haddders-Algra M, Prechtl HFR. Developmental course of general movements in early infancy. I. Descriptive analysis of change in form. Early Hum Dev 1992; 28: 201–213.S
13. Hadders-Algra M, Prechtl HFR. EMG correlates of general movements in healthy preterm infants (abstr). J. Physiol 1993; 459:330.
14. Hadders-Algra M, Klip-Van den Nieuwendijk AWJ, Martijn A, Van Eykern LA. Assessment of general movements: towards a better understanding of a sensitive method to evaluate brain function in young infants. Dev Med Child Neurol 1997; 39:88–98.
15. Einspieler C, Prechtl HFR, Ferrari F, Cioni G, Bos AF. The qualitative assessment of general movements in preterm, term, and young infants—review of the methodology. Early Hum Dev 1997; 50:47–50.
16. Heriza CB. Implications of dynamical systems approach to understanding infant kicking behavior. Phys Ther 1991; 71:222–235.
17. Thelen E, Spencer JP. Postural control during reaching in young infants: a dynamic systems approach. Neuro Sci Biobehav Rev 1998; 22:507–514.
18. Sheridan M. Developmental Progress in Infants and Young Children. London: Her Majesty's Stationary Office, 1968.
19. Bobath K. The Motor Deficit in Patients with Cerebral Palsy. Little Club Clinics in Developmental Medicine. London: Heinemann, 1966.
20. Peyser A. Cerebral Function in Infancy and Childhood. New York: Consultants Bureau, 1963.
21. Prechtl H, Beintema D. Neurological Examination of the Full Term Infant. Little Club Clinics in Developmental Medicine. London: Heinemann, 1964.
22. Milani-Camparetti A. Spasticity versus patterned postural and motor behavior of spastics. Excerpta Med. Int. Congr. Ser.107. IV International Congress of Physical Medicine, Paris, 1964.
23. Ounce of Prevention Fund. Starting Smart: How Early Experiences Affect Brain Development. Chicago: Ounce of Prevention Fund, 1996.
24. Greenough WT, Black JE, Wallace CS. Experience and brain development. Child Dev 1987; 58:539–559.
25. Kempermann G, Kuhn HG, Gage FH. More hippocampal neurons in adult mice living in an enriched environment. Nature 1997; 386:493–495.

26. Greenspan S. Infancy and Early Childhood: The Practice of Clinical Assessment and Intervention with Emotional and Developmental Challenges. Madison, CT: International Universities Press, 1992.

27. Medalie JH. Growth and development, Tables 3–12, 3–13. In: Behrman RE, Kleigman RM, eds. Nelson Textbook of Pediatrics, 14th ed. Philadelphia: Saunders, 1992: 41–42.

28. Hadders-Algra M. Assessment of general movements: a valuable technique for detecting brain dysfunction in young infants. Acta Paediatr 1996; 416(suppl):39–43.

29. Drillien CM. Abnormal neurologic signs in the first year of life in low birth weight infants: Possible prognostic significance. Dev Med Child Neurol 1972; 14:575–584.

30. Dargassies SS. Neurological Development in the Full Term and Premature Neonate. New York: Excerpta Medica, 1977.

31. Bobath B, Bobath K. Motor Development in Different Types of Cerebral Palsy. London: Heinemann, 1975.

32. Jennett RJ, Warford HS, Kreinick C, Waterkotte GW. Apgar Index: A statistical tool. Am J Obstet Gynecol 1981; 140:206–212.

33. Apgar V. A proposal for a new method of evaluation of the newborn infant. Anesth Analgesia 1953; 32:260–267.

34. Nelson KB, Ellenberg J. Apgar scores as predictors of chronic neurologic disability. Pediatrics 1981; 68:36–44.

35. Socol ML. Depressed Apgar scores. Am J Obstet Gynecol 1994; 170:991–998.

36. Hegyi T, Carbone T, Anwar M, Ostfeld B, Hiatt M, Koons A, Pinto-Martin J, Paneth N. The Apgar score and its components in the preterm infant. Pediatrics 1998; 101:77–81.

37. Beeby PJ, Elliott EJ, Henderson-Smart DJ, Rieger ID. Predictive value of umbilical artery pH in preterm infants. Arch Dis Child 1994; 7:F93–96.

38. Committee on the Fetus and Newborn, American Academy of Pediatrics, and Committee on Obstetric Practice, American College of Obstetrics and Gynecology. Use and abuse of the Apgar score. Pediatrics 1996; 98:141–142.

39. Perlman JM, Risser R. Can asphyxiated infants at risk for neonatal seizures be rapidly identified by current high risk markers? Pediatrics 1996; 97:456–462.

40. Martin-Ancel A, Garcia-Alix A, Pascual-Salcedo D, Cabanas F, Valcarce M, Quero J. Interleukin-6 in the cerebrospinal fluid after perinatal asphyxia is related to early and late neurological manifestations. Pediatrics 1997; 100:789–794.

41. Perlman JM, Tack ED. Renal injury in the asphyxiated newborn infant: relationship to neurologic outcome. J Pediatr 1988; 113:875–879.

42. Huang CC, Wang ST, Chang YC, Lin KP, Wu PL. Measurement of the lactate: creatinine ratio for the early identification of newborn infants at risk for hypoxic-ischemic encephalopathy. N Engl J Med 1999; 341:328–335.

43. Wald NJ, Watt GH, Hackshaw AK. Integrated screening for Down's Syndrome based on test performed during the first and second trimesters. N Engl J Med 1999; 341:461–467.

44. Hoon AH Jr. Neuroimaging in the high risk infant: relationship to outcome. J Perinatol 1995; 15:389–394.

45. Murphy DJ, Hope PL, Johnson A. Ultrasound findings and clinical antecedents of cerebral palsy in very preterm infants. Arch Dis Child Fetal Neonatal Ed 1996; 74: F105–F109.

46. Mercuri E, Gazzetta A, Haataja L, Cowan F, Rutherford M, Counsell S, Papadimitriou M, Cioni G, Dubowitz L. Neonatal neurological examination in infants with hypoxic ischaemic encephalopathy: correlation with MRI findings. Neuropediatrics 1999; 30:83–89.

47. Amess PN, Wylezinska M, Lorek A, Townsend J, Wyatt JS, Amiel-Tison C, Cady EB, Stewart A. Early brain proton magnetic resonance spectroscopy and neonatal neurology related to neurodevelopmental outcome at 1 year in term infants after presumed hypoxic-ischaemic brain injury. Dev Med Child Neurol 1999; 41:436–445.

48. Amiel-Tison C. Neurological evaluation of the maturity of newborn infants. Arch Dis Child 1968; 43:89–93.

49. Bayley N. Bayley Scales of Mental and Motor Development, as used in the Collaborative Perinatal Research Project. Bethesda, MD: National Institute of Neurological Diseases and Blindness, 1961.

50. Brazelton T, Nugent K. Neonatal Behavior Assessment Scale, 3rd ed. Clinics in Developmental Medicine, No. 137. London: Spastics International Medical Publications, 1995.

51. Dubowitz L, Dubowitz V, Goldberg C. Clinical assessment of gestational age in the newborn infant. J Pediatr 1970; 77:1–10.

52. Dubowitz L, Mercuri E, Dubowitz V. An optimality score for the neurological examination of the term newborn. J Pediatr 1998; 133:406–416.

53. Haataja L, Mercuri E, Regev R, Cowan F, Rutherford M, Dubowitz V, Dubowitz I. Optimality score for the neurological examination of the infant at 12 and 18 months of age. J Pediatr 1999; 135:153–161.

54. Reed H. Review of Peabody Developmental Motor Scales and Activity Cards. In: Mitchell J, ed. The Ninth Mental Measurements Yearbook. Lincoln: University of Nebraska Press, 1985:1119.

55. Frankenburg WK, Dodds J, Archer P, Shapiro H, Bresnick B. The Denver II: A major revision and restandardization of the Denver Developmental Screening Test. Pediatrics 1992; 89:91–97.

56. Glascoe F, Byrne KE. The usefulness of the Battelle Developmental Inventory Screening Test. Clin Pediatr (Phila) 1993; 32:237–280.

57. Leppert MLO, Shank TP, Shapiro BK, Capute AJ. The Capute Scales: CAT/ CLAMS–a tool for the early detection of mental retardation and communicative disorders. Ment Retard Devel Disabl Research Rev 1998; 4:14–19.

58. Knobloch H, Stevens F, Malone A. The Revised Developmental Screening Inventory. Houston, Texas: Gesell Developmental Test Materials, 1980.

59. Prechtl HF. State of the art of a new functional assessment of the young nervous system. An early predictor of cerebral palsy. Early Human Dev 1997; 24:1–11.

60. Prechtl HF, Einspieler C, Cioni G, Bos AF, Ferrai F, Sontheimer D. An early marker for neurological deficits after perinatal brain lesions. Lancet 1997; 349: 1361–1363.

61. Piper MC, Pinnell LE, Darrah J, Maguire T, Byrne PJ. Construction and validation

of the Alberta Infant Motor Scale (AIMS). Can J Publ Health 1992; 83(Suppl 2): S46–S50.

62. Morgan A. Early diagnosis of cerebral palsy using a profile of abnormal motor patterns (abstr). Dev Med Child Neurol 1988; 30(suppl 57):12.

63. Russell D, Palisano R, Walter S, Rosenbaum P, Gemos M, Gowland C, Galuppi B, Lane M. Evaluating motor function in children with Down Syndrome: validity of the GMFM. Dev Med Child Neurol 1998; 40:693–701.

64. Kaye L, Whitfield MF. The eight month movement assessment of infants as a prediction of cerebral palsy in high risk infants (abstr). Dev Med Child Neurol 1988; 30(suppl 57):11.

65. Campbell S, Osten E, Kolobe T, Fisher AG. Development of the test of infant motor performance. Phys Med Rehabil Clin 1993; 4:541–550.

66. Katelaar M, Vermeer A, Helders PJ. Functional motor abilities of children with cerebral palsy: a systematic literature review of assessment measures. Clin Rehabil 1998; 12:369–380.

67. Majnemer A, Mazer B. Neurologic evaluation of the newborn infant: definition and psychometric properties. Dev Med Child Neurol 1998; 40:708–715.

68. Liptak GS. The child who has severe neurologic impairment. Pediatr Clin N Am 1998; 45:123–144.

69. Wissow LS, Roter DL, Wilson, ME. Pediatrician interview style and mothers' disclosure of psychosocial issues. Pediatrics 1994; 93:289–295.

70. Allen MC, Alexander GR. Using motor milestones as a multi-step process to screen pre-term infants for cerebral palsy. Dev Med Child Neurol 1997; 39:12–16.

71. Vadasz AG, Epstein LG. Degenerative central nervous system disease. Pediatr Rev 1995; 16: 426–431.

72. Rosenthal R, Scherzer A, Cooper W. Unusual etiologies in congenital cerebral palsy. Rev Hosp Spec Surg 1971; 1:36–41.

73. Nellhaus G. Head circumference from birth to eighteen years: practical composite international and interracial graphs. Pediatrics 1968; 41:106–114.

74. Braddock SR, Braddock BA, Graham J. Rett Syndrome. An update and review for the primary pediatrician. Clin Pediatr 1993; 32:613–626.

75. Hadders-Algra M, Nakae Y, Van Eykern LA, Klip-Van den Nieuwendijk AWJ, Prechtl HFR. The effect of behavioral state on general movements in healthy full-term newborns. A polymyographic study. Early Hum Dev 1993; 35:63–79.

76. Cioni G, Ferrari F, Einspieler C, Paolicelli PB, Barbani MT, Prechtl HFR. Comparison between observation of spontaneous movements and neurologic examination in preterm infants. J Pediatr 1997; 130:704–711.

77. Dargassies SS. Le nouveau-Ne a terme. Aspect neurologique. Biol Neonate 1962; 4:174.

78. Thomas A, Chesni Y, Dargassies SS. The Neurological Examination of the Infant. Little Club Clinics in Developmental Medicine. London: Heinemann, 1960.

79. Paine R. The early diagnosis of cerebral palsy. R I Med J 1961; 44:522.

80. Paine R, Oppe T. Neurologic Examination of Children. Philadelphia: Lippincott, 1971.

81. Capute A, Accardo P, Vining E, Rubeinstein J, Harryman S. Primitive Reflex Profile. Baltimore: University Park Press, 1978.

82. Gupta V. Manual of Developmental and Behavioral Problems in Children. New York: Marcel Dekker, 1999.
83. Paine R. The evolution of infantile postural reflexes in the presence of chronic brain syndromes. Dev Med Child Neurol 1964; 6:345.
84. Casaer P. Postural Behavior in Newborn Infants. Clinics in Developmental Medicine No. 72. London: Heinemann, 1979.
84a. Paine RS. Neurological examination of infants and children. Pediatr Clin North AM 1960; 7: 471.
85. Molnar GE. Motor deficit of retarded infants and young children. Arch Phys Med Rehab 1974; 55:393–398.
86. Gingold MK, Jaynes ME, Bodensteiner JB, Romano JT, Hammond MT. The rise and fall of the plantar response in infancy. J Pediatr 1998; 133:568–570.
87. Hogan GR, Milligan JE. The planter reflex of the newborn. N Engl J Med 1971; 285:502–503.
88. Paine R, Oppe T. Neurological Examination of Infants and Children. Little Club Clinics in Developmental Medicine. London: Heinemann, 1966:187.
89. Msall ME, DiGaudio K, Rogers BT, LaForest S, Catanzaro NL, Campbell J, Wilczenski F, Duffy LC. The Functional Independence Measure for Children (Wee-FIM). Conceptual basis and pilot use in children with developmental disabilities. Clin Pediatr (Phila) 1994: 33:421–430.
90. Volkmar FR, Nelson DS. Seizure disorders in autism. J Am Acad Child Adolesc Psychiatry 1990; 29:127–129.
91. Lewine JD, Andrews R, Chez M, Arun-Angelo P, Devinsky O, Smith M, Kanner A, Davis JT, Funke M, Jones G, Chong B, Provencal S, Weisend M, Lee R, Orrison Jr. W. Magnetoencephalographic patterns of epileptiform activity in children with regressive autism spectrum disorders. Pediatrics 1999; 104:405–418.
92. First LR, Palfrey JS. The infant or young child with developmental delay. N Engl J Med 1994; 330:478–483.
93. Nelson KB, Ellenberg J. The asymptomatic newborn at risk of cerebral palsy. Am J Dis Child 1987; 141:1333–1335.
94. Hadders-Algra M, Groothuis AMC. Quality of general movements in infancy is related to neurological dysfunction, ADHD, and aggressive behavior. Dev Med Child Neurol 1999; 41:381–391.
95. Burke RE, Fahn S, Gold AP. Delayed onset dystonia in patients with 'static' encephalopathy. J Neurol 1980; 43:789–797.
96. Nelson KB, Ellenberg J. Children who "outgrew" cerebral palsy. Pediatrics 1982; 69:529–536.
97. Piper MC, Mazer B, Silver KM, Ramsey M. Resolution of neurological symptoms in high risk infants during the first two years of life. Dev Med Child Neurol 1988; 30:26–35.
98. Aicardi J, Bax M. Cerebral Palsy. In: Aicardi J. Diseases of the Nervous System in Childhood, 2nd ed. London: MacKeith Press, 1998:210.
99. Palisano R, Rosenbaum P, Walter S, Russell D, Wood E, Galuppi B. Development and reliability of a system to classify gross motor function in children with cerebral palsy. Dev Med Child Neurol 1997; 39:214–223.
100. Ford GW, Rickards AL, Kitchen WH, Lissenden JV, Keith CG, Ryan MM. Handi-

caps and health problems in 2 year old children of birth weight 500 to 1500 grams. Aust Paeditr 1985; 21:15–22.

101. Capute A, Biehl RF. Functional developmental evaluation: Prerequisite to habilitation. Pediatr Clin North Am 1973; 20:3–26.

102. Bobath B, Bobath K. Motor Development in Different Types of Cerebral Palsy. Little Club Clinics in Developmental Medicine. London: Heinemann, 1975.

103. Sinha G, Corry P, Subesinghe D, Wild J, Levene MI. Prevalence and type of cerebral palsy in a British ethnic community: the role of consanguinity. Dev Med Child Neurol 1997; 39:259–262.

104. Mitchell S, Bundy S. Symmetry of neurological signs in Pakistani patients with probable inherited spastic cerebral palsy. Clin Genet 1997; 51:7–14.

105. Nimityongskul P, Anderson LD, Sri P. Hereditary spastic paraplegia. Orthoped Rev 1992; 21:643–646.

106. Hughes I, Newton R. Genetic aspects of cerebral palsy. Dev Med Child Neurol 1992; 34: 80–86.

107. Molnar GE, Gordon SC. Cerebral palsy: predictive value of selected clinical signs for early prognostication of motor function. Arch Phys Med Rehabil 1976; 57:153–158.

108. Rapin I. Autistic children: diagnosis and clinical features. Pediatrics 1991; 87:751–760.

109. Happe F, Frith U. The neuropsychology of autism. Brain 1996; 119:1377–1400.

110. Kurita H. Specificity and developmental consequences of speech loss in children with pervasive developmental disorders. Psychiatry Clin Neurosci 1996; 50:181–184.

111. Connolly AN, Chez MG, Pestronk A, Arnold ST, Shobbna M, Deuel RK. Serum autoantibodies to brain in Landau-Kleffner variant, autism, and other neurologic disorders. J Pediatr 1999; 134:607–613.

112. Nyhan W, Oliver W, Lesch M. A familial disorder of uric acid metabolism and central nervous system function. J Pediatr 1965; 67:257.

113. Scherzer A, Ilson J. Normal intelligence in the Lesch-Nyhan Syndrome. Pediatrics 1969; 44:116–120.

114. Dubowitz V. The floppy infant: a practical approach to classification. Dev Med Child Neurol 1968; 10:706–710.

115. Leyton QH, Gabreels FJ, Renier WO, ter Laak HJ. Congenital muscular dystrophy: a review of the literature. Clin Neurol Neurosurg 1996; 98:267–280.

116. Voit T. Congenital muscular dystrophies: 1997 update. Brain Dev 1998; 20:65–74.

117. Aicardi J. Diseases of the Nervous System in Childhood, 2nd ed. London: Mac-Keith Press, 1998:751–752.

118. Amlar B, Ozdirim E, Renda Y, Yalaz K, Aysun S, Topsu M, Topaloglu H. Myasthenia gravis in childhood. Acta Paediatr 1996; 85:838–842.

4

Management and Treatment Planning for the Abnormally Developing Child

Alfred L. Scherzer
*Joan and Sanford I. Weill Medical College, Cornell University,
New York, New York*

I. INTRODUCTION

Early diagnosis of cerebral palsy will reveal an infant with significant delays in many important areas of growth and developmental maturation long before a recognizable pattern of motor deficit is apparent. There will be abnormalities of tone and patterns of motor behavior that are associated with difficulties in maintaining the body in space, restricting movement, and affecting the ability to interact with the environment. The motor difficulties will lead to limitations in movement that may, in time, result in fixed deficits that will further reduce function and participation. Early diagnosis provides an opportunity to assess these problems and the individual needs of the infant, and should lead to initiation of the habilitation process.

Habilitation must consider both *management* and *treatment* needs. The affected child will, first, be unable to participate well in daily care. The parent or guardian will have various responses to the state of the abnormal infant and will need guidance and direction in optimal ways to effectively manage daily care.

The neuropathological state of the infant will delay progression of motor development. Appropriate treatment is essential to reduce deficits, assist in motor progression, and help maintain appropriate levels of physical fitness. Similarly, the infant may have limitations in speech and cognitive development that must be addressed by relevant and coordinated treatment programs.

These needs and unique requirements can be best appreciated through considering the consequences of abnormal neurological development in the infant starting life with cerebral palsy.

Review of current treatment options for children in this age group can then be considered in the broadest developmental perspective.

II. CONSEQUENCES OF ABNORMAL NEUROLOGICAL DEVELOPMENT

A. Discordant Neurological Maturation

As we have seen, a nonprogressive deficit of the CNS may initially affect the brain stem and influence tone, as well as expression and integrity of primitive or postural motor patterns. Motor development and sensory response may equally be impaired. There is considerable variability in the expression of these deficits and *uneven developmental growth* is frequent. Thus, a child may respond reasonably well to the environment, yet be extremely floppy and demonstrate exaggerated primitive motor patterns. Variable maturational strengths and weaknesses are often a source of confusion in determining whether the child is normal or possibly has cerebral palsy. The apparent discrepancy in response, movement, posture, and patterns of motor behavior are often the initial basis for a parental concern.

The uneven nature of neurological maturation may also become more apparent with *physical growth.* Varying combinations of deficit may be encountered including floppy or exaggerated tone, immature posture, and abnormal motor patterns. Often these characteristics will be present in association with emerging motor problems or asymmetry. Such children are a puzzle to parents. They have some strengths but seem unable to progress in the usual stages. Or perhaps they are seriously limited in all areas, but from time to time seem to be making some progress, only to fall back and again be the cause for concern. This pattern may be the basis for initial anxiety, often the reason for referral, and generally at the root of tension that may greatly influence family relationships.

B. The Influence of Abnormal Tone

Excessive floppiness or stiffness of the young child may often be the precipitating cause of concern by the family. An intuitive sense of abnormality frequently occurs when the child is somehow recognized to be too flexible and difficult to handle or too rigid to accommodate in various usual positions.

1. Hypotonicity

Hypotonicity is associated with postural limpness and generally severe head lag. Often head, neck, and trunk control are also poor. Difficulties in handling and positioning the child are apparent early. This is initially seen in finding a comfortable, secure posture for feeding, whether by breast or bottle. There is excessive head lag and considerable support is generally necessary for the neck and trunk. This is true in a variety of postures including burping, dressing, bathing, and carrying the child. Floppy infants are immediately at a disadvantage also because they are greatly limited in their physical ability to maintain a secure posture in which to interact with the environment. This limitation could be the start of a long unbroken period of deprivation of contact and stimulation that may add to existing deficits.

2. Hypertonicity

Hypertonicity may have similar effects on the child, contact with family, and the environment. It differs in that excessive stiffness is more likely to be viewed as obstinacy by the parent or may be considered causally related to irritability. The possibility of a behavioral factor and emotional stress could thus be introduced early to complicate the picture further. At times, the stiffness enables some degree of ''standing'' at a very early age and may lead to the erroneous conclusion that the child is excessively mature and advanced in development.

Often tone will change greatly as the infant develops. As indicated in Chapter 3, it is not infrequent for the infant with hypotonia to later develop spasticity, or for the infant with initial hypertonus to appear ultimately as a child with dystonia. Change in tone patterns further confuses the daily problems in management. This is particularly true when the family is sensitive and responsive in adapting to the child.

There is often variable tone of the trunk and extremities. A hypotonic trunk may be associated with stiff upper extremities as seen in dystonia. Change in position may affect this relationship as well as postural motor patterns. The effect is to present much perplexity and many frustrations to those who deal with the child on a daily basis.

Finally, as the infant grows and matures, abnormalities of tone will increasingly restrict muscle range and movement. The resulting muscle contractures, particularly in the child with spasticity, will further restrict movement and function (1).

C. Sensory Deficit and Function

1. Visual

The infant with visual impairment may have a peripheral deficit such as cataract, congenital glaucoma, or other structural eye anomaly. On the other hand, the deficit may be central—within the optic tract—or may involve the optic cortex and result in some degree of cortical blindness. Both types of lesions may also be present. The effect of visual deprivation will be closely related to the complexity of involvement. An intact child with peripheral visual loss alone will obviously not respond to visual stimuli, but will respond to other sensory modalities. In this situation, it may be more difficult to identify early that sight is impaired since the child may interact fairly well with the environment.

A central lesion affecting vision is more likely to be associated with other sensory or motor deficits that limit the child's interaction with or appreciation of the surroundings. The limited overall reaction of the child may call attention to developmental abnormality at a very early age. While the infant may not see in either case, the presence of a peripheral lesion alone does not necessarily block other avenues for contact and learning.

Visual cues expected early, such as parental recognition, are missed initially, although a smile or verbal response to contact may occur. Within a fairly short time, the lack of visual response in feeding confirms the underlying parental anxiety. If a central lesion is present, there are likely to be associated abnormalities of tone and reflex behavior as well, further affecting development. At times, it may be quite difficult to determine on observation alone whether visual loss exists, either because the child otherwise interacts well or is totally globally limited. Examination by electroretinography or visually evoked electroencephalography (EEG) may be indicated to ascertain retinal function (2).

2. Auditory

Auditory loss is comparable in potentially restricting major environmental contact and the stimulation needed for early development. Extent of overall effect relates to the complexity of deficit, ranging from conductive and sensorineural to central lesions involving auditory pathways. Often hearing loss is not clinically recognized early and also may not be adequately considered in the globally involved child who interacts poorly. A variety of diagnostic procedures may be utilized to delineate the condition, including galvanic skin techniques (3) and the auditory-evoked EEG (4).

Recent data on hearing loss and emotional and social development confirm a much wider effect than had previously been recognized (5). This effect may be beyond the physical and developmental deprivation experienced as a result of limited environmental contact.

3. Other Sensory Deficits

The effect of tactile, proprioceptive, and gustatory loss on the young child has yet to be fully identified. One may speculate that individually, or in conjunction with a more complex central lesion, they each could contribute to further deprivation and raise the issue of an appropriate remedial approach. Perceptual and cognitive deficits, as seen in children with learning disabilities and mental retardation, respectively, are limiting factors that restrict the child's options for experience and learning. Those children with the greatest deficit have the least resources to utilize other strengths for development. The child who is more mildly involved, however, may be able to use other abilities effectively. Early identification of limitations in these areas is more difficult, and the question of how to remediate effectively remains open.

D. Abnormal Motor Patterns of Behavior and Deprivation

In conjunction with other initial neurological deficits, abnormalities of primitive and postural motor patterns may become major limiting influences on development. The child who roots and sucks poorly will feed poorly. Indeed, a first indication of deficit may be expressed as "colic" and irritability associated with the feeding process related to poor sucking and swallowing, with air trapping and inadequate intake. A strong asymmetric tonic neck will limit reaching out, bringing the hand to the mouth, and having contact with textures, shapes, and objects in the environment. Rolling from supine will be delayed or difficult, and progression to sitting, crawling, and ambulation will be greatly impeded. Similarly, persistence of the tonic labyrinthine, with associated truncal extension, will delay and limit sitting. Crawling will be restricted by a persistent symmetric tonic neck pattern in which position of the head and upper extremities correspond so that extension of the head will result in extension of the upper limbs and may obstruct movement. Strongly active and continued primitive motor patterns will also influence parents' ability to perform child-care activities. Marked influence is inevitable on positioning, holding, bathing, dressing, and feeding because of abnormal postures and associated easily elicited motor pattern responses. The implications for management as well as parent–child interaction are obvious and far-reaching. The continued active influence of these and other primitive motor patterns serves to "trap" the child in an immature state and intrinsically limit possibilities for self-initiated contact with the environment. Thus, by virtue of the early neurological deficit, the child suffers deprivation of experience and possibly social interaction as well. These problems exist in addition to frequent physical limitations in tone abnormalities and specific motor disorder.

For the slightly older child, similar concerns relate to delayed or incomplete appearance of the postural motor patterns. Late neck and body righting restricts efforts to roll, sit, and crawl. Limited or incomplete righting reactions affect trunk control, weight bearing, and walking. Here, too, delayed expression of motor patterns occurs in conjunction with other function-restricting neurological deficits that impair the ability to interact with and actively participate in the environment.

These deficits have an immediate and continuing impact on the child's ability to learn actively from the environment and participate in the process of socialization. Hence, the child with neurologic impairment may remain passive, dependent, and out of active contact unless his or her specific developmental needs are recognized and an active stimulation process is individually constructed. Implications for both education and socialization of the affected infant relate directly to the inherent restriction from the very beginning of development.

E. Specific Motor Abnormality: Posture and Movement

The child with a focal motor lesion, such as hemiplegia, may show signs of asymmetry. This may be apparent in limited expression of the Moro or startle response. Paucity of movement on the affected side will be seen as the infant is handled, positioned, and dealt with in all areas of child care.

More subtle and generalized motor limitations may be present and will affect movement and affect progression toward the upright posture. Moreover, the normal progression from the initial obligatory symmetric movements to voluntary, asymmetric, and localized ones will be delayed (6). The presence of actual motor signs and restriction will be associated with deficits of tone and patterns of motor behavior. Such a child may well be further limited in physically moving effectively in the environment, increasing with growth as the persistent limitations of muscle stretch and movement result in muscle contracture (7). Deprivation of environmental contact and inability to participate actively in surroundings are serious consequences that may further affect the child's development.

F. Oral Development Deficits

Of the many parameters impinging on early maturation, oral development has perhaps the most far-reaching influence. Many dimensions must be considered and full details of evaluation are delineated in Chapter 6. The rapidly emerging literature in this field gives some indication of the extensive areas that must be considered (8–11). From a functional point of view, the initial concerns relate to abnormality of rooting and sucking motor patterns, with frequent concomitant inadequate swallowing mechanism. This problem is not unusual when associated with fixed CNS deficit. Inefficient feeding with poor intake and frequent air trapping often results, accompanied by marked irritability and the infant's inability to be satisfied. This clinical picture is often confused with ''colic'' and may result in frequent formula changes or alterations in breast feeding. In fact, this pattern is often the first "soft sign" that neurological abnormality exists, and will call for changing the approach in handling, positioning, and managing the child.

As the child grows, the oral development problems may involve inability to chew and swallow solids or to drink from a cup. Complicated multiple deficits in taste and proprioception of tongue, lips, and jaw may all play a part (12). Restrictions in head, neck, and trunk control may further limit maintenance of the upright posture in sitting, which will affect the infant's ability to participate actively in the feeding process (13).

Abnormality in development of speech itself relates to hearing, intelligence, development of receptive and expressive language, integration of motor mechanisms of the tongue, palate, lips, and associated musculature (14). Maturation of the breathing pattern from initially nasopharyngeal to predominantly abdominal in the young infant, to thoracic in the normally developing child, may also be impaired and affect the speech mechanism (15).

Thus a fixed CNS lesion may influence all areas of oral development through direct effect on the structures of the oral cavity itself, as well as indirectly through abnormality of tone and patterns of motor behavior involving the head and neck. The major consequence is a restriction of normal active experience with the mouth, its relation to other parts of the body, and to the surrounding environment. As in other areas already discussed, the net effect is to place the child at an experiential disadvantage; to make him or her a passive participant; and to compel a role of dependency. In this sense, the neurological lesion serves to entrap such children at an immature stage where they may remain unless some active intervention process alters their relation to the environment.

II. MANAGEMENT AND TREATMENT CONSIDERATIONS

The functional consequences outlined above provide a perspective that must also be considered in planning for the daily needs and treatment requirements of the infant. As well as a systematic examination of the neurological and developmental levels, particular attention must be directed to problems in child management arising out of the deficits identified in the evaluations. For example, persistent primitive motor patterns and hypotonia will have obvious consequences for posture, movement, and motor development. They will also affect many aspects of daily care of the child for which the parent will require management assistance and guidance. Appropriate daily care procedures will have important consequences for infant interaction with the environment and for learning, and must be given equal consideration with the specific treatment procedures that are undertaken.

A. Management Assistance

Management concerns should cover at least the following major areas: handling, positioning, and daily care, including, bathing, dressing, and feeding.

1. Handling

Handling refers to awareness of special requirements for carrying the child, for adequate support, and for supervision necessitated by abnormalities of tone, motor behavior, or motor limitations. Various postures may exaggerate abnormal tone or accentuate immature motor patterns, for example. Others may enable the child to assume a more physiological pattern yet be consistent with the tasks required of the parent, and these need to be emphasized.

2. Positioning

Positioning is similar but relates to specific adaptations that may be necessary in order to deal with the child. What is the best position, given the specific limitations, for cleaning, bathing, dressing, or feeding? The individual needs will determine how these can best be accomplished and simultaneously promote the level of development.

3. Daily Care

Daily care includes all of the demands for infant management that are made more stringent when the child is developmentally delayed. Physical organization of equipment and space is a primary consideration with special attention needed for adaptations of crib, high chair, layette, bathing, and other equipment (16). Where there are problems of positioning and handling, the parent must be aware of steps that can be taken in preparation for care and of how the child can be helped to be a more secure participant.

(a) *Bathing.* Bathing is a good example of a daily activity requiring special handling and positioning for the infant. Without adequate preparation, the child may be totally unstable for support and sitting in a wash basin or tub, which could lead to an increase in tone and exaggeration of startle or other primitive motor patterns. Moreover, under these circumstances, a potential opportunity for positive contact with the environment and learning could be lost. A more optimum experience could be achieved with stabilization of the child from behind in a midline position. A safe, upright posture would then enable comfort and freedom of the arms and trunk, allowing the child to participate actively in a more productive learning and socializing experience.

(b) Dressing. Dressing, similarly, is an essential activity with many opportunities for interaction between parent, child, and the environment. Problems of abnormal tone and pathological motor patterns, for example, could totally influence the effect of this activity. Specific attention to details of positioning, handling, and movement patterns as dressing is performed will enable guidelines to be formulated for the best possible dressing experience. As with other areas of management, a guiding principle should be to assist the child to a secure position so that the youngster can observe and participate actively, if possible, in the entire process. For example, it may involve obtaining supported seating, so the child can be guided from behind when putting on articles of clothing (17). Functional evaluation must provide an insight into the child's specific deficits that have to be considered in working toward this goal.

(c) Feeding. Feeding is the child's most complex functional activity. It directly incorporates problems of tone, posture, motor abnormality, and patterns of motor behavior with the head, neck, and oral mechanisms. As with other areas of management in the infant diagnosed with cerebral palsy, specific associated abnormalities must be identified as they relate to the normal feeding process (18), or where tube feeding is required (19, 20). In either situation, the goal is to afford a positive, active experience for the child, to enable ease of care, as well as maximize potential for learning and social development. Specific management and treatment techniques concerned with feeding are reviewed in detail in Chapters 8 and 9.

B. Current Treatment Options

1. Therapy

For the infant and young child up to age 3, the treatment of choice most frequently is a therapy program. The starting point is a detailed evaluation of tone, patterns of motor behavior, motor and sensory status, and posture conducted by the physical and occupational therapist upon referral following diagnosis. In addition, involving an interdisciplinary team including speech therapists and early education specialists is essential for evaluation and early intervention planning (21). The evolving dynamic systems approach now increasingly focuses upon improving function and maintaining physiological conditioning, rather than primarily attempting to change abnormal neurological motor patterns (22).

In the actual management/treatment situation, the approach of the therapist should be as advisor or coach to caregivers, emphasizing daily carryover at home. The aim is to help develop compensatory mechanisms that will enhance the child's function. Suggested evaluation procedures are outlined in detail in Chapter 6.

(a)   Overview of Therapy Methods.   Definitive approaches to therapy for the young child with cerebral palsy have been evolving since the turn-of-the-century attempts of Jennie Colby (23). The trend toward very early diagnosis and intervention has greatly shifted initial emphasis away from orthopedic surgery and placed priority on global remediation of the existing developmental deficits, building on strengths, use of technology, and much more emphasis on cognitive needs. The physical therapy modalities in current use reflect a continuum of approaches that have evolved over the past 50 years or more for some and more recently for others (see Chapter 5). Unequivocal benefit or superiority of any given method, including those now based on the most recently evolved dynamic systems approach, has not been clearly established by current follow-up studies (24–26). However, there are data on the relevance of therapies in providing family support (27) and their potential for strengthening and maintaining physiological function (28, 29). In addition, there are increasing data on multimodal early intervention programs in effecting developmental change (30–32). Chapters 6 through 9 will deal with the therapeutic approach to the young child, with particular emphasis on function.

(b)   Early Intervention Programs.   Treatment of cerebral palsy by definition must deal with the developmental needs of the child with multiple handicaps. The areas of disability go far beyond motor development and maturation alone. Moreover, there are finite limitations in what can practically be expected of therapy programs as the child grows and develops. Therapy should be offered as the earliest approach to habilitative treatment, but is now among many other available modalities that have been shown by past experience to be acceptable for the complex needs of the growing child (33). Moreover, emphasis has shifted from a concentration on individual systems of treatment modalities to widespread programs of early intervention that incorporate physical, occupational, and speech therapy with infant/childhood development and early education methods (34). These early intervention programs for cerebral palsy and other developmental disabilities are now proliferating within the United States and throughout the Western world. The models vary considerably; some are home-based and totally individualized, while others utilize group methods with therapists and educational specialists in a center-based setting. The current United States Individuals with Disabilities Education Act (IDEA) of 1997 (PL 105-17) has provisions enabling early intervention programs for children up to age 3 in all 50 states (35). It is the result of a progressive involvement of younger children from legislation dating back to the Education for All Handicap Act of 1975 (PL 94-142) (36).

The early intervention programs offer the earliest form of special education for the child and a major opportunity for active involvement of the parent. Whenever possible, the therapy program should be integrated into such a total educational effort enabling contact with other infants and families. This contact can greatly influence early learning and social maturity of the child and provide the support and direction needed by many families (37) (Chapter 9). However, current data do not demonstrate long-term effectiveness of early intervention in maintaining developmental change. This may reflect the need for more intensive exposure, especially to families requiring considerable information and support (38). How these early intervention programs further develop and are used, and their relationships to other types of intervention, will depend upon needed changes to improve long-term effectiveness as well as availability.

2. Adaptive Equipment

A variety of assistive and functional aids are available to be used in association with therapy programs for the infant and very young child. The prone or supine stander, corner chair, feeding chair, other adaptive seating arrangements, sensory and motor stimulating toys, and specialized feeding equipment are a few of the many innovations that both the therapist and the parent can use to deal with individual requirements. Such equipment is increasingly being devised with an awareness of its potential value in assisting with daily living (39) and in motor development. Considerably less emphasis is now being placed on use of standing tables and other rigid, essentially passive, structural devices that merely contain the child.

3. Orthotics

The use of orthotics in cerebral palsy has a long history and was often employed alone as the definitive modality because of obvious clinical benefit. Tardieu, for example, showed that there was no progressive contracture of the soleus muscle when an ankle foot orthosis was worn for at least 6 h daily (40). However, the use of orthoses as a treatment procedure in itself is not usually recommended today since experience has shown they may be restrictive, passive, and without maximum benefit unless part of an active therapy program (41). Current practice emphasizes the initial use of therapy to help achieve functional head control, sitting, and weight bearing. With growth, restriction in range of motion, and persistent functional dependence, many clinicians would then consider offering some form of orthotic for the lower extremities in the hope of overcoming deforming forces, preventing contracture, and stabilizing posture and gait (42). As an adjunct to therapy or in conjunction with orthopedic surgery procedures, the use of orthoses can effectively maintain position and improve function (43, 44). Complementary use of therapy and orthoses need not be in conflict, but may be mutually supplemental in helping to achieve functional development. It should be kept in mind that orthoses have a definite effect on sensation as well as motor functioning. Also, their use should be task oriented (i.e., in sitting, standing, or weight bearing). Functional orientation will enable better integration into the overall therapy program.

4. Inhibitive Casting

Inhibition or serial casting can be used effectively as an alternative or in conjunction with orthotics in the growing infant (45). The child with an obvious hemiplegia, for example, might be a suitable candidate for initial serial casting to prevent or reduce contracture and enable earlier weight bearing. The use of an ankle-foot orthosis (AFO) could precede or follow a trial of serial casting, depending on clinical circumstances. Again, there need not be conflict with a therapy program if functional goals are clear (46).

5. Mobility Aids

As the child progresses toward weight bearing and ambulation, appropriate use and progression to walkers, crutches, and canes must be carefully considered. In addition, shoe insert orthoses may be very useful in compensating for foot deformity and stabilizing gait (47).

Wheelchairs are also becoming more functional. Many types are now available and are suitable for even very young children. They offer better maneuverability and ease of handling for the parent, together with improved stability for the child. Use of manual or powered wheelchairs augment mobility and provide self-controlled locomotion that can promote a greater degree of independence, reduce feelings of helplessness, and increase possibilities for socialization and opportunities for cognitive development. Children as young as 18 months have demonstrated ability to learn to use powered mobility quickly and safely (48). With active involvement in a therapy program, there is less concern about early dependency on a wheelchair, especially if it forms part of a functional treatment program.

6. Orthopedic Care and Management

In conjunction with other medical specialists and therapy staff, the orthopedist should provide early guidance and direction in the use of conservative approaches, such as serial casting and orthoses, to limit or prevent motor abnormality, and the use of special equipment (49). As the child grows, limited orthopedic surgical procedures may be considered in this age group, including adductor lengthening to prevent hip subluxation and dislocation, and possible gastrocnemius lengthening for the severely deformed foot (50). In general, orthopedic surgery should be avoided until gait matures (51). Because of the enormous potential for growth in the infant and child up to age 3, the judgment of when and how extensively to operate is the key to proper orthopedic care. Early and continuous involvement of the orthopedist with the child provides the best hope for the most realistic and appropriate future surgical intervention.

7. Treatment of Spasticity

The last several years have seen the emergence of medical and surgical approaches to improve or correct the motor deficit in cerebral palsy itself. The emphasis has been primarily on spasticity (52), but some attempts are being focused on dystonia as well (53). The extent to which this type of treatment will result in functional change remains to be seen. Indications for use in the actively growing infant up to age 3 are yet to be well established, and clearly require broad clinical standards of uniformity and consistency.

(a) Oral Medication. The use of drugs given orally to alter the motor deficit of childhood cerebral palsy and improve movement has a relatively recent and generally unsuccessful history (54, 55). Their use with infants and young children under age 3 is not generally recommended, and has usually been limited to patients in at least the later preschool years. However, one experienced group has reported them to be helpful in conjunction with therapy and to improve ease of care (M. Barry, personal communication, 1999).

The ability of oral baclofen to significantly reduce spasticity has been seriously questioned (56), and it has shown definite central nervous system side effects, including lethargy and irritability, in some children (57). Intrathecal baclofen (ITB), on the other hand, is now being widely used in reducing spasticity in generalized cerebral palsy, but there is little experience at the preschool level (58). See below for further discussion of ITB.

Dantrolene sodium has generated conflicting claims of benefits and may be associated with weakness and possibly serious liver dysfunction (59, 60). Its use in childhood cerebral palsy has not been demonstrated to be effective (61).

Tizanidine, which has been used to reduce spasticity in spinal cord injury (62) and in multiple sclerosis (63), has been introduced recently to reduce muscle tone in the child with cerebral palsy (64). There are no studies regarding its use in patients with cerebral palsy at this time, and it is not approved for children under 12 years of age. Its many serious side effects, including lethargy, hallucinations, and liver damage, have been documented previously (65).

Tranquilizers, such as chlordiazepoxide and diazepam, have been used with some effect in relieving increased tone and movement, particularly in the older child with dystonia (66). In conjunction with an active therapy program, tranquilizers are considered by some to be a useful and a temporary adjunct (67).

A variety of muscle relaxants have also been tried in this age group with little benefit (68). As with all of the oral drugs available, none can be documented to offer effective and sustained relief from motor, tone, and postural deficits by itself in the infant up to 3 years of age.

(b) Neurolytic Blocks. A variety of local blocking agents have been in use for many years in temporary management of focal spasticity, including 45% alcohol and 4 to 6% aqueous phenol (69). Phenol blocks may be difficult to administer, can be painful, and are associated with numerous complications. The effects, however, may last up to 9 to 12 months (70). The more recent advent of botulinum toxin A has led to its widespread use as a neurolytic blocking agent in cerebral palsy.

Botulinum toxin A. Since the nineteenth century, the toxin produced by the anaerobic bacterium, *Clostridium botulinum*, has been identified as the causative agent of botulism (71). This often deadly infection occurs following ingestion of contaminated food or as the result of a wound infection. The discovery in 1949 that the toxin acted through blocking neuromuscular transmission (72) has led to its purification as commercially available botulinum toxin A. Initial success with its use in strabismus (73) has stimulated application to a wide variety of abnormal neuromuscular conditions. Selective intramuscular injection of botulinum toxin A has now been shown to be effective in short-term (12 to 30 weeks) reduction of spasticity in children with cerebral palsy (74, 75), as well as in prevention of contracture in the experimental animal (76). In children with spasticity, botulinum toxin A has been shown to delay shortening of the gastrocnemius muscle, and may have a role in delaying early orthopedic surgery (77). Similar effect on hip adductors, with possible reduction in hip subluxation, has also been suggested (M. Barry, personal communication, 1999).

At the present time, its use with individually affected muscle groups is being refined in relation to other nonsurgical treatment components including physical therapy, occupational therapy, use of orthotics, and serial casting (78). The decision to employ botulinum toxin A in conjunction with limited orthopedic surgery in this age group (see above) remains a matter of individual clinical judgment. However, potential for rapid changes in motor deficits with growth alone raises concern about its use in children up to age 3. Other limiting factors include the potential for pain, bruising, and weakness (79) and the short-term effects that necessitate repeat procedures. Its use under 18 months of age is considered to be contraindicated by one experienced group (80), but has been successfully tried with hamstring spasticity as early as 12 months (81). Other groups have no age limit and use botulinum toxin A selectively for individual muscle groups where needed, as in a 4-month-old with torticollis (82). The manufacturer refers to ''juvenile cerebral palsy'' as the treatment focus (83), but the U.S. Food and Drug Administration (FDA) has not yet approved this indication. At the present time, the consensus among clinicians is to employ botulinum toxin A in

this age group to "buy time" while the child grows, and before the use of permanent procedures such as selective dorsal rhizotomy or orthopedic surgery.

(c) Intrathecal Baclofen. Baclofen administered intrathecally using a
pump implanted within the abdomen has FDA approval in generalized cerebral
palsy for the child older than 4 years (84). Delivery of medication is adjustable
on a continuous basis to provide central control of spasticity, but can be associated
with many side effects and complications, including the potential for seizures
(85). Clinical experience with patient selection and indications for use in relation
to other modalities is evolving at the present time (86). Potential functional benefits, especially in younger children, need extensive study.

(d) Selective Dorsal Rhizotomy. A procedure that has gained considerable attention is selective dorsal rhizotomy (87). SDR is generally considered
appropriate for the preschool age child at the earliest (88). Using lumbar laminectomy, the procedure attempts to identify and then divide out nerve rootlets that
are associated with an abnormal motor response, leaving intact those that function
normally. Intensive postoperative physical therapy is generally employed as part
of the total program. Definite reduction in spasticity is reported as compared to
the use of physical therapy alone (89). When surgery is followed by physical
and occupational therapy, improved function was noted at 12 months by Wright
(90), while McLaughlin found an equivalent improvement in mobility between
the group receiving SDR plus physical therapy, and those on PT alone at 12 and
24 months (91). One 10-year follow-up study has shown improved range of motion and gait (92). However, sustained or long-term effects are yet to be consistently achieved or results regularly replicated. Weakness of affected muscle
groups is seen frequently (93), and there continue to be concerns regarding potential for later abnormal bladder function (94), lordosis, and scoliosis (95). Clearly,
it remains to be seen whether reduction in spasticity, or improvement in gross
motor function beyond therapy alone, will be sustained on long-term follow-up,
and particularly if the cost/benefit ratio is favorable for the child with cerebral
palsy.

8. Treatment of Associated Conditions

It is essential to monitor the general health of the infant and young child with
cerebral palsy, looking particularly to remediate early any conditions that may
be associated with additional deficits. Examples include seizure disorders, visual,
and hearing impairment. Anticonvulsants are mandatory in the management of
seizure disorders and must be continuously reevaluated. Eye surgery for strabismus should be performed as early as appropriate to prevent amblyopia. Correction
of any hearing impairments must be considered a priority. Other types of correc-

tive procedures may be necessary and should be planned in conjunction with the ongoing therapy program.

9. Behavior Modification

This is a system with roots in developmental psychology that is used to stimulate new or alter previous behavior (96). A specialized aspect, biofeedback, involves voluntary change that can even affect physiological parameters such as blood pressure or heart rate (97). Data from the psychology literature confirm effectiveness of the technique for many discrete types of behaviors, especially for short time periods (98). It has been utilized in the infant with cerebral palsy to improve head control and sitting (99), with the preschool child to overcome equinus (100), and in gait training to develop symmetry (101). Planning the target behavior and developing the reward or reinforcement procedure requires a joint effort of therapist and psychologist. Sometimes the procedure can be used to condition the child to the therapy session itself to obtain better cooperation and participation. The technique may have much to offer in a broader way than presently recognized and deserves wider application. For example, its use in dealing with self-abusive or other unacceptable social behaviors is increasingly apparent (102). This type of behavior may be seen in children with various levels of mental retardation and organic brain deficits. It can greatly affect management both in the home, therapy, or school situations, and referral for an appropriate behavior management program should be considered part of the total interdisciplinary approach that can be offered.

C. Social and Mental Health Services

A major advantage of working with the affected infant up to age 3 is the opportunity it provides for becoming totally involved with the family. Often the child is identified only after a period of diagnostic confusion and a long search for the appropriate referral agency. The family frequently feels anxiety and guilt. Conflicting information and advice about care or treatment may be overwhelming. Problems concerning finances and transportation may prevent needed participation. These and other problems require an active social service program with involvement in the home when needed. Counseling and definitive psychiatric referral and care must also be available. Parental discussion groups in conjunction with the therapy program can offer the support and direction to assure carryover at home and an atmosphere conducive to growth. Professionals should not lose sight of the fact that early appropriate supportive care for the family is the major ingredient reported by older patients, in long-term follow-up studies, to have influenced their functioning and development (103).

D. Controversial/Alternative Treatments

Management and treatment programs clearly require continual use of a variety of modalities. Timing, emphasis, and application will vary with the strengths and orientation of professionals, outcome experience, and hopefully now with evidence-based practice (104). Programs will differ in approach, and there will always be some variance with parental expectation. This is a natural consequence of continual change in technology, experience, and the realistic limitations of what can be achieved at any given time for children with chronic disabilities. In addition, the current universal media attention, easy access to unlimited Internet information, and aggressive commercial interests all add to increasing demands for more immediately gratifying treatment results. Cerebral palsy and other developmental disorders are, therefore, prime targets for controversial and alternative treatments (105).

Some procedures are in use and may have appeal, yet are strongly questioned, because of unacceptable theory, methods employed, demands on the family, or outcomes claimed. This is true, for example, with patterning therapy (Fay-Doman), which has been strongly criticized (106), and not recommended for referral by the major medical specialty societies (107).

Hypnosis has been used with older children (108) and acupuncture has also been advocated without any evidence of meaningful benefit (109). Optometric exercises are widely prescribed for perceptual motor deficits, coordination, and balance, without any evidence of long-term effects (110). Diet therapy is commonly employed for behavioral and perceptual problems, including the Feingold regime and use of megavitamins. Neither has been substantiated as having relevance (111, 112). Vestibular stimulation has been studied in a control design and was found to have no significant effect (113), although Chee et al. had previously shown positive results (114). Use of neuromuscular electrical stimulation, likewise, remains controversial (115–117).

Hyperbaric oxygen therapy also has its proponents. A Canadian Foundation for Hyperbaric Oxygen for Children with Cerebral Palsy (HOT 4 CP) has been in existence since 1998. It has reported on the Internet a preliminary study of 25 children aged 3 to 8 that showed significant post-treatment functional improvement with the use of 1.75 atm for 2 weeks, using the GMFM, the Jebsen test for fine motor, and the modified Ashworth Test for spasticity (118). On the other hand, a 1999 unpublished study at Cornell Medical Center using 1.50 atm daily for 1 month found no significant functional benefits among a group of 24 children with moderate/severe cerebral palsy aged 1 to 5, using Peabody testing and a parent questionnaire (M. Packard, personal communication, 1999). No other documentation of studies is currently available.

A field dealing with chronic disability always requires the search for new and better approaches, and there is no doubt that affected families and professionals are ever on the lookout for simple solutions to the complex problems of the infant with cerebral palsy. In this quest, the basic principles of objective evaluation and relevance to existing treatment must be kept in mind. As we enter the twenty-first century, the following poem is also a reminder of the need to maintain a historical perspective and avoid "reinventing the wheel":

> A Short History of Medicine
> "Doctor, I have an earache."
> 2000 BC "Here, eat this root."
> 1000 AD "That root is heathen. Say this prayer."
> 1850 AD "That prayer is superstition. Drink this potion."
> 1900 AD "That potion is snake oil. Swallow this pill."
> 1950 AD "That pill is ineffective. Take this antibiotic."
> 2000 AD "That antibiotic doesn't work anymore. Here, eat this root."
> (From Ref. 119.)

III. DEVELOPING A PLAN FOR TREATMENT AND EVALUATION

Identification of the child with significant developmental delay or with a definite diagnosis of cerebral palsy should lead to team referral for appropriate care without delay. The physician and other professionals should be familiar with relevant resources within the community that can provide needed services, or at least be able to refer the patient to a source of information. The present accepted practice of early evaluation and intervention will be helpful in obtaining parental understanding and acceptance, even if a specific diagnostic label cannot be given. Professional direction in finding the appropriate resource can help avoid "shopping" among agencies, ensure good communication, and avoid unnecessary delay in treatment. It is also essential that, following referral, the physician maintain active contact with the treatment agency to enable close follow-up of the patient and guidance for the family.

The referral for therapy is essentially a team undertaking and should include the basis for concern, diagnosis, if possible, specific functional evaluation, and need for further workup. First consideration should be given to management problems to assist the family with daily care of the child. A full examination of sensory and motor development would then be expected so that the child can be placed in an appropriate treatment program. The elements of management and treatment should both be included to ensure the most appropriate planning for the atypically developing child.

Generally, the local medical society, health department, or educational authority will have information concerning early intervention services for the young child. Search of the Internet will also enable reference to a multitude of voluntary agencies providing relevant services.

REFERENCES

1. Little JW, Merritt JL. Spasticity and associated abnormalities of muscle tone. In: DeLisa JA, ed. Rehabilitation Medicine Principles and Practice. Philadelphia: Lippincott, 1988.
2. Tomita Y, Shichida K, Takashita K, Takishima S. Maturation of blink reflex in children. Brain Dev 1989; 11:389–393.
3. Vlach V, Bermuth H. von, Prechtl H. State dependency of exteroceptive skin reflexes in newborn infants. Dev Med Child Neurol 1969; 11:353–362.
4. Graziani L, Weitzman E, Velasco M. Neurological maturation and auditory evoked responses in low birth weight infants. Pediatrics 1968; 41:483–494.
5. Cavins G, Butterfield E. Assessing infant's auditory functioning. In: Friedlander B. Exceptional Infant, Vol. III. New York: Brunner, Mazel, 1973: 84–108.
6. Blasco PA. Normal and abnormal motor development. Ped Rounds 1992; 1:1–6.
7. O'Dwyer NJ, Nelson PD, Nash J. Mechanisms of muscle growth related to muscle contracture in cerebral palsy. Dev Med Child Neurol 1989; 31:543–547.
8. Stevenson RD, Allaire JH. The development of normal feeding and swallowing. Ped Clin North Am 1991; 38:1439–1453.
9. Logan W, Bosma J. Oral and pharyngeal dysphagia in infancy. Pediatr Clin North Am 1967; 14:47–61.
10. Brown J. Feeding reflexes in infancy. Dev Med Child Neurol 1969; 11:641–643.
11. Bosma F. ed. Second Symposium on Oral Sensation and Perception. Springfield: Charles C Thomas, 1970.
12. Haruki Kanomi R, Morita H, Kawabata J. Oral morphology and tongue habits. Int J Orofacial Myol 1995; 21:4–8.
13. Robbins J, Klee T. Clinical assessment of oropharyngeal motor development in young children. J Speech Hear 1987; 52:271–277.
14. MacNeilage PF. The frame/content theory of evolution of speech. Behav Brain Sci 1998; 21:299–511.
15. Hutchison AA. Respiratory disorders of the neonate. Curr Opin Pediatr 1994; 6: 142–153.
16. Finnie NR. Handling the Young Cerebral Palsied Child at Home, 3rd ed. Oxford: Butterworth-Heinemann, 1997.
17. Connor F, Williamson G, Siepp J, eds. Program Guide for Infants and Toddlers with Neuromotor and Other Developmental Disabilities. New York: Teachers' College Press, 1978.
18. Sholl C, Scherzer A. Feeding problems of the cerebral palsied infant. Ped Dig 1974; 16:19–25.
19. Plioplys AV, Kasnicka I, Lewis S, Moller D. Survival rates among children with severe neurologic disabilities. South Med J 1998; 91:161–172.

20. Naureckas SM, Christoffel KK. Nasogastric or gastrostomy feedings in children with neurologic disabilities. Clin Ped (Phila.) 1994; 33:353–359.
21. Haynes U. A Developmental Approach to Case Finding with Special Reference to Cerebral Palsy, Mental Retardation, and Mental Disorders. Washington, D.C.: Public Health Service Publication No. 2017, 1970.
22. Whitall J, Spezzano C. What's new in physical therapy? 53rd Annual Meeting of the American Academy for Cerebral Palsy and Developmental Medicine, Washington, D.C., Sept 15–18, 1999.
23. Colby J. Massage and remedial exercises in the treatment of children's paralysis: their difficulties in use. Boston Med Surg J 1915; 173:696.
24. Palmer FB, Shapiro BK, Wachtel RC, Allen MC, Hiller JE, Harryman SE, Mosher BS. The effects of physical therapy on cerebral palsy. A controlled trial in infants with spastic diplegia. N Engl J Med 1988; 318:803–808.
25. Piper MC, Kunos VI, Willis DM, Mazer BL, Ramsay M, Silver KM. Early physical therapy effects on the high risk infant: a randomized controlled trial. Pediatrics 1986; 78:216–224.
26. Weindling AM, Hallam P, Gregg J, Klinka H, Rosenbloom L, Hutton JL. A randomized controlled trial of early physiotherapy for high risk infants. Acta Paediatr 1996; 85:1107–1111.
27. Scherzer A, Mike V, Ilson J. Physical therapy as a determinant of change in the cerebral palsied infant. Pediatrics 1976; 58:47–52.
28. Damiano DL, Abel MF. Functional outcomes of strength training in spastic cerebral palsy. Arch Phys Med Rehabil 1998; 79:119–125.
29. Bower E. Physiotherapy for cerebral palsy: a historical review. Baillieres Clin Neurol 1993; 2:29–54.
30. Tjossem T, ed. Intervention Strategies for High Risk Infants and Young Children. Baltimore: University Park Press, 1976.
31. Resnick MB, Armstrong S, Carter RL. Developmental intervention program for high risk premature infants: effects on development and parent–infant interactions. J Dev Behav Ped 1988; 9:73–78.
32. McCormick MC, McCarton C, Tonascria J, Brooks-Gunn J. Early intervention for very low birth weight infants: results from the Infant Health and Development Program. J Pediatr 1993;123:527–533.
33. Silver L. Acceptable and controversial approaches to treating the child with learning disabilities. Pediatrics 1975; 55:406.
34. Graves P. Therapy methods for cerebral palsy. J Paediatr Child Health 1995; 31:24–28.
35. Dept. of Education. Assistance to States for the Education of Children with Disabilities and the Early Intervention Program for Infants and Toddlers with Disabilities. Fed Reg, 1999; 64:34047–34100.
36. Adams RM. P.L. 94–142: Education for All Handicapped Act, 1975. J Sch Health 1980; 50:242–243.
37. Parry TS. The effectiveness of early intervention: a critical review. J Paediatr Child Health 1992; 28:343–346.
38. Guralnick MJ. Effectiveness of early intervention for vulnerable children: a developmental perspective. Am J Ment Retard 1998; 102:319–345.

39. Korpela R, Seppanen RL, Koivikko M. Technical aids for daily activities: a regional survey of 204 disabled children. Dev Med Child Neurol 1992; 34:985–998.

40. Tardieu C, Lespargot A, Tabary C, Bret MD. For how long must the soleus muscle be stretched each day to prevent contracture? Dev Med Child Neurol 1988; 30:3–10.

41. DeLuca PA. The musculoskeletal management of children with cerebral palsy. Ped Clin North Am 1996; 43:1135–1150.

42. Wilson H, Haideri N, Song K, Tilford D. Ankle–foot orthoses for pre-ambulatory children with spastic diplegia. J Ped Orthoped 1997; 17:370–376.

43. Carlson WE, Vaughan CL, Damiano DL, Abel MF. Orthotic management of gait in spastic diplegia. Am J Phys Med Rehabil 1997; 76:219–225.

44. Radtka SA, Skinner SR, Dixon DM, Johanson ME. A comparison of gait with solid, dynamic, and no ankle-foot orthoses in children with spastic cerebral palsy. Phys Ther 1997; 77:395–409.

45. Sussman MD. Casting as an adjunct to neurodevelopmental therapy for cerebral palsy. Dev Med Child Neurol 1983; 25:804–805.

46. Watt J, Sims D, Harckham F, Schmidt L, McMillan A, Hamilton J. A prospective study of inhibitive casting as an adjunct to physiotherapy for cerebral palsied children. Dev Med Child Neurol 1986; 28:480–488.

47. Rosenthal RK. The use of orthotics in foot and ankle problems in cerebral palsy. Foot Ankle 1984; 4:195–200.

48. Butler C. Effects of powered mobility on self-initiated behaviors of very young children with locomotor disability. Dev Med Child Neurol 1986; 28:325–332.

49. Hoffer MM, Koffman M. Cerebral palsy: the first three years. Clin Orthoped 1980; 151:222–227.

50. Rang M, Silver R, Ganza J. Cerebral Palsy. In: Lovell WW, Winter RB, eds. Pediatric Orthopedics. Philadelphia: Lippincott, 1989.

51. Dormans JP. Orthopedic management of children with cerebral palsy. Ped Clin North Am 1993; 40:645–657.

52. Dabney KW, Lipton GE, Miller F. Cerebral palsy. Curr Opin Ped 1997; 9:81–88.

53. Albright AL, Barry MJ, Fasick P, Barron W, Shulz B. Continuous baclofen infusion for symptomatic generalized dystonia. Neurosurgery 1996; 38:934–938.

54. Badell A. The effects of medications that reduce spasticity in the management of spastic cerebral palsy. J Neuro Rehab 1991; 5(suppl 1):S13–S14.

55. Davidoff RA. Antispasticity drugs: mechanisms of action. Ann Neurol 1985; 107–116.

56. Albright AL. Baclofen in the treatment of cerebral palsy. J Child Neurol 1996; 11:77–83.

57. Gracies J, Nance P, Elovic E, McGuire J, Simpson DM. Traditional pharmacological treatments for spasticity Part II: General and regional treatments. Muscle Nerve Suppl 1997; 6:S92–S120.

58. Albright AL. Intrathecal baclofen in cerebral palsy movement disorders. J Child Neurol 1996; 11(suppl 1):S29–S35.

59. Herman R, Mayer N, Mecomber S. Clinical pharmaco-physiology of dantrolene sodium. Am J Phys Med 1972; 51:296–311.

60. Chyatte S, Birdsong J, Roberson D. Dantrolene sodium in athetoid cerebral palsy. Arch Phys Med Rehabil 1973; 54:365–368.

61. Mayer N, Mecomber S, Herman R. Treatment of spasticity with dantrolene sodium. Am J Phys Med 1973; 52:18.

62. Nance PW, Bugaresti J, Shellenberger K, Sheremata W, Martinez-Arizala A, North American Tizanidine Study Group. Efficacy and safety of tizanidine in the treatment of spasticity in patients with spinal cord injury. Neurology 1994; 44(suppl 9):44–53.

63. Nance PW, Sheremata WA, Lynch SG, Vollmer T, Hudson S, Francis GS, O'Connor P, Cohen JA, Schapiro RT, Witham R, Mass MK, Lindsey JW, Shellenberger K. Relationship of antispasticity effect of tizanidine to plasma concentration in patients with multiple sclerosis. Arch Neurol 1997; 54:731–736.

64. Edgar TS. Effective management of spasticity. Presented during the 52nd Annual Meeting of the American Academy for Cerebral Palsy and Developmental Medicine, San Antonio, TX, Sept. 16–19, 1998.

65. Knuttsson E, Martensson A, Gransberg L. Antiparetic and antispastic effects induced by tizanidine in patients with spastic paresis. J Neurol Sci 1982; 53:187–204.

66. Keats S, Morgese A, Nordlund T. The role of diazepam in the comprehensive treatment of cerebral palsied children. Western Med J 1963; 4:22.

67. Denhoff E. Cerebral palsy: pharmacologic approach. Clin Pharmacol Ther 1964; 5:947.

68. Denhoff E. Drugs in Cerebral Palsy. Little Club Clinics in Developmental Medicine. London: Heinemann, 1964.

69. Koman LA, Mooney JF 3rd, Smith BP. Neuromuscular blockade in the management of cerebral palsy. J Child Neurol 1996; 11 (Suppl 1):S23–S28.

70. Gormley Jr ME. Decision making in spasticity management: Oral medication and neurolytic blocks. 53rd Annual Meeting of the American Academy for Cerebral Palsy and Developmental Medicine, Washington, D.C., Sept. 15–18, 1999.

71. Jankovic J, Brin MF. Botulinum toxin: historical perspective and potential new indications. Muscle Nerve Suppl 1997; 6:S129–S145.

72. Burgen ASV, Dickens F, Zatman LJ. The action of botulinum toxin on the neuromuscular junction J Physiol 1949; 109:10–24.

73. Scott AB. Botulinum toxin injection of eye muscles to correct strabismus. Trans Am Ophthalmol Soc 1981; 79:734–770.

74. Calderon-Gonzalez R, Calderon-Sepulveda RF, Rinconreyes M, Garciaramirez J, Minoarango E. Botulinum toxin A in management of cerebral palsy. Ped Neurol 1994; 10:284–288.

75. Koman LA, Mooney JF, III, Smith PB. Botulinum toxin: potential role in the management of cerebral palsy during childhood. In: Jankovic J, Hallett M, eds. Therapy with Botulinum Toxin. New York: Marcel Dekker, 1994:511–522.

76. Cosgrove AP, Graham HK. Botulinum toxin A prevents the development of contractures in the hereditary spastic mouse. Dev Med Child Neurol 1994; 36:379–385.

77. Eames NWA, Baker R, Hill N, Graham K, Taylor T, Cosgrove A. The effect of

botulinum toxin A on gastrocnemius length: magnitude and duration of response. Dev Med Child Neurol 1999; 41:226–232.

78. Leach J. Children undergoing treatment with botulinum toxin: The role of the physical therapist. Muscle Nerve Suppl 1997; 6:S194–S207.

79. Wong V. Use of botulinum toxin injection in 17 children with spastic cerebral palsy. Paed Neurol 1998; 18:124–131.

80. Russman BS, Tilton A, Gormley Jr. ME. Cerebral palsy: A rational approach to a treatment protocol, and the role of botulinum toxin in treatment. Muscle Nerve Suppl 1997; 6:S181–191.

81. Graham HK. Botulinum toxin A in the treatment of hamstring spasticity. 52nd Annual Meeting of the American Academy for Cerebral Palsy and Developmental Medicine, San Antonio, TX, Sept 16–19, 1998.

82. Gormley Jr ME. Botulinum toxin: how much is enough? 53rd Annual Meeting of the American Academy for Cerebral Palsy and Developmental Medicine, Washington, D.C., Sept. 15–18, 1999.

83. Allergan, Inc. BOTOX: Indications and Usage. Physicians' Desk Reference, 52nd ed. Oak Brook, IL: PDR, 1998:490–491.

84. Symposium II. Management of Spastic Diplegia: Moving Toward a Critical Path. 52nd Annual Meeting of the American Academy for Cerebral Palsy and Developmental Medicine, San Antonio, TX, Sept 16–19, 1998.

85. Armstrong RW, Steinbok P, Cochrane DD, Kube SD, Fife SE, Farrell K. Intrathecally administered baclofen for treatment of children with spasticity of cerebral origin. J Neurol Surg 1997; 87:409–414.

86. Gerszten PC, Albright AL, Johnstone GF. Intrathecal baclofen infusion and subsequent orthopedic surgery in patients with spastic cerebral palsy. J Neurosurg 1998; 88:1009–1013.

87. Vaughan CL, Subramanian N, Busse ME. Selective dorsal rhizotomy as a treatment option for children with spastic cerebral palsy. Gait Posture 1998; 8:43–59.

88. Peacock W, Arens L, Berman, B. Cerebral palsy spasticity. Selective posterior rhizotomy. Ped Neurosci 1987; 13:61–66.

89. Steinbok P, Reiner AM, Beauchamp R, Armstrong RW, Cochrane DD, Kestle J. A randomized clinical trial to compare selective dorsal rhizotomy and physiotherapy with physiotherapy alone in children with spastic diplegia. Dev Med Child Neurol 1997; 39:178–184.

90. Wright FV, Sheil EM, Drake JM, Wedge JH, Naumann S. Evaluation of selective dorsal rhizotomy for the reduction of spasticity in cerebral palsy: a randomized controlled trial. Dev Med Child Neurol 1998; 40:239–247.

91. McLaughlin JF, Bjornson KF, Astley SJ, Graubert C, Hays RM, Roberts TS, Price R, Temkin N. Selective dorsal rhizotomy: efficacy and safety in an investigation-masked, randomized trial. Dev Med Child Neurol 1998; 40:220–232.

92. Subramanian N, Vaughan CL, Peter JC, Arens LJ. Gait before and ten years after rhizotomy in children with cerebral palsy spasticity. J Neurosurg 1998; 88:1014–1019.

93. Abbott R. Complications with selective dorsal rhizotomy. Ped Neurosurg 1992; 18:43–47.

94. Steinbok P, Schrag C. Complications after selective dorsal rhizotomy for spasticity in children with cerebral palsy. Ped Neurosurg 1998; 28:300–313.
95. Peter JC, Hoffman EB, Arens LJ. Spondylolysis and spondylolisthesis following five–level lumbosacral laminectomy for selective dorsal rhizotomy in cerebral palsy. Child Nerv Syst 1993; 9:285–287.
96. Bandura A. Principles of Behavior Modification. New York: Holt, Rinehart, and Winston, 1969.
97. Green E, Green A, Walters E. Voluntary control of internal states: psychological and physiological. Trans Pers Psychol 1970; 2:1.
98. Hawkins R, Peterson R, Schweid E, Bijou S. Behavior therapy in the home. Amelioration of problem parent-child relations with the parent in a therapeutic role. J Exp Psychol 1966; 4:99–107.
99. Silverstein L. Biofeedback with young cerebral palsy children. In: Feingold B, Bank D, eds. Developmental Disabilities of Early Childhood. Springfield: Charles C Thomas, 1978:142–147.
100. Campbell SK. Efficacy of physical therapy in improving postural control in cerebral palsy. Ped Phys Ther 1990; 2:135–140.
101. Seeger BR, Caudrey DJ. Biofeedback therapy to achieve symmetrical gait in children with hemiplegic cerebral palsy: long-term efficacy. Arch Phys Med Rehabil 1983; 64:160–162.
102. McGee J. Bonding as pedagogical phenomenon. A data based analysis of how children and adults with severe behavioral problems learn to interact with their care givers. Cathleen Lyle Murray Lecture. 41st Annual Meeting American Academy for Cerebral Palsy and Developmental Medicine, Boston, MA, Oct. 7–10, 1987.
103. Symposium: People with cerebral palsy talk for themselves. 25th Annual Meeting American Academy for Cerebral Palsy, New York, NY, Nov. 29–Dec 12, 1971.
104. Sackett DL. Evidence-based medicine. Semin Perinatol 1997; 21:3–5.
105. Matthews DJ. Controversial therapies in the management of cerebral palsy. Ped Ann 1988; 17:762–764.
106. Freeman, R. Controversy over ''patterning'' as a treatment of brain damage in children. JAMA 1967; 202:385–388.
107. American Academy of Pediatrics. The treatment of neurologically impaired children using patterning. Pediatrics 1999; 104:1149–1151.
108. Nieburgs T, Goldenson R, Nieburg H, Kline M. Hypnotic approaches to neuromuscular impairment: speech rehabilitation of the cerebral palsied. 31st Annual Meeting American Academy for Cerebral Palsy and Developmental Medicine, Atlanta, GA, Oct. 5–9, 1977.
109. Sanner C, Sundequist U. Acupuncture for the relief of painful muscle spasms in dystonic cerebral palsy. Dev Med Child Neurol 1981; 23:544–545.
110. American Academy of Pediatrics. Learning disabilities, dyslexia, and vision: a subject review. Committee on Children with Disabilities, American Academy of Pediatrics (AAP), and American Academy of Ophthalmology (AAO), American Association for Pediatric Ophthalmology and Strabismus (AAPOS). Pediatrics 1998; 102:1217–1219.
111. Conners C, Goyette C, Southwick D, Lees J, Andrulonis P. Additives and hyperkinesis: A controlled double-blind experiment. Pediatrics 1976; 58:154–166.

112. American Academy of Pediatrics, Committee on Nutrition. Megavitamin therapy for childhood psychoses and learning disabilities. Pediatrics 1976; 58:910–912.

113. Sellick K, Over, R. Effects of vestibular stimulation on motor development of cerebral palsied children. Dev Med Child Neurol 1980; 22:476–483.

114. Chee F, Kreutzberg J, Clark D. Semicircular canal stimulation in cerebral palsied children. Phys Ther 1978; 58:1071.

115. Dubowitz L, Finnie N, Hyde SA, Scott OM, Vrbova G. Improvement of muscle performance by chronic electrical stimulation in children with cerebral palsy. Lancet 1988; 1:587–588.

116. Carmick J. Managing equinus in children with cerebral palsy: electrical stimulation to strengthen the triceps surae muscle. Dev Med Child Neurol 1995; 37:965–975.

117. Hazelwood ME, Brown JK, Rowe PJ, Salter PM. The use of therapeutic electrical stimulation in the treatment of hemiplegic cerebral palsy. Dev Med Child Neurol 1994; 36:661–673.

118. www.hot4rcpkidsfoundation.on.ca/page69.html

119. Lange RH, Rogers CE. In my opinion: alternative medicine no substitute for evidence-based medicine. Medical Society of the State of New York. News of New York 1999; 54:4.

5

Historical Perspective to Current Practice
Habilitative Services

Margaret J. Barry
Department of Physical Therapy, Youngstown State University, Youngstown, Ohio

I. INTRODUCTION

Therapy for children with cerebral palsy (CP) began almost 100 years ago. Treatment has evolved from focusing on impairments (such as spasticity and contractures) to activities (such as walking), and then to considerations of participation (such as a child's family role as a sibling) (1). The assumption that "more is better" guided therapists in the past, but today there is more judicious use of resources and implementation of services. The concept of family-centered care has changed the paternalistic role of the medical team forever. In the past, the therapist determined the goals of treatment; today, the child and family identify their goals and direct their programs based on the family's needs. Over the years, therapists have implemented a great variety of treatment interventions with different theoretical bases. There are few clear standards of care. The move toward evidence-based medicine means careful analysis of the best available evidence combined with clinical judgment (2) to determine the most appropriate care for an individual child. This chapter provides a historical perspective of therapy interventions, from past to present, allowing us to understand where we have been, where we are, and where we are going.

II. EARLY HISTORY OF THERAPY IN THE UNITED STATES

Jennie Colby, a gymnast, was among the first to initiate physical therapy for children in the United States at Children's Hospital in Boston. She used massage and exercise to help a variety of patients with movement disorders. Her techniques were incorporated into the treatment approach of the neurologist Bronson Crothers (3). Crothers believed active movement and stimulation were key concepts, even for children with severe involvement. He supported the idea of independence and individual treatment plans. Winthrop Phelps, an orthopedic surgeon, went on to further expand the idea of interdisciplinary treatment (4). In the late 1930s, Phelps developed a pediatric rehabilitation center in Maryland. The center followed a team approach, with specific functional goals for treatment set by the team. All treatment began with relaxation and progressed to active movement. Phelps emphasized the use of strengthening and massage, as well as rhyming activities to promote active movement. He felt that the use of orthoses was important in maintaining appropriate alignment and promoting control. As control developed, the level of bracing decreased. His teams were innovative in their use of adaptive equipment to maintain postural control and to assist with functional tasks. Many of the concepts that Phelps promoted continue to be seen in today's practice.

Another pioneer in the treatment of children with CP was a physiatrist, George Deaver (5). Deaver was an advocate for promoting functional abilities, especially the use of wheelchairs and the performance of activities of daily living. He also advocated the extensive use of orthoses, but moved toward less bracing as the child developed control. Cosmetic appearance was a concern for Deaver, and in some cases, he advocated orthopedic procedures that resulted in cosmetic improvements without functional improvements. As the treatment approaches of Phelps and Deaver evolved in the United States, other treatments originated in Europe.

III. TREATMENT INTERVENTIONS

A. Neurodevelopmental Treatment

Perhaps the most renowned of all interventions addressing the movement and posture of children with CP is neurodevelopmental treatment (NDT). The treatment, developed by Karel and Berta Bobath (6), began in the 1940s. Karel was a neuropsychiatrist, and his wife, Berta, was a physical therapist (7). Attempting to explain the clinical observations of his wife, Dr. Bobath based his theories on the hierarchical and maturational theories of neuroscience at the time (8). The

Bobaths promoted the use of handling techniques to inhibit abnormal tone and primitive reflexes and to facilitate normal movement (6). They believed that children with CP needed the experience of normal movement. For children unable to move, a therapist's hands provided the experience. Quality of movement was considered very important. Initially, the Bobaths also used reflex-inhibiting positions to reduce the effects of the tonic reflexes. However, they later felt that these positions limited opportunities for movement and did not change reflexes. They believed that they had overemphasized the importance of the primitive reflexes. Treatment progression centered on the normal developmental sequence, assuming carryover to functional tasks. However, with clinical experience, they did not find functional carryover.

The Bobaths continued to update their theories and techniques as they gained experience and as additional knowledge of neuroscience became available. Today, NDT emphasizes functional goals (9). Principles of treatment include weight shifting, weight bearing, and normalizing muscle tone. Quality of movement is still important and may reduce abnormal stresses on joints, possibly preventing secondary impairments and deformity. Modalities include the use of balls, bolsters, horseback riding, and swimming. Therapists combine NDT principles with a variety of other approaches, such as strengthening and the use of adaptive equipment. An 8-week certification course is available, as well as numerous shorter courses. Throughout their lives, the Bobaths stressed the importance of parental involvement and a level of comfort in caring for the child (6). With advances in science and clinical experience, NDT continues to evolve, making it difficult to define and to research (see Chapter 11 for a discussion of the evidence regarding NDT and the implications for practice and future studies).

B. Vojta

In Germany, Dr. Vaclav Vojta developed another early intervention treatment method based on the maturational and hierarchical theories. The Vojta method, used in Europe and Asia, never became popular in the United States. Vojta attempts to activate postural and equilibrium reactions to guide normal development (10). Reflex locomotor patterns and proprioceptive input are the basis for treatment. The therapist develops a treatment plan that is implemented by parents. The therapist monitors the program on a weekly basis for infants, and on a monthly basis for older children. Treatment is uncomfortable, and children often cry (11). A Japanese study of Vojta found that children who initiated treatment at 3 months of age began walking earlier and with a steadier gait pattern (12). Proponents of Vojta suggest that very early intervention does not allow the development of abnormal crawling patterns, and subsequently promotes normal walking patterns.

C. Patterning

Perhaps the most controversial figure in the early history of the treatment of children with CP is Temple Fay, a neurophysiologist. Fay believed that "ontogeny recapitulates phylogeny," or that individual development follows the evolutionary process (13). According to Fay, a child's brain evolves as that of a fish, reptile, mammal, and, ultimately, a human. If there is an injury to the brain, development stops at that level of maturation. Further maturation is not possible without intervention to stimulate the brain.

Doman and Delacato based a treatment method, called patterning, on Fay's principles. They suggested that patterning facilitates normal development in undamaged areas of the brain and leads to changes in the damaged areas, which allows more normal movement (14). The idea of the program is neurological organization and respiratory control. Parents who consult The Institutes for the Achievement of Human Potential receive instruction in the very strict patterning treatment regimen (15).

Doman and colleagues described the treatment, with different regimens for nonambulatory and ambulatory children (14). For children unable to walk, they spend the day on the floor in prone position, encouraged to creep or crawl. For all children, a team of at least three adults provides patterning for 5 min four times a day, every day. With the child lying on his stomach, the head, arms and legs are moved in the appropriate patterns. The head is turned, and the extremities are flexed and extended. Sensory stimulation, activities to promote dominance of one hemisphere, and a breathing program are other components of the treatment regimen.

This treatment is potentially harmful to children and their families (15,16). Besides the time and expense of providing the intensive program, there are many psychosocial issues to consider. Instead of accepting the child's disability and learning to cope with it, families may harbor false hope for a cure. The demanding regimen also interferes with the child's opportunities for appropriate social interactions and overall development. In the 1980s, in separate policy statements, the American Physical Therapy Association and the American Academy of Pediatrics expressed concerns regarding the effectiveness of patterning and the promotional methods of the Institutes for the Achievement of Human Potential (15). Although there is no evidence to support this treatment, failure is blamed on the parents. Our current knowledge of neuroscience does not support a theory that involves the patient as a passive participant. Learning requires active involvement.

D. Rood

Rood utilized both the sensory and motor systems to facilitate movement with her treatment techniques (17). She felt that preventing the development of abnormal movement patterns was important. She used sensory input to activate or relax muscles to promote normal movement. For example, she applied heat or cold, along with stroking or brushing the skin over a muscle, to activate the muscle. Movements in the developmental patterns were then encouraged for function. Brushing continues to be utilized by some therapists, either as a method of relaxation or stimulation.

E. Sensory Integrative Therapy

Sensory integrative (SI) therapy, developed by Jean Ayres, is based on promoting the organization and processing of sensory information (18). Proponents believe that information coming into the body from the proprioceptive, tactile, and vestibular systems is disorganized and not processed well. This lack of cognitive processing is considered a perceptual problem (17). These processing problems cause difficulties with motor planning and motor control. Therapy focuses on movement and environmental awareness. The use of swings, scooters, and other moving objects helps the child process sensory input and use sensory information to plan movement and gain postural control (18). Traditionally, occupational therapists are more involved in the use of SI treatment.

F. Strengthening

As previously mentioned, Colby, Crothers, and Phelps advocated the use of strengthening exercises. Although the Bobaths revised their opinions on the importance of following the developmental sequence and primitive reflexes, their feelings toward activities requiring a great deal of effort did not change (6). They felt that these activities would result in increased spasticity and associated reactions. Thus they did not support the use of strengthening exercises. Several researchers have looked at the effects of strengthening, and no study identified increased spasticity as an adverse effect (19–21). However, some NDT therapists are still reluctant to do resistive exercises (20).

Herman Kabat recognized the importance of strengthening, demonstrated by his development of proprioceptive neuromuscular facilitation (PNF). Kabat was a physician and a neurophysiologist, interested in the treatment of patients with CP (22). He teamed with Margaret Knott, a physical therapist, and the popularity of PNF grew as she presented the method to other therapists. The technique is hands-on, using diagonal patterns of movement to activate muscles and gain strength and control.

Today we have evidence that children with CP are weak. One study compared leg strength in children with diplegia, hemiplegia, and age-matched peers (23). The children with CP demonstrated weakness, with the greatest weakness in the distal muscles. In children with hemiplegia, even the less involved side was weak when compared to typical children. All children in this study were all able to walk; it is possible that weakness is even more significant in children who are not as active.

Damiano and colleagues are strong advocates of strength training for weakness in children with CP (19,24,25). They recommend using loads at least 65% of the maximum voluntary contraction. They suggest 6-week programs, performing four sets of five repetitions of each exercise, at a frequency of three times per week. They used this protocol for 14 children with CP who gained strength in the quadriceps, with most attaining normal strength (19). Gait analysis demonstrated reduced crouch and increased stride length. There were only two missed sessions for the entire program, indicating that children were very compliant. Damiano's most recent study also found improved muscle strength, as well as improved gross motor skills and walking speed (25). These functional gains may result in reduced disability for these children.

There is no evidence that strengthening increases spasticity. There is evidence that weakness is a problem in this population of children, and strengthening is effective in reducing weakness and improving function. For very young children, weight training may not be appropriate, but therapists can incorporate strengthening activities into the child's therapy program through games and repetition of functional movements.

G. Electrical Stimulation

Another treatment approach that is sometimes used for strengthening is electrical stimulation. This treatment can be controversial. Therapists use electrical stimulation for children with CP for several reasons. In addition to building strength, it may be used to improve function, gain or maintain range of motion, facilitate voluntary muscle control, and/or reduce spasticity. Electrical stimulation is used in young children, but tolerance is sometimes an issue.

Most often, stimulation is at an intensity great enough to cause muscle contraction. In the literature, there are case reports of improvements after stimulation of either spastic muscles or their antagonists. In a randomized, controlled study, investigators matched ten pairs of children with hemiplegia (26). They stimulated the tibialis anterior muscle to increase range of motion, hoping subsequently to improve gait. The treatment group received electrical stimulation to elicit dorsiflexion 1 h per day for 1 month. The researchers found increased strength and range of motion, but the gait pattern did not change. Improvements in the gait pattern may have required more time and therapy. The researchers felt that electrical stimulation may be helpful in the prevention of contractures. It may be advantageous to use this modality during growth spurts.

One of the more recent applications of electrical stimulation is termed threshold electrical stimulation (TES), previously referred to as therapeutic electrical stimulation. Karen Pape developed the TES method in Toronto (27), which involves very low intensities of stimulation that do not cause a visible muscle contraction. Treatment is done during sleep. The youngest recommended age for beginning TES is 2 years. Children must have enough surface area to place electrodes far enough apart to carry current. Safety is also a concern when TES is being considered for the very young. Although most of the studies on TES are case series, there was one randomized, controlled trial in children who had undergone selective dorsal rhizotomy. In that study, children on TES made significantly greater gains in gross motor function than children who did not receive TES (28). However, they found no differences in strength. Pape claims TES improves muscle bulk, but there is no published evidence supporting this claim (27). One of the dangers of this intervention is the presumption by proponents that the treatment is always effective if applied as directed. Failure is blamed on the parents, although research does not to support the notion that the treatment is effective for every patient.

H. Stretching

Some therapists spend a great deal of time stretching tight muscles. Others incorporate stretching in home programs where parents perform stretching exercises or children are placed in positioning devices, such as long-sitters, to stretch the hamstrings. Serial casting is another method of stretching, which seems to be effective in young children. Therapists apply a cast with the joint held in a stretched position, as far as tolerated by the child. After a week or two, the therapist removes the cast and then applies another cast, providing additional stretch. Therapists may repeat this process until there is no further gain in range of motion, or they reach full range of motion. Casting may prevent or delay the need for orthopedic surgery to lengthen muscles, such as the calf muscles.

One use of orthoses (braces) is to provide stretching. Tardieu and colleagues did a study to determine the amount of time typical children and children with CP stretch the soleus muscle each day (29). Children's ages ranged from 9 to 15 years; the study period was 7 months. Researchers found that, during daily activities, five typical children spent an average of 7 h stretching the soleus. For children with CP, those who maintained their ankle range of motion wore ankle foot orthoses 6 h per day; those who wore orthoses only 2 h per day developed contractures.

In terms of preventing contractures at other joints, there is not as strong a scientific basis for appropriate intervention. More studies need to describe the amount of stretching performed by typical children and children with disabilities and the outcomes of stretching programs.

Orthoses are also used to compensate for deformity and to optimize function. Early in their careers, the Bobaths disapproved of orthoses and adaptive equipment (30), which caused some therapists to resist using them. But eventually the Bobaths accepted orthoses. They also felt that inhibitive casting reduced tone and abnormal foot reflexes. Knutson and Clark (31) provide a reference for the indications for the use of a variety of orthoses. Studies suggest ankle foot orthoses and inhibitive casts improve stride length and balance in gait, and maintain heel cord length if worn at least 6 h per day (29,32,33).

I. CONDUCTIVE EDUCATION

Andras Peto developed conductive education in Hungary (34,35). Conductive education is not specifically a therapy approach, but rather an integration of cognitive, motor, self-care, and social training. The conductor is the one professional responsible for the child's daily program, including education, nursing, and habilitation (34,36). The goal of conductive education is independent function without aids or assistance. In Hungary, children must walk and function independently to attend typical schools; thus, achieving such independence is extremely important (37,38). In other areas of the world, intervention may focus on different goals, depending upon accessibility for persons with disabilities. Education of the conductor is a 4-year program. Conductors spend the first 2 years in a teacher training college, then spend two-thirds of their remaining time training directly with a conductor. There is very little formal training in occupational, physical, and speech therapies (37).

Children initiate and carry out tasks to rhythms and songs, often working together in groups (34,36,39,40). Ladder-back chairs and plinths are used for functional activities (40). Conductors choose tasks that are goal-oriented and meaningful to the child, providing minimal assistance (41). Children with severe cognitive deficits are not considered appropriate candidates because following directions is part of the program. Children must be capable of communication and have some intentional function (39,40,42). Other conditions, such as uncontrolled seizures, hearing and visual impairments, and fixed deformities are also considered contraindications (34). The residential program allows little opportunity for family and social interaction, other than in the educational setting (35). Visitors to the Peto Institute in Hungary report that the children and the conductors demonstrate enthusiasm and enjoyment (37,39). It is not known how well these children integrate into their communities (43), but the Peto Institute reports that 73% of their students achieve independent function (37). The success of the program may be due in part to their selection criteria, since they only admit children with good potential for functional independence (34).

Conductive education is becoming increasingly popular in many parts of the world, including the United Kingdom, Australia, Japan, Canada, and the

United States (42,44). Despite its popularity, there is little evidence to support conductive education over other interventions. An Australian study randomized children to conductive education or standard treatment and found little difference between the groups (45).

J. Assistive Technology

Increasingly, opportunities for using assistive technology are becoming available to very young children. Computer applications, powered mobility, myoelectric prostheses, and augmentative communication devices have been utilized in research studies (46). Infants as young as 3 months have purposefully interacted with computers; 18-month-old toddlers have safely driven powered mobility devices; and 2-year-olds have communicated with speech synthesizers.

Investigation of the early introduction of assistive technology results from an increasing awareness in child psychology of the relationship between physical and psychological development. When development is delayed in any domain, other domains also suffer adverse effects. Motor skills allow the young child to learn, socialize, and develop a sense of independence. Through motor interactions, infants and toddlers learn about their environment and the concept of cause and effect. Young children with CP who are unable to move and interact with people and their environment tend to become passive, unable to actively initiate and participate in experiences. With assistive technology, children have the chance to be more successful in directly controlling their environment, and may thereby reduce potential secondary social–emotional and cognitive impairments.

The equipment options available to families today continue to expand with advances in technology, especially tools designed for young children. Children with speech and language difficulties have numerous options in augmentative communication devices. Charlene Butler supports the early use of augmentative mobility devices in children with limited mobility (47–50). In six young children from 18 months to 3 years of age, Butler studied the effects of powered mobility and found increased self-initiated behaviors (50). Parents reported satisfaction and there were positive psychosocial outcomes. In reviewing the literature, Butler stated that ''the availability of mobility options does not impede the development of ambulatory potential, nor do children 'give up' walking when they have alternatives available'' (47).

Despite technological advances, the emphasis on early intervention continues to be centered on the family. The family's goals are the priority, with their resources and needs taken into consideration. Therapists, along with other medical and educational team members, want to empower families to make treatment decisions and plan for the future of their children with disabilities. Part of the planning process is the consideration of treatment outcomes across many aspects of life. Disablement models define dimensions for the assessment of treatment outcomes.

IV. DISABLEMENT MODELS

There are several frameworks for considering the effects of disablement, planning treatment approaches, and evaluating the effects of interventions. The latest model comes from the World Health Organization (WHO) International Classification of Impairment, Disability and Handicap (ICIDH-2), which describes the consequences of disease. The ICIDH-2 is similar to the National Center for Medical Rehabilitation Research model, which was originally adopted by the American Academy of Cerebral Palsy and Developmental Medicine (AACPDM) (1). However, the ICIDH-2 model puts a more positive light on the framework, moving away from terms such as handicapped and disabled. When this revised WHO model became available, the AACPDM incorporated its concepts and terminology into its framework for evaluating treatment outcomes. The ICIDH-2 framework covers the body level, the person, the social situation, and environmental or contextual factors. Throughout this book, these levels will be considered in the evaluation and treatment of young children, and the research evidence supporting these interventions. The four dimensions of the ICIDH-2 model will be introduced here, beginning at the body level.

A. Body Level

The first level is functional and structural integrity of the body, which, in a more negative sense, is referred to as impairment. In the past, changing impairments was the basis for treatment. Therapists believed that if they changed impairments, the patient would demonstrate changes in function. Today there is still a concern for body structures, but the major emphasis of intervention is functional. Therapists try to prevent deformity, thus they are concerned with impairments such as decreased range of motion. They also consider impairments, for example, decreased range of motion and weakness, which may interfere with functional abilities.

B. Person Level

Activities, referring to functioning at the person level, are another dimension in the framework. Tasks like walking, talking, and toileting fall under this category. Therapists work on these tasks, but there is also a greater awareness of the environment in which these tasks are performed in daily life. Therapists consider not only walking, but also helping families decide on the most appropriate means of mobility.

C. Social Level

Participation at the social level is the next dimension to consider. Therapists are becoming more attuned to this dimension. Participation refers to the ability to become involved in the situation and to carry out social roles. For instance, for a 3-year-old boy who has a new baby sister, one role would be big brother. The issue of social participation has been largely ignored in the past. Today, the ultimate goal of intervention is minimizing disability to allow the child to participate in society as fully as the child's potential allows. In early intervention, the social roles of family members are also important to consider. For instance, a mother who is returning to school may need support in her new role as a student.

D. Environmental Level

The fourth level involves contextual factors, covering cost of intervention, acceptance by society of interventions such as technology, and accessibility. The prevalent attitude in the United States that more services are always more optimal than fewer services, for example, may be a limitation when considered from the aspect of societal cost.

The traditional focus on body structure and function and on impairments such as spasticity is no longer the primary consideration in providing services. The disablement model allows us also to consider the effects of an intervention on a child's functional abilities and social roles. We want to consider the young child crawling not only in the hallway of the clinic, but also at home and in day care. Past research rarely focused on issues of participation, but awareness of the importance of outcomes at this level is growing (51–53).

V. Theoretical Considerations

The first theories of motor development and control were the hierarchical and maturational theories, based on reflexes and development of the central nervous system (CNS). Treatments such as NDT, Vojta, and patterning evolved under this theoretical framework. Movement was thought to be the result of a stimulus–response mechanism: a sensory stimulus led to a motor response. As the nervous system matured, the levels of control moved from the spine to the brain stem to the subcortex to the cortex (54). The complexity of movement and integration of primitive reflexes depended on the maturation process. Therapy aimed to change the CNS through stimulation. Treatment progression followed the typical attainment of motor milestones, from sitting to crawling to standing to walking. Normal movement patterns were thought to change through facilitation, and abnormal tone and reflexes could be inhibited. These changes were thought to lead to independent motor control.

Dynamic systems theory is the "new" basis for therapeutic interventions. This theory suggests that the nervous system is one system that influences a person, but it is not the only system responsible for motor development and motor control. There are numerous complex systems that interact (54). The musculoskeletal and sensorimotor systems, as well as the environment, are considered as important as the nervous system. The person, the task, and the environment all interact (55). The therapist identifies the constraints interfering with the task, which could involve changing an impairment, modifying the task, or the environment. For example, the therapist may determine that a child may not be able to learn to carry a lunch tray with a glass of milk, but may be able to carry a carton of milk, so the task is modified to promote a successful outcome. In another case, the child may need to gain strength in her arms in order to be able to carry the tray, so a body system needs to be addressed.

The motor learning approach advocates teaching problem-solving skills, a cognitive process (54,56). The idea of repetition is important, varying the task to allow problem solving and learning, as the task is practiced over and over again (55). The therapist provides feedback. The research regarding the appropriate amount and timing of feedback is still evolving, but random feedback that is provided after a short delay may be most effective (57). Allowing several seconds before giving feedback may give the person time to process the intrinsic feedback as to what occurred before providing additional input. Intrinsic feedback is the body's own sensory feedback, including input from the kinesthetic, visual, and auditory systems. The concept is the same as an athlete learning a movement like a backhand swing of a tennis racket. The movement must be practiced, there must be intrinsic and extrinsic knowledge of performance and results. A consistent backhand swing becomes automatic only after hours, even years, of practice. A coach may facilitate the process by providing feedback at appropriate intervals and also providing opportunities for the person to integrate his or her own sensory information.

This theory supports working with children in their natural environment because the environmental system is an important component in achieving a task. For example, working on mobility on the playground may be more effective than working in the therapy gym. There is also the concept of a "hands-off" approach, allowing children to move and learn from their own mistakes and successes. Children initiate movement, thus the tasks must be meaningful to them. The therapist must identify when a child is in a transitional state, ready to learn a new skill, and apply the appropriate intervention at the time (58). The dynamic systems theory is influencing pediatric therapy practice. Therapists are working with children in their natural environments, including the home and day-care center. Children are being given augmentative communication and mobility devices at an earlier age, modifying their tasks, allowing them to learn and explore their environments. The traditional hands-on NDT approach, originally based on early neuroscience theories, now considers current concepts of motor learning.

VI. MEDICAL TEAM APPROACH

With the increasing use of pharmacological and surgical interventions in young children with CP, the team approach becomes increasingly important. Therapists play an important role in the decision-making process. Therapists often know the children and families more intimately than any other medical team member does. These close relationships often mean that families place their trust in therapists. Therapists need to be aware of the available evidence supporting and refuting various interventions so that they can provide appropriate information and advice.

Therapists have several roles in the use of oral and intrathecal medications, botulinum toxin, and selective dorsal rhizotomy. The community therapist may refer a family to a clinic for possible intervention to reduce a movement disorder, such as spasticity. The therapist refers children who have involuntary movements that interfere with function or care. For example, the child may demonstrate extensor posturing of the trunk that interferes with sitting. Or a child may be walking up on his toes. The clinic therapist examines the child, discusses the family's needs and desires, and presents findings to the team. The team should make recommendations that allow for the facilitation of care, improved comfort, and/or functional gains. If an intervention is recommended, the community therapist needs to be aware of the decision, potential benefits and adverse effects, and appropriate therapy to maximize the effects of the medical treatment. Good communication between the clinic and community team members reduces family anxieties and confusion and promotes optimal care for the child.

VII. CONCLUSIONS

Habilitation professionals today have a responsibility to provide family-centered care to young children with CP. The family identifies goals and therapists provide guidance, keeping future considerations for the child in mind. The therapist may also provide information regarding the different types of interventions available and the types of service delivery, such as home- and center-based treatment. Therapy involves assisting the family with management issues in terms of daily care as well as developing the treatment plan directed to the therapy goals. Aug-

mentative communication and augmentative mobility are a part of early intervention, allowing children to interact with their environment, to learn, to play, to
promote self-esteem, and to reduce learned helplessness. For some children,
walking may be the primary goal, but independent power mobility may be of
greater overall benefit than limited mobility at a high energy cost. Secondary
conditions such as musculoskeletal problems are considerations in the decision
to use orthoses, assistive devices, and adaptive equipment. The goal of therapy
is not to provide a lifetime of therapy, but rather to facilitate living, enjoying the
best possible quality of life (59).

From this historical perspective, we move on to consider the practical application of therapeutic principles in the following chapters. We also consider the
evidence for our interventions in Chapter 11 as we strive for evidence-based
practice. As we weigh the evidence, we must also take the focus of treatment
into account, including body systems, activities, and participation. The present
era of health care requires therapists to carefully discern the most appropriate
intervention in the most efficient and effective manner. We take the lessons of
our history with us as we move forward, caring for infants and children with CP
in the twenty-first century.

REFERENCES

1. National Advisory Board. Research Plan for National Center for Medical Rehabilita-
    tion Research. Washington, DC: U.S. Dept of Health and Human Services, 1993.
2. Sackett DL, Richardson WS, Rosenberg WMC, Haynes RB. Evidence-Based Medi-
    cine: How to Practice and Teach EBM. New York: Churchill Livingstone, 1997:1–
    20.
3. Crothers B. Disorders of the Nervous System in Childhood. New York: Appleton,
    1926.
4. Slominski AH. Winthrop Phelps and the Children's Rehabilitation Institute. In:
    Scrutton D, ed. Management of the Motor Disorders of Children with Cerebral Palsy.
    Philadelphia: JB Lippincott, 1984:59–74.
5. Deaver G. Methods of treating the neuromuscular disabilities. Arch Phys Med Reha-
    bil 1956; 37:363.
6. Bobath K, Bobath B. The neuro-developmental treatment. In: Scrutton D, ed. Man-
    agement of Motor Disorders in Children with Cerebral Palsy. Philadelphia: JB Lip-
    pincott, 1984:6–18.
7. Semans S. A neurophysiological approach to treatment of cerebral palsy: introduc-
    tion to the Bobath method. Phys Ther Rev 1958; 38:598–604.
8. Keshner EA. Reevaluating the theoretical model underlying the neurodevelopmental
    theory. Phys Ther 1981; 61:1035–1040.
9. Bly L. A historical and current view of the basis of neurodevelopmental treatment.
    Pediatr Phys Ther 1991; 3:131–135.

10. Vojta V. The basic elements of treatment according to Vojta. In: Scrutton D, ed. Management of the Motor Disorders of Children with Cerebral Palsy. Philadelphia: JB Lippincott, 1984:75–85.
11. Jones RB. The Vojta method of treating cerebral palsy. Physiotherapy 1975; 61: 112–113.
12. Kanda T, Yuge M, Yamori Y, et al. Early physiotherapy in the treatment of spastic diplegia. Dev Med Child Neurol 1984; 26:438–444.
13. Fay T. The use of pathological and unlocking reflexes in the rehabilitation of spastics. Am J Phys Med 1954; 33:347.
14. Doman RJ, Spitz EB, Zucman E, Delacato CH, Doman G. Children with severe brain injuries. JAMA 1960; 174:257–262.
15. American Academy of Pediatrics. Policy Statement: The Doman-Delacato treatment of neurologically handicapped children. Pediatrics 1982; 70:810–812.
16. Golden GS. Nonstandard therapies in developmental disabilities. Am J Dis Child 1980; 134:487–491.
17. Lunnen KY. Children with severe and profound retardation. In: Campbell SK, ed. Pediatric Neurologic Physical Therapy, 2nd ed. New York: Churchill Livingstone, 1991:276–279.
18. White R. Sensory integrative therapy for the cerebral-palsied child. In: Scrutton D, ed. Management of the Motor Disorders of Children with Cerebral Palsy. Philadelphia: JB Lippincott, 1984:86–95.
19. Damiano DL, Kelly LE, Vaughn CL. Effects of quadriceps femoris muscle strengthening on crouch gait in children with spastic diplegia. Phys Ther 1995; 75:658–671.
20. Giuliani C. Dorsal rhizotomy for children with cerebral palsy: support for concepts of motor control. Phys Ther 1991; 71:248–259.
21. Holland LJ, Steadward RD. Effects of resistance and flexibility training on strength, spasticity/muscle tone, and range of motion of elite athletes with cerebral palsy. Palaestra 1990; Summer:27–31.
22. Voss DE, Ionta MK, Myers BJ. Proprioceptive Neuromuscular Facilitation, 3d ed. Philadelphia: Harper & Row, 1985.
23. Wiley ME, Damiano DL. Lower-extremity strength profiles in spastic cerebral palsy. Dev Med Child Neurol 1998; 40:100–107.
24. Damiano DL, Vaughan CL, Abel MF. Muscle response to heavy resistance exercise in children with spastic cerebral palsy. Dev Med Child Neurol 1995; 37:731–739.
25. Damiano DL, Abel MF. Functional outcomes of strength training in spastic cerebral palsy. Arch Phys Med Rehabil 1998; 79:119–125.
26. Hazlewood ME, Brown JK, Rowe PJ, Salter PM. The use of therapeutic electrical stimulation in the treatment of hemiplegic cerebral palsy. Dev Med Child Neurol 1994; 36:661–673.
27. Pape K. Therapeutic electrical stimulation (TES) for the treatment of disuse muscle atrophy in cerebral palsy. Pediatr Phys Ther 1997; 9:110–112.
28. Steinbok P, Reiner A, Kestle JRW. Therapeutic electrical stimulation following selective posterior rhizotomy in children with spastic diplegic cerebral palsy: a randomized clinical trial. Dev Med Child Neurol 1997; 39:515–520.
29. Tardieu C, Lespargot A, Tabary C, Bret MD. For how long must the soleus muscle

be stretched each day to prevent contracture? Dev Med Child Neurol 1988; 30:3–10.

30. Cintas HM. Neurodevelopmental treatment: the legacy of Berta and Karel Bobath. Pediatr Phys Ther 1991; 3:117–118.

31. Knutson LM, Clark DE. Orthotic devices for ambulation in children with cerebral palsy and myelomeningocele. Phys Ther 1991; 71:947–960.

32. Bertoti DB. Effect of short leg casting on ambulation in children with cerebral palsy. Phys Ther 1986; 66:1522–1529.

33. Harris SR, Riffle K. Effects of inhibitive ankle-foot orthoses on standing balance in a child with cerebral palsy. A single-subject design. Phys Ther 1986; 66:663–667.

34. Bairstow P, Cochrane R, Rusk I. Selection of children with cerebral palsy for conductive education and the characteristics of children judged suitable and unsuitable. Dev Med Child Neurol 1991; 33:984–992.

35. Beach RC. Conductive education for motor disorders: new hope or false hope? Arch Dis Child 1988; 63:211–213.

36. Titchener J. A preliminary evaluation of conductive education. Physiotherapy 1983; 69:313–316.

37. Robinson RO, McCarthy GT, Little TM. Conductive education at the Peto Institute, Budapest. Br Med J 1989; 299:1145–1149.

38. Anonymous. Physical therapy in spastic diplegia. Lancet 1988; 2:201–202.

39. Todd JE. Conductive education: the continuing challenge. Physiotherapy 1990; 76:13–16.

40. Reddihough D. Conductive education. J Paed Child Health 1991; 27:141–142.

41. Bax M. Conductive education. Devel Med Child Neurol 1991; 33:941–942.

42. Sutton A. Conductive education. Arch Dis Child 1988; 63:214–217.

43. Ross E. Conductive education at the Peto Institute, Budapest. Br Med J 1989; 299:1461.

44. Catanese AA, Coleman GJ, King JA, Reddihough DS. Evaluation of an early childhood programme based on principles of conductive education: the Yooralla project. J Paed Child Health 1995; 31:418–422.

45. Reddihough DS, King J, Coleman G, Catanese T. Efficacy of programmes based on conductive education for young children with cerebral palsy. Dev Med Child Neurol 1998; 40:763–770.

46. Butler C. High tech tots: technology for mobility, manipulation, communication, and learning in early childhood. Infants and Young Child 1988; 1:66–73.

47. Butler C. Augmentative mobility: Why do it? Pediatr Rehabil 1991; 2:801–815.

48. Butler C, Okamoto GA, McKay TM. Powered mobility for very young disabled children. Devel Med Child Neurol 1983; 25:472–474.

49. Butler C, Okamoto GA, McKay TM. Motorized wheelchair driving by disabled children. Arch Phys Med Rehabil 1984; 65:95–97.

50. Butler C. Effects of powered mobility on self-initiated behaviors of very young children with locomotor disability. Devel Med Child Neurol 1986; 28:325–332.

51. Brown K. They are improved, but are they better? Devel Med Child Neurol 1997; 39:213.

52. Butler C. Outcomes that matter. Devel Med Child Neurol 1995; 37:753–754.

53. Butler C, Chambers H, Goldstein M, Harris S, Leach J, Campbell SK, et al. Evaluating research in developmental disabilities: a conceptual framework for reviewing treatment outcomes. Devel Med Child Neurol 1999; 41:55–59.
54. Horak FB. Motor control models underlying neurologic rehabilitation of posture in children. In: Forssberg H, Hirschfeld H, eds. Movement Disorders in Children. Basel: Karger, 1992:21–30.
55. Valvano J. Applications of Concepts from a Dynamical Systems Perspective, Instructional Course. American Academy of Cerebral Palsy and Developmental Medicine Annual Meeting, 1998.
56. Lee TD, Swanson LR, Hall AL. What is repeated in a repetition? Effects of practice conditions on motor skill acquisition. Phys Ther 1991; 71:150–156.
57. Winstein CJ. Knowledge of results and motor learning—implications for physical therapy. Phys Ther 1991; 71:140–149.
58. Kamm K, Thelen E, Jensen JL. A dynamical systems approach to motor development. Phys Ther 1990; 70:763–775.
59. Campbell SK. Therapy programs for children that last a lifetime. Phys Occupat Ther Pediatr 1997; 17:1–15.

6
Clinical Assessment of the Infant

Gay L. Girolami
Pathways Center, Glenview, Illinois

Diane Fritts Ryan and Judy M. Gardner
DuPage Easter Seals, Villa Park, Illinois

I. INTRODUCTION

In this chapter, a model for infant evaluation will be presented. We are defining evaluation as the entire information-gathering process (1). The potential purposes of the evaluation process are to:

1. Determine the infant's developmental levels.
2. Answer the family's questions about their infant's development.
3. Determine eligibility for early intervention services.
4. Identify the infant's strengths and needs.
5. Gather information to use in setting goals and treatment planning.
6. Determine appropriate intervention strategies.
7. Measure progress over time
8. Obtain data for evaluation of program effectiveness.
9. Collect data for research, if applicable (2).

Assessment is a major part of that information-gathering process and may include discipline-specific standardized testing and/or clinical observations. The assessment data, together with the medical history, parental concerns, and reports from other professionals, are then analyzed and used to make intervention recommendations. In the infant evaluation process, the type of assessment often varies according to the reason for the evaluation and the discipline evaluating the infant. Both standardized tools and clinical observation have value. Standardized assessments are objective, structured tools that have been validated and measure prog-

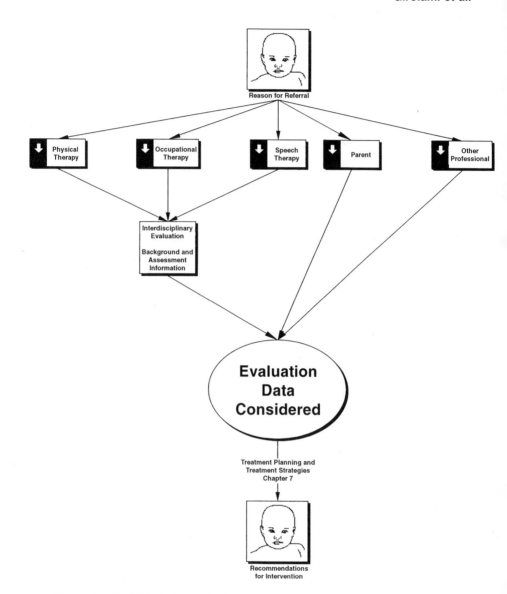

Figure 1 Model for infant evaluation.

ress over time (3–6). Each test focuses on specific performance areas and age ranges, and has its own time frame, reliability, and validity parameters.

Clinical observations are the more subjective and flexible tools of assessment. When clinical observations are done to accompany a standardized assessment, quality of movement and behavior can be looked at in more depth. For example, an infant may pass a sitting item on a standardized test, but the therapist may have concerns about posture, symmetry, and the use of upper extremities. Further assessment, through clinical observations in a variety of positions, may reveal that the child has a mild motor deficit (e.g., spastic hemiplegia).

When clinical observations are used as the sole assessment tool in the evaluation process, the therapist's skills and clinical experience must be well developed. Therefore, an intimate knowledge of the performance areas of development for both the preterm and full-term infant in discipline-specific domains is essential. Knowledge of skill expectations, quality of movement, and behaviors are important prerequisites for the therapist.

Whether standardized testing or clinical observations are chosen to obtain discipline-specific assessment data, the evaluation model presented in this chapter can be of use in using the information to develop appropriate recommendations for the infant and his family. Because there are may resources available for selecting and administering standardized tests, we will focus in greater detail on the assessment process using clinical observations to obtain comprehensive information about the infant's sensorimotor function and developmental skills.

This model for infant evaluation is interdisciplinary. The infant is observed by all disciplines in each position and in each activity. The interdisciplinary evaluation facilitates an integrated understanding of the infant's strengths and needs, and reduces the fatigue factor commonly observed in young infants. After gathering all of the information, the professionals involved discuss their combined observations, sharing information from discipline-specific points of view. This allows them to present unified and comprehensive recommendations for intervention to the family (Fig. 1).

II. EVALUATION MODEL

A. A Model for Clinical Assessment

Assessment and treatment planning for children with cerebral palsy (CP) is a very complicated process. Cerebral palsy impacts on a number of physiological systems, and the therapist must have an organized model to insure that all systems are adequately assessed. The information gathered during the assessment is used to develop a treatment plan, set goals, design appropriate treatment strategies, and document baseline functional skills from which to assess treatment outcomes.

In this chapter, we will present a model for assessment. It is based on the disablement model developed by the National Center for Medical Rehabilitation Research (NCMRR) (7). The NCMRR Advisory Board rejected the traditional linear view of disability in favor of a systems approach that considers organic, psychosocial, and environmental issues that contribute to disability.

The World Health Organization (WHO), the Public Health Service (PHS), Institute of Medicine (IOM), and S. Naghi have also developed disability classification models. Recently, the ICIDH-2 Advisory Board of the World Health Organization reviewed all of these models and revised the terms that best represented all aspects of their proposed systems approach. We have used a combination of both models to define the categories for our assessment process. Chapters, 6 through 9 will refer to this structure as the "Disability Model." Definitions and examples of these terms as they relate to infants with cerebral palsy will be defined in the following sections (Fig. 2).

B. Disability Terminology Defined

1. Pathophysiology

Pathophysiology is defined as interruption of, or interference with, normal physiological and developmental processes or structures. In the case of CP, one infant may sustain an intraventricular hemorrhage resulting in spastic hemiplegia or quadriplegia, while another infant may be diagnosed with periventricular leukomalacia resulting in spastic diplegia.

In another situation, a single infant may have both motor and visual or motor and respiratory pathologies that must be assessed and addressed. These multiple pathophysiologies may cause impairments in the motor, cognitive, perceptual, or sensory systems of the infant. And, while the treating therapists do not directly intervene at the level of the pathophysiology, knowledge of type of injury may provide insight into the resultant impairments and assist the therapist in determining how to best manage treatment planning and therapeutic intervention.

2. Impairments

Impairments are a loss or abnormality at the organ or organ system level. Impairments may be of cognitive, emotional, physiological, or anatomical (abnormalities in structure or function) (8). Some of the most common organ systems are: neuromuscular; musculoskeletal; gastrointestinal; sensory; and cardiopulmonary.

When a clinician assesses an infant, the observations result in a list of movement patterns and descriptions of *how* the infant moves. To determine the impairments and eventual treatment strategies, the clinician must take another step and hypothesize *why*. Armed with the knowledge that impairments may be

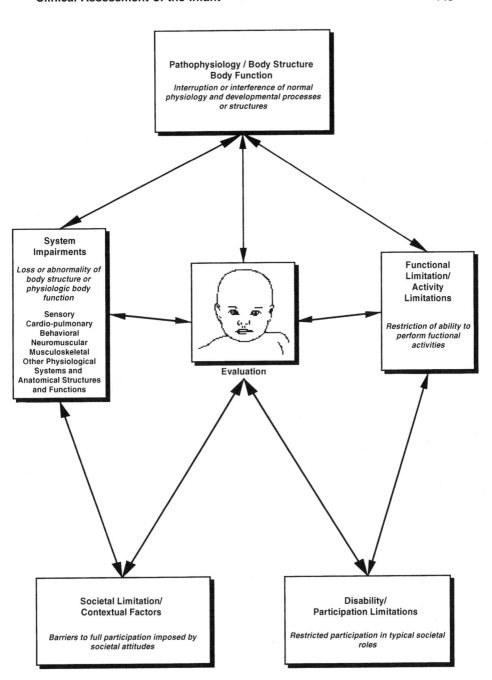

Figure 2 Disability model.

a result of pathology in a variety of systems, the clinician mentally reviews the systems that may be involved and hypothesizes and prioritizes potential impairments that must be considered. Once the impairments are identified, the clinician can begin to see how they interfere with function.

3. Functional Limitations/Activity Limitations

Functional limitations are defined as the restriction of ability to perform functional activities. These are secondary to impairments in body structure or function. Functional limitations are atypical performance or inability to perform functional tasks such as eating, walking, or sitting. Functional limitations are directly related to an impairment or combination of impairments, but they are not descriptions of movement patterns such as poor head control or thoracic rounding. Determining the most critical functional limitations is the key, so that realistic goals can be set with the family and intervention protocols planned to assist the infant in achieving developmentally appropriate function. In the infant, early therapeutic intervention may minimize the long-term effects of the impairments and prevent or reduce disability.

4. Disability/Participation Limitations

In this model, a limitation in performing tasks, activities, and roles to levels expected within the physical and social contexts is considered a disability. Early referral of infants with suspected neuromotor conditions could optimize functional outcomes and minimize disabilities. Also consider adaptive equipment and assistive technology to minimize the disability.

The clinician must consider the possible resultant disabilities associated with each functional limitation. Additionally, disabilities must be assessed within the context of the age and environment of the infant.

5. Societal Limitations/Contextual Factors

In the disability model, this is defined as restrictions attributable to social policy or barriers, structural and/or attitudinal, that limits fulfillment of roles or denies access to services and opportunities that are associated with full participation in society. Infants with CP may be exposed to societal limitations, and therefore it is imperative that the clinician assist the family in understanding their child's rights. It is also important to support parents and encourage them to advocate for their infant whether in the health care or societal arena.

Based on the disability model and definitions presented, we have developed a framework for assessing impairments and defining functional limitations, setting goals, and developing a treatment plan and intervention strategies for infants with cerebral palsy (Fig. 3). The following sections will present an overview of the data-gathering process and the performance areas to be assessed. Chapter 7 will focus on how all of the information gathered during the assessment process can be used to develop goals, a treatment plan, and intervention strategies.

III. GATHERING INFORMATION FOR THE INTERDISCIPLINARY ASSESSMENT

We are advocating that the assessment format be interdisciplinary. This can also be called an arena assessment (9). In the arena format, physical, occupational, and speech therapists assess the infant simultaneously. Generally, there is one lead person handling the case, although there may be instances throughout the assessment when each professional is specifically interacting with the infant.

The data obtained during assessment is gathered through observation and handling. In an arena assessment, it is not practical to perform standardized testing in all of the discipline-specific areas, although normative data from standardized tests are often used as a guide to clinical observations of performance areas.

A. Background Data

Before assessing the infant, it is important for the evaluating team to familiarize themselves with any available background information. This information may include reasons for referral and medical information from other health professionals who have already seen the infant. Parental information can be obtained prior to the assessment through a written intake process or telephone contact. Each of these areas should specifically be addressed in the summary and recommendations.

It is also important to understand the birth and medical history and any hospitalizations or illnesses that may have impacted on the infant's development. Current medical issues and management should also be considered. Additional information from other health professionals who have assessed or treated the infant should also be included.

B. Assessment Data

In this section of the assessment, data from the therapy-specific performance areas are collected. A performance area refers to a category of functions or behav-

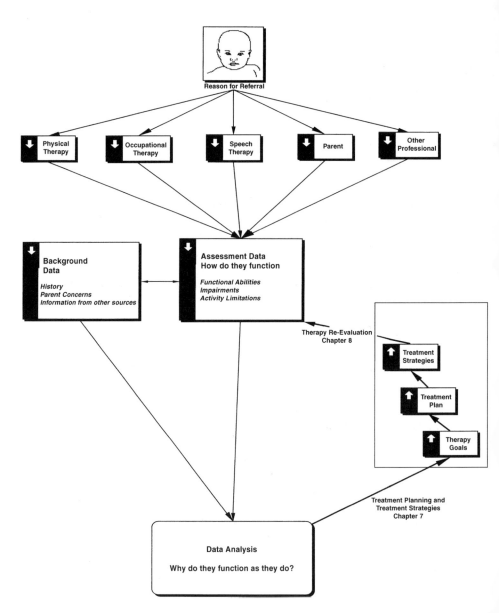

Figure 3 Multidisciplinary assessment.

iors that have something in common (10). The main performance areas for each discipline are:

Physical therapy—gross motor functions, gait, activities of daily living and equipment

Occupational therapy—reaching and upper extremity supporting abilities, hand function, play behaviors, and activities of daily living

Speech therapy—communication, oral motor/feeding, respiratory, and phonatory skills.

In the process of collecting the assessment data, each therapist should note the strengths of the infant and the family. The infant's responses to handling, as well as their behavior and interactional style, are also observed. Parent input should continue to be solicited throughout the assessment for clarification of the infant's responses.

Within the performance areas, each therapist observes the infant's spontaneous movements, motor and behavioral responses in different environmental contexts, and the ability to organize and perform structured tasks. Observation of spontaneous movements allows the therapist to assess the infant's ability to adjust posture and alignment relative to a specific motor activity or functional task. By altering the environmental context, the therapist is able to determine whether the infant can adapt behavior and motor performance in novel situations. The use of structured tasks allows the therapist to determine whether the infant can produce the appropriate movement patterns to perform expected activities that are not spontaneously observed.

We have just defined and discussed two of the major information-gathering sections of this arena assessment model. The next section of this chapter focuses more specifically on what to assess in each of the major organ systems to assist in determining *why* the infant moves or behaves in a particular manner. Therapists from each discipline may look at the various organ systems with a somewhat different emphasis or in greater detail; however, each organ system must be assessed by each of the disciplines to insure that no interfering variables are overlooked.

IV. OVERVIEW OF THE SYSTEMS TO ASSESS

As we look at the discipline-specific performance areas, each therapist assesses contributing factors from the various systems. These systems are looked at from the unique perspective of each discipline and with regard to how they affect discipline-related functions (Fig. 4). Common systems to consider include: regu-

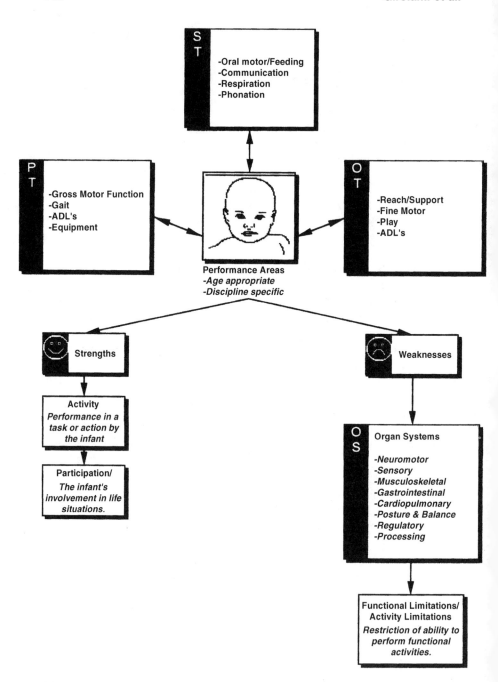

Figure 4   The assessment process.

latory system; sensory processing system; neuromuscular system; musculoskeletal system; cardiopulmonary system; and gastrointestinal system.

A. Regulatory

Therapists evaluating the infant, must all be keenly aware of the regulatory system and its impact on every area of development. Degangi and Greenspan (11) refer to self-regulation as the internal capacity to tolerate sensory stimulation from individuals, as well as from the environment. It involves the capability to modulate the intensity of arousal experienced while remaining engaged in the interaction/activity. The infant has an evolving capacity to self-regulate.

Als and colleagues are well known for their research concerning regulatory function in the infant. Als' synactive theory outlines five subsystems of an organism that are continuously interactive and interdependent in terms of behavioral organization. One of these subsystems is regulation, and it is critical to behavioral organization in the infant (12).

Regulation is the ability to maintain and regain well-modulated subsystem balance. This includes behaviors that the infant uses and the facilitation that the infant requires from the environment to achieve and sustain this balance (12). The baby uses the other four subsystems (sensorimotor, autonomic, and state and attention) to communicate both self-regulation and disorganization.

Regulatory dysfunction is the presence of persistent symptoms that interfere with adaptive functioning (i.e., sleep, feeding, arousal, mood, and transitions). Parental insights relative to their infant's regulatory abilities during daily activities are valuable to the therapist in determining the most significant concerns interfering with function. Some of the typical areas to observe or inquire about include:

Sleep patterns and routines

Presence of feeding issues

Calming/coping strategies used by parents (e.g., rocking, visual distraction, etc.)

Infant's ability to self-calm using a variety of sensory strategies (e.g., hand to mouth, visual and auditory attending, etc.)

Infant's ability to handle movement transitions and position changes during activities of daily living (e.g., feeding, bathing, etc.)

Infant's physiological responses to movement and handling as an indicator of state organization

Infant's ability to attend to and process sensory input for play, transitions, imitative behaviors, vocalizations, gross and fine motor movements, etc.

Assessment of the level of stimuli needed to elicit and sustain infant arousal

Visual engagement and attention to objects and to people
Any regulatory concerns affecting possibilities in other performance areas.

B. Sensory Processing

Sensory processing is defined as the ability to receive, register, and organize sensory input for use in generating the body's adaptive responses to human and object interactions and to the surrounding environment (12–14). Sensory processing is the umbrella that encompasses the sensory systems. It includes the awareness of and the ability to orient to sensory information, as well as integrating combinations of multisensory input for functional behavior.

When we assess sensory processing in the infant, we observe our discipline-specific performance areas, keeping in mind the impact of the five primary sensory systems: tactile/somatosensory, proprioceptive, vestibular, visual, and auditory. The ability to use these systems to process information provides body-oriented perception and has critical importance in the developing sense of self (14–17). The sensory systems contribute to the planning and execution of purposeful goal-directed movements. They are used to guide, modify, and adapt movements to achieve desired outcome (15). In addition, these sensory systems are important in early self-regulation and in the development of caregiver attachment (16). Sensory processing is evidenced in the infant's movement, play, and daily living and interaction skills.

When assessing sensory processing, illnesses, tiredness, hunger, medications, teething, and other unusual, transient conditions that may be contributing to an atypical response should be ruled out. Parent input is vital to the sensory-processing assessment. They provide perspective on usual behaviors or concerns experienced outside the evaluation setting. Also, it is often necessary to observe an infant over time to discern the magnitude of the suspected areas of sensory-processing concerns.

Infants with cerebral palsy often have sensory-processing impairments that impact on their ability to effectively utilize incoming sensory input. It is important for therapists of all disciplines to assess the sensory subsystems to determine how they might impact on the infant's ability to function in their environment. What follows are brief descriptions of each of the sensory subsystems.

1. Tactile/Somatosensory

The sense of touch is believed to be the most mature sensory system at birth. Receptor sites are primarily located in the skin. Touch has an important role in balancing social–emotional security, protective versus discriminative input, and central nervous system organization (18). Some of the typical areas to observe or inquire about are included in Table 1.

2. Proprioceptive

This system provides information about the orientation of our body parts, our movement, and where our bodies are in relation to gravity. It provides information regarding force, timing, and speed of muscle contraction and movement. Receptor sites are in the muscle spindles, ligaments, tendons, and joints (14,17). Some of the typical areas to observe or inquire about are included in Table 1.

3. Vestibular

The vestibular system is considered the first sensory system to develop in utero and is fully myelinated by 27 to 29 weeks gestation (19). Although the vestibular system begins to develop early, it becomes mature during the first couple years and actually continues to mature through early adolescence (18). The receptor sites of the vestibular system are the semicircular canals and the utricle located in the inner ear. The vestibular system registers speed, force, and direction of head movement. It contributes to muscle tone, reflex maturation, balance, ocularmotor, attention, and emotional state.

Together, the proprioceptive and vestibular systems coordinate body movement in response to the earth's gravitational pull (16). With somatosensory input, these systems plays a vital role in creating the accurate body image needed to guide the infant's orientation to perform a task (11,18). Observations that relate to the infant's ability to process vestibular information are included in Table 1.

4. Visual

The visual system develops later than the three sensory systems just described (20). It is considered the window to the brain. Unlike the other systems, vision is a distant receptor that allows increased reaction time (21). Structural development of rods (light perception) and cones (acuity) begins in utero during the 25th gestational week, but oculomotor skills are not fully functional until the sixth month of life (20).

Visual motor and visual perceptual skills become more apparent during the sixth to twelfth month and can be assessed during play behaviors with objects/toys or people (i.e., pointing, in/out container play, discriminating between foods, object permanence, cause–effect, etc.). Some of the typical areas to observe or inquire about are included in Table 1.

5. Auditory

The auditory system consists of hearing, speech and language, responses to environmental sounds, and the infant's ability to perceive speech and follow direc-

Table 1 Sensory Processing

Tactile	Proprioceptive	Vestibular	Visual	Auditory
Does the infant tolerate and/or enjoy handling, dressing, and bathing?	Does the infant tolerate movement and position changes?	Is there comfort with and enjoyment of supported movement in all planes and with varying speeds?	Is the head and trunk control adequate to support use of vision?	Does the infant alert to variation in the pitch, tone, and rhythm of speech?
Can touch be used as a means of comforting?	Does the infant exhibit age-expected gross motor skills and independence in transitional movements?	Does the infant tolerate imposed weight shift?	Is oculomotor control age appropriate in all positions expected for the infant's age including:	Can the infant tolerate progressing from a quiet, monotone voice to a louder, enthusiastic voice?
	Do they demonstrate a variety of movement strategies?		The ability to use the eyes to fixate, localize and track objects in all fields?	
	Can the infant modulate sensory input from other sensory systems?		Use eyes together? Dissociate eyes from head? (4–6 mos.)	
Is the infant able to tolerate and accommodate to contact with various surfaces?	Are righting and equilibrium reactions present?	Does the infant react to weight shift with appropriate protective or balance reactions?	Can the infant attend to visual stimulation age appropriately?	How does the infant respond to different types of music?
Is there approach or avoidance exploration when different textured objects or toys are presented?	Does the infant exhibit appropriate anticipatory responses to changes in position?	Does the infant initiate movement with their ability?	Is there any hyperresponsiveness to visual stimulation such as tuning out, becoming irritable, overting eyes from stimulus, excessive widening of eyes, upon presentation of stimuli?	Does the infant demonstrate attention to people through Changes in affect, vocalization, or motor patterns Gestures Signs, words, or symbols?

Is there appropriate mouthing of toys, objects, hands, and feet?	Is their body play and body image appropriate for their age or motor development?	Are head righting responses appropriate?	Is there hyporesponsiveness to visual stimulation such as no reaction, no movement toward, or attention for the visual input?	Does the infant demonstrate attention to activity through Changes in affect, vocalization, or motor patterns? Gestures? Signs, words, or symbols?
Does the infant engage in body exploration (i.e., hand to mouth, hands to feet, hands together, hands to chest)?	Can they initiate, plan, and sequence body movements within the limits of their motor control?	Are balance and equilibrium responses present?	Does the infant visually engage with people?	
Are the reflexes (i.e., rooting, finger, and plantar grasps) caused by tactile input appropriate?	Can they imitate basic motor movements consistent with their developmental age?	Can a nystagmus response from rotary movement be elicited?		
Does the infant conform to being held or cuddled?	Does the infant demonstrate the ability to grade weight bearing through his extremities?	Can vestibular input be used for comforting, such as rocking, bouncing, and walking?		
Is there appropriate use of the infant's hands to explore objects?	Can they adapt their body posture to novel situations? Is excessive practice necessary?			

tions (22). The auditory system detects aspects of sound and provides the brain with information regarding frequency, intensity, and spatial location of sound (23). Some infants with cerebral palsy may have hypo- or hyperresponses to auditory stimuli. Some of the typical areas to observe or inquire about are included in Table 1.

Additional inquiries regarding sensory processing that is *not* specific to any one sensory system (and not included on Table 1) are:

1. Has the infant been exposed to unusual or negative sensory experiences that may affect behavior, but are not true sensory processing impairment?
2. Do motor abilities/concerns affect sensory processing?
3. Does sensory processing impact on motor performance?
4. Do the infant's sensory responses affect regulatory behaviors?
5. Does the regulatory system affect sensory experiences?
6. Do the infant's sensory responses affect interactions?
7. How often are any atypical responses elicited and under what circumstances?
8. How atypical is the response?
9. Can atypical responses be managed with specific structuring, environmental alterations, or handling by the therapist, parent, or other caregivers?

In summary, processing information from the five primary sensory systems (tactile, proprioceptive, vestibular, visual, and auditory) collectively contributes to the development of body scheme and the ability to organize and plan movement. It also impacts on regulatory and emotional development (16). In addition, the sensory feedback generated by the movements themselves permits adaptation of motor actions to changes in environmental and task demands. This, in turn, facilitates motor learning (24). Clearly, the importance of sensory issues transcends all disciplines and all should be assessed.

C. Musculoskeletal

Even though the pathophysiology occurs in the central nervous system, impairments may develop in the musculoskeletal system (25). Exaggerated stretch reflexes, muscle hypoextensibility, and insufficient force production are major impairments in the muscular system and can lead to abnormal postural alignment, range of motion restrictions, and eventual contractures and deformities in the skeletal system. All of these impairments can have a significant impact on postural control and neuromuscular function in children with cerebral palsy (26).

Spasticity is defined as hyperexcitability of the stretch reflex resulting in a velocity-dependent increase in muscle tone (27). Clinically, the term muscle tone is used to describe this resistance to passive movement associated with cerebral palsy. However, this is more correctly a combination of two impairments: spasticity and hypoextensibility (25).

Secondary to the brain lesion, there are also mechanical changes in the muscles of children with cerebral palsy. The muscles produce more force for a given change in length, and therefore feel stiff and resist passive lengthening. This is referred to as muscle hypoextensibility or stiffness (28).

Hypoextensibility makes it difficult for the infant to actively move through complete ranges of motion and interferes with postural control and function. In fact, the muscles of infants with cerebral palsy resist passive lengthening at shorter ranges than those of nondisabled children (28). Over time, this may compromise normal skeletal alignment, which may lead to muscle contractures and bony deformities.

Inability to produce sufficient muscle force is another muscular system impairment seen in children with cerebral palsy. It has been shown that maximal muscle force is lower in children with cerebral palsy and occurs earlier in the range, secondary to the hypoextensibility of the muscle (25). Another limiting factor that impacts on the capacity to produce power is the impaired facility to recruit an adequate number of motor units from the motor neuron pool (29).

Insufficient force production results in decreased ability to produce power during active contraction, for example, vertical jumping or push-off during gait. Reduced power is also associated with the inability to sustain adequate force production for a specific functional task. This is also known as muscle endurance.

The muscular system impairments described above can have a detrimental impact on the skeletal system. Therefore, it is important to obtain good baseline measurements of joint range of motion and to adequately assess how restrictions in normal muscle length may contribute to abnormal alignment in age-appropriate positions. Muscle shortening may be observed even in very young infants, and, if addressed early, may decrease the atypical impact on alignment and function.

Manual muscle testing may be used to obtain a baseline measurement of strength. There is, however, some doubt that muscle testing provides reliable results in children with neurological disorders. However, Damiano and colleagues (30) have had success using hand-held dynamometers to test muscle strength in children with cerebral palsy. They have been able to correlate the increase in strength with changes in gait parameters.

It is extremely important for the therapist to evaluate the musculoskeletal system to assess muscle tone and stiffness, and to document baseline strength and range-of-motion measurements. This information is useful in determining how restrictions and impairments in this system impact upon the infant's function.

Some questions to ask when assessing the musculoskeletal system follow.

1. Is the muscle tone altered? Too high? Too Low?
2. Are the muscles stiff and difficult to move passively?
3. Does the infant have range of motion restrictions?
4. Does the infant have any obvious or suspected contractures? Deformities?
5. Can the infant actively move through the expected range of motion when performing functional activities?
6. Does the infant have adequate muscle strength?
7. Does the infant have difficulty producing adequate force for functional activities?
8. Does the infant have difficulty sustaining adequate muscle activity for functional activities?
9. Is normal alignment compromised by range of motion, muscle tone, or strength issues?

D. Neuromuscular

Components of the neuromuscular system include timing and sequencing of muscle activity, agonist and antagonist muscle control, and grading of eccentric and concentric muscle activity. Through these neuromuscular functions, we are able to selectively control and regulate muscle activity, anticipate postural changes, and learn to execute unique movements (25).

The ability to selectively control movement is characterized by the capacity to sequence and time muscle activity. For example, electromyography has shown that in individuals with an intact central nervous system, there are specific sequences and timing of muscle activity for repetitive functional tasks (e.g., standing balance and gait) (31). In children with cerebral palsy, impaired neuromuscular control results in poor timing and sequencing, often accompanied by irradiation of muscle activity into antagonist muscle groups causing muscle coactivation and limiting the excursion of free movement (29).

The ability to anticipate and prepare for movement is necessary for transitions and to sustain balance (26). Nashner and colleagues (32) demonstrated that children with cerebral palsy have difficulty sequencing appropriate strategies for muscle activation during standing balance activities. The strategies selected were inefficient and very different from those used by nondisabled children. Their efficiency was also compromised by coactivation of antagonists, limiting available movement to produce adequate balance reactions.

This impaired neuromuscular control also interferes with the ability to learn new movement patterns and to adapt available movement patterns for novel tasks and different environmental contexts (33). Consequently, children with cerebral palsy seem to have movement patterns that are restricted in range, limited in variety, and stereotypical (34,35).

These neuromuscular impairments contribute to the poor motor control and subsequent postural issues seen in children with cerebral palsy. When assessing movement in various positions, it is not enough to describe how the child moves, but to hypothesize what neuromuscular impairments may be contributing to what is observed. By doing this the therapist can begin to apply more specific and innovative treatment strategies to reduce the impact of those impairments. As more information is learned about motor control, there is the potential to devise and implement more sophisticated technology, pharmacology, and handling strategies to alter the impaired movement patterns associated with cerebral palsy.

Some questions to ask when assessing the neuromuscular system follow:

1. Does the infant demonstrate a variety of movement patterns?
2. Can the infant selectively control individual limb movements?
3. Can the infant selectively control individual muscle groups?
4. Is the infant able to move limb segments without overflow of muscle activity into adjacent segments?
5. Does the infant have increased cocontraction during active movements?
6. Can the infant efficiently grade movements producing smooth, controlled eccentric and concentric muscle contractions?
7. Is the infant able to initiate, sustain, and terminate movement?
8. Can the infant control speed, timing, and sequencing according to task demands?

E. Cardiopulmonary

Infants with cerebral palsy often have impaired cardiopulmonary function particularly as it relates to physiological control and endurance. It is important for therapists in each discipline to be aware of potential impairments that may affect the performance areas they are assessing.

1. Physiological Control

The infant's physiological and autonomic responses to movement must be considered during the assessment process. Parameters such as heart rate, respiratory rate, and oxygen saturation, as well as autonomic and visceral indicators of stress, should be addressed (36).

Als (11) refers to these physiological changes as stress cues. If these stress cues are present during interactive or motor behaviors (e.g., eating), it may be an indication that the task is too difficult for the infant. Many of the common indicators of stress are: sighing; yawning; sneezing; sweating; hiccuping; trem-

oring; startling; gasping; straining; coughing; spitting up; gagging/choking; color
change; respiratory pauses; and irregular respirations.

2. Endurance

When the infant fatigues easily or has poor intake and poor weight gain, this can
be caused by decreased endurance. This results in a circular effect and the poor
intake and failure to gain weight contribute to greater impairments in endurance.
Some of the diagnoses associated with poor endurance include prematurity, bron-
chopulmonary dysplasia (BPD), congenital heart disease, diaphragmatic hernia,
or structural abnormalities like tracheal stenosis or Pierre-Robin malformation.

    The resultant clinical characteristic of impaired endurance is muscle weak-
ness and poor cardiovascular function, and yet, strengthening and aerobic conditioning are rarely advocated in treatment of cerebral palsy (37–39). With regard
to aerobic capacity, correlation studies document a 30 to 50% difference in sub-
maximal heart rate between children with cerebral palsy and their nondisabled
peers (39–41). Descriptive information about cerebral palsy is rich with observations describing the slow and labored movements necessary to complete simple
tasks (42,43).

    It is clear that impairments in the cardiopulmonary system can have a dev-
astating impact on the infant's ability to interact with the environment and to
perform functional tasks. A fragile cardiopulmonary system can limit an infant's
ability to perform; conversely, the system can become weak secondary to the
poor movement capabilities inherent in cerebral palsy.

    Some questions to ask when assessing the cardiopulmonary system follow:

1. Does the infant exhibit any stress cues during interactions with the
   examiner?
2. Does the infant exhibit any stress cues during handling or position
   changes?
3. How frequently are the stress cues observed and what are the antecedents?
4. Does the infant fatigue easily?
5. Can the infant sustain normal activity levels without cardiopulmonary
   compromise?
6. Does the infant have sufficient motor function to develop adequate
   endurance?

F. Gastrointestinal

Gastrointestinal (GI) problems are frequently seen in infants with cerebral palsy,
including motility disorders, gastroesophageal reflux (GER), peptic ulcer disease,

and constipation (44). These problems may appear as disorders of motor behavior. For example, increased arching observed following feeding could be a result of abdominal pain or reflex rather than overactivity of the back extensors. Therefore, a careful history is essential to determine whether abnormal movement patterns are influenced by impairments in the GI system.

This importance of assessing issues related to this system is often overlooked. However, GI impairments can have a significant effect on posture, movement, and infant behavior. Some questions to ask when assessing the gastrointestinal system follow:

1. Does the infant show abnormal extensor tone following feedings?
2. Does the infant frequently refuse feeding or take small amounts of food during feedings?
3. Is the infant extremely irritable following feedings?
4. Does the infant have excessive vomiting following meals?
5. Does the infant have excessive GI discomfort (e.g., gas or burping) during or following feedings?
6. Does the infant demonstrate gastric distention?
7. Does the infant dislike prone positioning?
8. Is the infant frequently constipated?

G. Postural Control and Balance

There are a variety of different system models that hypothesize how impairments in the various systems impact on postural control, an identified task, or a selected goal. Each of these system theories implies that the emphasis shifts among the contributing systems to produce the desired posture, task, or goal (45). This section emphasizes postural control as the primary outcome of a systems model.

Postural control is the ability to adjust the body's position in space for the purposes of orientation, stability, anticipatory control, and alignment (46). Contributions from all systems play a role in maintaining postural control. If any system is impaired, postural control may be compromised, and alternative, less efficient strategies will be developed.

Postural orientation is important in maintaining the appropriate relationship between body segments in a specific environment for a specific task. Input from the sensory system provides valuable information about the body in space and the environment. The neuromuscular and musculoskeletal systems synchronize the timing, force, and movements needed to successfully complete the task.

Postural stability or balance requires the infant to maintain the center of mass (COM) over the base of support (BOS). If balance cannot be maintained, and the COM is displaced outside the BOS, a variety of protective reactions can be used to prevent a fall. To maintain balance, the infant relies on vestibular, visual, tactile, and proprioceptive information, and the neuromuscular system must be intact to appropriately coordinate the selection of the most efficient muscles, as well as the timing and sequencing of the muscle activity. An intact musculoskeletal system insures adequate range of motion, muscle strength, and muscle tone to carry out the task in variety of environments.

Alignment contributes to both postural orientation and stability. It assists the infant in maintaining the most optimal posture with respect to gravity and the base of support. This permits the infant to use the input from various systems to maintain or alter posture dependent on the task and the environment. Children with cerebral palsy often have inefficient postural alignment (35). This can be a result of system impairments that interfere with reception or processing of information or ability to activate and sustain muscle activity and selectively control movement. Abnormal alignment may lead to joint limitations and eventual deformities that will permanently compromise the infant's function.

Anticipatory postural control is the ability to modify the sensory and motor systems in response to changing task and environmental demands (46). Studies have shown that normal individuals preset their posture in anticipation of the task and not as a feedback response (47). Anticipatory control is dependent on previous experiences and learning. Children with cerebral palsy, who have impairments in the sensory and motor systems, may lack the opportunity to explore and learn from their experiences, and therefore initiate inefficient strategies for anticipatory control.

Postural control is required for every task we perform and is dependent on the interaction of the infant with the task and the environment (46). Research has shown that, in normal children, there are very definite sequences of muscle recruitment that are task and environment dependent (48). In children with cerebral palsy, alternative muscle sequences and timing are utilized, which are less efficient and interfere with postural control (49).

The therapist must observe the infant performing a variety of tasks within different environmental contexts to determine the integrity of the infant's postural control. It is also essential for the therapist to observe the infant performing age-appropriate tasks and moving about the environment. This insures a greater depth of understanding regarding how the infant uses and adapts his postural system for stability and balance.

Postural control is possible because of complex interactions among the all of the individual systems. Without postural control, the infant cannot efficiently and successfully function. Assessing the infant's ability to maintain and regain postural control forms the foundation of the discipline-specific performance areas.

V.   ASSESSMENT OF THE DISCIPLINE-SPECIFIC
PERFORMANCE AREAS

In the last section, information about each of the systems was presented, detailing how impairments may contribute to the abnormal postural control and functional limitations associated with cerebral palsy. In the following section, the assessment considerations related to the discipline-specific performance areas will be presented. The information in each discipline performance area details how impairments in each system should be assessed to determine the impact on the function of the infant.

As stated earlier in the chapter, standardized testing will not be specifically addressed. The purpose of this chapter is to provide a framework for assessment that will enable the therapist to develop treatment plans and intervention strategies aimed at optimizing the motor performance of infant's with cerebral palsy. However, there are many excellent test tools available that enable the therapist to evaluate gross, fine, and oral motor skills, as well as receptive and expressive language levels (3–6). In addition, there is an excellent overview of infant assessment tools in the third chapter of Pediatric Occupational Therapy and Early Intervention (50).

A.   Physical Therapy Assessment

Considering each of the systems discussed previously, the physical therapist assesses the infant in the following performance areas: gross motor functions; Gait; activities of daily living; and equipment. A list of questions that may assist you in assessing each of these performance areas can be found in Table 2.

1.   Gross Motor Functions

The physical therapist looks at age-appropriate gross motor functions to determine how the infant performs within varying environmental contexts. For each of the gross motor functions, the physical therapist must observe the infant's postural control and the ability to transition from one position to another. In addition, the influence of range of motion, skeletal alignment, reflexes, postural reactions, and cardiopulmonary function must also be considered.

To do this efficiently, the therapist should have an organized approach. Köng (51) recommends looking at the infant in eight positions: prone; supine; sidelying; pull to sit; sitting; horizontal suspension; vertical suspension; and standing.

Based on her experience evaluating and diagnosing infants with cerebral palsy, Köng has found these positions provide a comprehensive view of the in-

Table 2   Physical Therapy Assessment of the Infant

1. Gross Motor Functions
   a. Posture and Transitions
      Assess patterns of movement in functional positions with and without assisted postural support.
      For each age-appropriate position, observe and evaluate the following:
      • What are the parental concerns?
      • How would you characterize the infant's muscle tone at rest?
      • Do movements, sensory stimuli, or emotional responses alter muscle tone?
      • Does the infant tolerate handling and interaction with a stranger?
      • Does the infant tolerate being placed in various positions?
      • Is the base of support appropriate for the activity?
      • Can the infant achieve good postural alignment for the activity?
      • Does the infant have adequate postural control to initiate weight shifting in all planes?
      • Can the infant initiate a variety of spontaneous and selective movements?
      • Does the infant have strategies to sequence movement?
      • Is the infant able to appropriately time muscle activity?
      • Can the infant generate adequate speed and force necessary for the activity?
      • Can the infant grade agonist and antagonist control of muscle activity?
      • Can the infant transition into and out of positions?
      • Does the infant have adequate strength and endurance to initiate and sustain gross motor activity?
      • Can the infant perform fine motor or feeding tasks in these positions?
      • Can the infant process sensory stimuli for postural control and movement?
      • Does the infant have strategies for problem solving?
      • Does the infant demonstrate intact body awareness?
      • Are there regulatory issues that interfere with gross motor function?
      • How does posture and movement affect respiration and endurance?
      • Does the infant have any GI issues that may interfere with gross motor function and transitions?
   b. Range of Motion and Structural Alignment
      • Are there joint range limitations?
      • How do ROM limitations interfere with postural responses or gross motor function?
      • Are there skeletal abnormalities?
      • Do bony alignment abnormalities interfere with postural responses or function?
   c. Reflexes
      • Are reflexes obligatory for movement or function?
      • Do reflexes interfere with function?
      • Do reflexes cause asymmetries that interfere or compromise movement?

Table 2 Continued

   d. Postural Reactions
- Are head and trunk right reactions observed in transitions to and from supine, prone, and sidelying?
- Does the infant demonstrate age-appropriate protective responses: forward, sideways, and backward?
- Are vertical and horizontal suspension responses adequate for the infant's age?
- Does the infant use equilibrium reactions to maintain balance and postural alignment?

   e. Cardiopulmonary Status
- Does the infant have a normal resting heart rate?
- Is the recovery heart rate within normal limits?
- Is the infant's endurance adequate to sustain an activity for an extended period of time?
- Are there changes in respiration secondary to movement or effort?

2. Gait
- Assess the infant's ability to ambulate with and without support
- Assess arm swing, stride length, and phases of gait
- Assess distance and speed
- Assess gait on different surfaces and ability to stop and change directions.

3. Activities of Daily Living
- Inquire about the infant's sleep patterns and daily routine?
- Inquire about feeding.
- What calming and coping strategies do the parents use?
- What calming and coping strategies does the infant use?
- Is the infant able to participate in activities of daily living: dressing, undressing, bathing, and diapering? (This may be obtained per parent report)
- Do impairments in any system interfere with performance or participation in ADLs?
- Assess positions used by the parents for carrying and sleeping.

4. Equipment
- Assess equipment used for positioning the infant.
- Assess day or night splinting used to maintain the infant's range of motion or alignment.

---

fant, allowing the examiner to correlate normal, atypical, and abnormal postural control among the positions. The importance is not in the position itself, but in knowing what the infant should be able to demonstrate in each position at any given age.

For the therapist, these same positions can be used to assess gross motor functions. However, this requires an intimate knowledge of normal motor development to determine whether the infant is able to perform the functions using age-appropriate components. Books on normal development are an excellent source of information, as well as videotapes and observation of normal infants (52–54).

(a) Postural Control and Transitions. The physical therapist assesses the infant's postural control, movement patterns, and ability to transition during the performance of age-appropriate gross motor functions. The therapist may place the child in a variety of positions or observe how the infant attains these positions independently. As part of this observation, the infant's muscle tone should be assessed and changes in tone related to movement, sensory stimuli, or emotional reactions should be noted.

The infant's alignment and weight bearing should be observed in each of the gross motor functions and during transitions and functional tasks. Weight-shifting capabilities in static postures, transitions, and during functional tasks are also assessed to determine whether the infant is able to move in all planes: frontal, sagittal, and transverse.

Selective motor control, the variety of available movements, and the infant's functional ability to perform functional tasks in each position are also observed. Neuromuscular control relative to timing, sequencing, and agonist/antagonist muscle activity should be assessed during spontaneous play and structured tasks. The infant's ability to generate adequate force production and sustain muscle activity should also be judged.

Transitions should also be observed, as the infant moves into and out of each position. Infant's with cerebral palsy may appear quite functional in one position, but be unable to independently move into other positions. It is important for the therapist to know what positions and transitions emerge at each age, and the postural and movement precursors required to support them.

The infant's response to sensory stimuli and its effect on gross motor function is another important observational area. This will provide insights concerning the infant's ability to process and use sensory input to plan, organize, and sequence movements for function. The therapist can use this information to hypothesize how sensory system impairments affect postural control and transitions.

(b) Range of Motion and Skeletal Alignment. Limitations in the musculoskeletal system can strongly impact movement and gross motor function. It is not uncommon for very young infants to have joint range limitations secondary to positioning or poor selective movement capabilities. When passive movement reveals joint restrictions, the physical therapist should assess and document joint range of motion, using a goniometer. This information should be reassessed frequently to insure that the interventions or positioning developed to prevent muscle shortening is effective.

Actual or potential skeletal abnormalities should also be assessed and noted. Insufficient muscle activity, asymmetries, or muscle weakness can all be contributing factors. The therapist has the potential to minimize the secondary effects of cerebral palsy when the infant is referred early. However, this requires critical observational skills, clinical reasoning, and creative intervention strategies.

(c) Reflexes. Reflexes are assessed to determine their impact on posture and movement. Generating a list of reflexes serves no purpose unless the therapist can determine whether the reflex activity interferes with function, causes asymmetries, or is simply appropriate for the infant's age. If the therapist observes redundant patterns that limit the variety of selective movement or interfere with function, this may be the influence of reflexes, but can also be related to sensory or neuromuscular impairments.

Knowledge of reflexes is important to the therapist if the information can be used to develop intervention strategies, which minimize or eliminate the negative effect of the reflex on movement or function. The goal is to provide the infant with the possibility to organize and perfect alternative movements that will produce more functional results.

(d) Postural Reactions. Testing and assessing the availability of righting, equilibrium, and protective reactions provides information regarding the infant's ability to align and orient the body in space, maintain the center of mass over the base of support, and prevent a fall when the center of mass moves outside the base of support. How the infant responds to the various stimuli used to elicit these responses can assist the therapist in identifying impairments in the sensory, neuromuscular, or musculoskeletal systems. This information may provide an insight into why an infant is having difficulty organizing and responding to intrinsic and extrinsic stimuli.

(e) Cardiopulmonary Status. Finally, the therapist should determine how gross motor function, transitions, and functional activities impact the infant's heart rate, endurance, and respiration. Decreased activity or prolonged hospitalization can have a detrimental effect on the cardiopulmonary system that may interfere with the infant's ability to initiate or sustain age-appropriate postures and functions. Conversely, compromised motor activity related to impairments in the musculoskeletal and neuromuscular systems can adversely affect status of the cardiopulmonary system. In either case, intervention strategies must be implemented to enhance the capacity of this system.

2. Gait

If the infant is walking, it is crucial for the therapist to assess gait. When looking at gait, the therapist assesses the same areas described in the section on postural control and transitions. Additionally, the therapist should assess gait parameters including arm swing, stride length, heelstrike, toe-off, and stance. There are many excellent resources available to assist the therapist in learning the normal gait parameters for infants and children (55,56).

3. Activities of Daily Living

This may technically be considered the domain of the occupational therapist, but it is also important for the physical therapist to determine how the infant participates or independently performs daily living skills. This will provide more in-depth insights concerning how impairments interfere with function. In addition, the information can be used to develop goals and intervention strategies that are directly associated with improved performance of relevant functional skills.

    The therapist should also inquire and observe how the infant is carried, dressed and handled by the family or caregiver. This knowledge will be helpful in working with the family to alter handling and positioning that may minimize neuromuscular, sensory, or musculoskeletal system impairments.

4. Equipment

The therapist should inquire about and, if possible, look at equipment used to position the infant to enhance function or to maintain optimal musculoskeletal alignment. Positioning is an important aspect of treatment intervention. Potential musculoskeletal contractures and deformities, as well as neuromuscular, sensory, and regulatory impairments can often be addressed through consistent positioning or changes in the environment.

B. Occupational Therapy Assessment

The occupational therapist assesses the performance areas of: reach and supporting abilities in the upper extremities; hand function; play behaviors; and activities of daily living.

    It is important for the therapist to have a comprehensive understanding of the developmental expectations in each performance area and how they interrelate. Assessment of the performance areas is based on impairments in each of the systems to determine how they interfere with upper extremity and fine motor function. A list of questions that may assist you in assessing each of these performance areas can be found in Table 3.

1. Reach and Upper Extremity Support

The occupational therapist looks at the infant's reach and supporting abilities in spontaneous play as well as during structured tasks. Postural control and sensory

Table 3 Occupational Therapy Assessment of the Infant

1. Reach and Supporting Abilities in the Upper Extremities
   - Are there parental concerns in this area?
   - In each position assessed, postural control adequate to support upper extremity functioning?
   - Are there joint range limitations in the upper extremity?
   - What reach patterns are used in each position? (If necessary to elicit reach, assistance in postural support is given in order to observe reach patterns available.)
   - Does the infant reach in a variety of planes (frontal, sagittal, transverse)?
   - Does infant use unilateral and bilateral approach as task demands?
   - Is the infant able to combine upper and lower arm movement patterns for functional reach, near and away from the body?
   - Are there preferences or asymmetries between right and left upper extremities?
   - Is there strength and endurance to initiate and sustain reach?
   - Is the infant's reach possible without the influence of grasp?
   - Can the infant support on upper extremities?
   - What is the quality of movement patterns throughout the upper extremity and body upper extremity supporting?
   - Is the infant able to weight bear and reach in a variety of planes as appropriate for age expectations?
   - What is the quality in movement patterns during upper extremity supporting?
   - Can the infant initiate placement, maintain the appropriate weight shift, and reach?
   - Is the infant able to adequately grade and control perceptual-motor aspects such as timing, speed, and the ability to orient to an object?
   - Is reach spontaneous upon presentation of stimuli?
   - Are there any sensory impairments (decreased awareness, poor registration, over reactivity to sensory input) contributing to upper extremity limitations?
   - Are play and interactional interests appropriate to support/motivate upper extremity function?
   - Does the infant appear to understand that the upper extremities, especially the hands, can affect the environment?
2. Fine Motor Function
   - Are there parental concerns in this area?
   - Is the infant's postural control and proximal upper extremity function adequate to support fine motor performance in all positions expected for their age?
   - Are regulatory abilities and sensory processing adequate to support fine motor development and opportunities?
   - What is the general appearance of the infant's hands?
   - Are there any joint range limitations in the infant's hands?
   - Are grasp, traction, and orienting reflexes appropriately integrated in the infant's hands?
   - Does the infant initiate a variety of grasps appropriate for their age?
   - Can the infant sustain a variety of grasps?

Table 3 Continued

- Are the thumbs active in various grasps and during spontaneous hand movements?
- What movement patterns are used during the different grasps?
- Can the infant release an object?
- What movement patterns are used in releasing an object?
- Does external support allow for higher level hand functioning?
- Is hand development symmetrical?
- Does the infant have a hand preference?
- Does the infant exhibit premanipulative skills such as: spontaneous movements in fingers and thumb, dissociated movements between fingers, dissociation of radial and ulnar sides of hands, and isolated finger use?
- Does the infant engage in bimanual fine motor ability as expected for his age?
- Is the infant's attention adequate for the fine motor task?
- Is the infant able to adequately grade and control perceptual-motor aspects such as timing, speed, and the ability to orient to an object?
- Does the infant exhibit adequate oculomotor control to support hand function?
- Does the infant display adequate eye–hand coordination?
- Can the infant combine hand function with reach?

3. Play
   - Is the infant motivated or interested in age-appropriate play?
   - Does the infant have adequate postural control to support expected play behaviors?
   - Does the infant have a variety of positions available to allow for independence and age-appropriate play experiences?
   - Are the infant's gross and fine motor abilities able to support expected play behaviors?
   - Are regulatory and sensory-processing abilities adequate to support play development?
   - Does the infant exhibit playfulness with objects and people?
   - Is the infant able to be entertained using a variety of objects?
   - Is the infant able to be entertained using social interaction with a variety of people?
   - What play schemes does the infant display with objects and people and are they age appropriate?
   - Is the infant independent in playing with regard to attention, intention, and problem solving?
   - How long is the infant able to entertain himself?

4. ADL
   - Do parents have any concerns in this area?
   - Does the infant tolerate or enjoy: feeding, dressing, bathing, diapering, and being carried?
   - Does the infant participate appropriately in: feeding, dressing, bathing, diapering, and being carried?
   - Are regulatory, sensory-processing, cardiopulmonary, gastrointestinal or postural control issues interfering with ADL performance?
   - Assess positions and routines used for: feeding, dressing, bathing, diapering, carrying, and sleeping.

processing provide the foundation for upper extremity function and hand skill development. In early development, the upper extremities are used to assist with postural stability and control (53,57). As the infant develops greater head and trunk control, arm function increases. The freedom to move the arms away from the head and trunk, as well as the quality of how this is done during both reaching and supporting activities, gradually improves with age.

In addition, the upper extremity is used to support partial body weight during transitional movements. Weight bearing, weight shifting, and reaching in the upper extremities also assist in the development of postural control as well as the development of scapula-humeral control necessary for reaching in space (53, 57).

Therefore, it is important to assess postural control as it relates to upper extremity skills in all functional positions. It is important to determine what the infant can do independently. When posture and balance are limited, providing external control may increase reaching and supporting abilities.

In the infant under 4 months of age, little voluntary reaching or transitional movements are present. However, prereaching behaviors should be assessed, and may include: (1) random, involuntary movement of the arms away and toward the body; (2) midline grasping of clothing, hand-to-hand play; (3) the ability to bring arms forward to support in prone on elbows; (4) the ability to push down against the surface with the upper extremities; and (5) the ability to initiate and sustain weight bear while lifting and turning the head.

By the time the infant is 4 months, head and trunk control are sufficient to allow initiation of voluntary swiping of objects. The occupational therapist assesses the spontaneity of arm placement, quality and functional use of reach and weight bearing in the upper extremity. This includes observation of movement patterns and range of motion in the spine, scapula, humerus, and lower arm. Reach is assessed for variety, symmetry, and planes of movement. These are continually related to alignment, weight bearing, and weight shifting in the body as a whole.

In addition to the motor components, other systems that may affect reach in the infant with cerebral palsy need to be considered, such as sensory processing and respiration. If oculomotor function, modulation of sensory stimuli, or body awareness is insufficient, then the infant's quality or ability to reach is also deficient. Similarly, if respiration is compromised, the infant often uses shoulder elevation to assist in breathing, thus limiting the arm's availability for reach experiences. Table 3 summarizes questions for assessing upper extremity functioning from perspectives of all systems.

2. Hand Function

Two responsibilities of the hand are the sensorimotor exploration of objects and the perceptual gathering of information. In its most obvious role, the hand provides infinite sensorimotor capabilities. The hand allows for simple motor patterns using power, precision, and coordination, as well as very complex combinations of in-hand manipulations and use of tools. The hand also affords a wealth of perceptual information about size, shape, contour, weight, density, texture, and temperature, all of which dramatically contribute to our environmental understanding and learning. There are many important contributing factors to the development of hand function in the child such as postural control, proximal upper extremity control, sensory functioning, cognition, and intention (58).

Proximal and distal upper extremity control develops almost simultaneously (59). However, hand skills are dependent on proximal control for both stability and mobility to allow placement of the hand for interaction with the environment, toys, and self (58). Forearm and wrist control are also important to orient the hand in space. This allows the optimal hand position and stability for prehension. Therefore, assessment of postural and proximal control, including the forearm and wrist, are necessary in evaluating fine motor function.

Hand function typically includes the use of voluntary grasp, release, and manipulation, which does not occur before 4 months. However, in the birth to 3-month-old infant, the occupational therapist observes pregrasp components that are important to later hand function (52). These include: (1) general appearance of the hands (relaxed, fisted, in-dwelling thumb); (2) emergence and integration of grasp and traction reflexes; (3) orienting and opening responses to touch; (4) spontaneous opening and closing of fingers and thumbs; (5) visual and tactile awareness to hands observed through hand-to-hand contact, hand-to-mouth contact, and opportunities for eyes to visualize the hands.

As the infant continues to gain early postural control in prone and supine positions, freedom of the fingers from fisting, early scratching, hands more often open with early reach and support are expected. By 5 to 6 months, grasp patterns can then be assessed from a developmental perspective looking at motor, perceptual, sensory, and play aspects while presenting objects of different sizes and in different orientations. These basic prehension patterns are interdependent upon sensory processing, cognitive intent, and play development, laying the foundation for manipulative functions of the infant's hand.

The infant is observed for abilities to both sustain a placed grasp and to initiate a variety of age-expected prehension patterns (57,60). The grasp of the infant is observed in combination with reaching and in various positions. As with reach, symmetry, strength, and selective motor control are assessed. Both unilateral and bilateral tasks are observed.

Adequate sensory registration and processing are necessary for optimal hand functioning (17,57,58). In particular, tactile, oculomotor development, and attention should be specifically noted (61). Sensory and perceptual aspects of grading, timing, orientation, and accommodation are also important to assess.

Table 3 summarizes questions for assessing fine motor functioning from perspective of all systems.

3. Play

Play is considered one of the primary roles of the child (62). It is the central focal point for learning about and interacting in the world. There is much information on perspectives, philosophies, scales, and play-based assessment tools in the literature (62). In the infant with cerebral palsy, motor control, schemes, and interactional behaviors are important components in assessing play.

Motor aspects include the postural control and the gross and fine motor skills necessary to support play experiences and development. Play schemes and behaviors assess what and how the infant explores and interacts with objects and people, for example, mouthing, clapping, poking, etc. It is important that the infant be able to play independently as well as engage in interactions with people. Infants with cerebral palsy have sensory and motor limitations that often decrease the opportunities for play development. Through play, the infant learns to problem solve and practices organizational and sequencing strategies. Table 3 summarizes questions for assessing play in the infant with cerebral palsy.

4. Activities of Daily Living (ADLs)

Activities of daily living are primarily assessed from the care-taking perspective. Interviewing the parents offers insights into areas of concern regarding dressing, bathing, handling, sleeping, and position tolerance. By 4 to 5 months, the typical infant is tolerating and even enjoying daily living tasks. In the 6- to 12-month old infant, increased participation in daily routines is present. Activities of daily living encompass sensory and motor experiences, self-regulatory functioning, and play development. Table 3 summarizes questions for assessing ADLs in the infant 0 to 12 months.

D. Discipline-Specific Speech Therapy Assessment

An infant's ability to get adequate nutrients required for normal growth and development is dependent on both physiological and environmental processes. The oral–motor ability to prepare a food bolus and swallow with coordination of the respiratory pattern is essential for feeding and speaking. This section will provide a comprehensive look at the interdisciplinary assessment of the infant for oral motor/feeding, respiration, phonation, and communication. Keep in mind that the speech therapist is looking at the discipline-specific performance areas with reference to posture and movement and how impairments in the various systems impact on function. A list of questions that may assist you in assessing each of the performance areas can be found in Table 4.

Speech therapy assesses the performance areas of: oral motor/feeding function; respiratory function; phonatory function; and communication function (receptive and expressive).

1. Oral Motor/Feeding

The clinical history of the infant will often characterize the type of feeding/oral motor problem that an infant manifests. The causes of feeding and respiratory disorders in infants are numerous. The feeding history needs to be taken in the context of each child's general health, developmental status, and environment. A complete history includes the type of feeding mode, diet, supplements, length of time of feedings, and amount of food being ingested. How the infant reacts to changes in movement, texture, temperature, and taste continue to influence the sensory and regulatory functions of the infant.

Posture and movement control in the head and trunk are the foundation for oral motor function and speech development. Dissociation of the head from shoulders and trunk from legs can determine the level of fine oral motor control the child may achieve. The ability to dissociate the jaw, tongue, and lips and coordinate it with respiration are strongly associated with the oral motor function the infant will develop in feeding. For example, if an infant does not have adequate postural control to clear the airway, oral feeding would be inappropriate.

During the clinical oral motor examination, the therapist must have a thorough understanding of the infant feeding mechanism. Determinations of the symmetry, structure, and patterns of oral motor function must be made. The speech therapist must ascertain whether the oral motor patterns are developmentally, transitionally, or abnormally present in the infant. Figure 5 is a feeding assessment form.

2. Respiratory Control

With regard to the cardiopulmonary system, the speech therapist focuses on respiration. Respiration is defined as the exchange of oxygen and carbon dioxide between the atmosphere and the cells of the body through the process of inhalation (inspiration) and exhalation (expiration) (52). All of the systems impact on the respiratory function of the infant. It is necessary to assess the structure, movement patterns, and coordination of the respiratory mechanism. The therapist should assess the infant in the most stable and functional position for respiratory control.

3. Phonatory Function

The ability to generate a voiced sound is a very complex area to assess. The speech therapist evaluates the infant's ability to vocalize and subsequently use

Table 4 Speech Therapy Assessment of the Infant

---

1. Oral Motor Function
   a. History
      - How is the infant fed? (NGT, GT, Oral(PO))
      - What is the infant fed?
      - Are there any supplemental feedings?
      - How long does it take for one feeding?
      - What is the quantity of liquids in a 24-h period?
      - Are the infant's nutrients being met?
      - What is the frequency of feedings?
      - How is the infant held for feeding?
      - Is there any distress on liquids?
      - Is there any distress on solids?
      - Are they using any special feeding techniques?
      - Are you using any special utensils/nipples for feeding?
      - Is the infant being fed at the age-appropriate level? (bottle, cup, spoon, finger food, etc.)
      - Is the child able to control oral secretions?
      - Has the child a history of respiratory disorders?
      - Does the child have other signs of distress?
      - Does the child have a past medical or surgical history?
      - Does the child have gastrointestinal or motility problems (vomiting, gastrointestinal reflux-GER, abdominal pain, constipation, failure to thrive)?
   b. Clinical Examination
      - Are there sensory or regulatory issues contributing to oral motor functions (see Table 2)?
      - Is there a presence or absence of the oral reflexes (rooting, sucking, etc.)?
      - What is the infant's reaction to touch in the oral area?
      - How does the infant react to changes in texture, temperature, and taste of food?
      - How does the infant react to soft toys around the mouth?
      - Is the infant's postural control adequate to support respiratory function?
      - How does the face look (symmetry, structure, tone, movement patterns)?
      - How do the lips look (symmetry, structure, tone, movement patterns)?
      - How does the mandible look (symmetry, occlusion, teeth, movement patterns)?
      - How does the tongue look (symmetry, structure, tone, movement patterns)?
      - How does the maxilla and palate look (symmetry, structure, tone, movement patterns)?
      - What does the sucking pattern look like (strength, suction, compression, coordination)?
      - What does the swallowing pattern look like (pattern, noisy, gulping, rhythm, etc.)?
      - What does the chewing pattern look like (movement, type, dissociation)?

Table 4 Continued

- How does the infant coordinate the suck/swallow/breathe function? And what impact does the infant's position have on this function?
- Does the infant have the ability to bring their hand to mouth and react?
- Is jaw clonus, grimacing, and/or drooling present?

2. Respiratory Function
   - Are there sensory or regulatory issues contributing to respiratory functions (Table 2)?
   - Is the infant's postural control adequate to support respiratory function?
   - What type of breathing pattern do you see (diaphragm vs. abdominal)?
   - What is the general appearance of the rib cage (sternal retraction, bulge at rectus, rib flaring)?
   - Is their rib cage movement?
   - Is their lower rib expansion?
   - Is their belly expansion?
   - What happens with respiration when there are changes in position?

3. Phonatory Function
   - Are there sensory or regulatory issues contributing to phonatory function?
   - Is the infant's postural control adequate to support respiratory function?
   - Is the infant's speech intelligible?
   - What is the rate of speech (timing)?
   - What is the voice quality (breathy, shrill, hypernasal, gurgly, weak, hyponasal)?
   - Is there nasal emission during speech?
   - What is the pitch (high, low, normal)?
   - What is the volume (normal, weak, overloud)?

4. Communication Function (receptive and expressive)
   - Are there sensory or regulatory issues contributing to phonatory function?
   - Is the infant's postural control adequate to support respiratory function?
   - What level of expressive language is the infant exhibiting (cooing, babbling, jargon, single words, etc.)?
   - What is the infant's level of play?
   - What level of receptive skills does the infant demonstrate with people and objects (auditory awareness, following directions, etc.)?
   - What is the mean length of vocal response in different positions and with active movement (verbal and nonverbal)?

(a)

Clinical Feeding Evaluation

Name:	Date of Evaluation:
Address:	Birthdate:
	Chronological age:
Telephone:	Birth weight:
Parents Names:	
Diagnosis:	Physician:

Recheck
CA:
CA:

Current Status: Comments:

0 = within normal limits
1 = concern
2 = abnormal

Feeding Mode: ☐ ngt ☐ gt ☐ oral				
Diet: Texture: ☐liquid ☐strained ☐semi-solid ☐ solid				
Supplements: ☐formula ☐additives ☐vitamins				
Feeding: Duration: ☐20 min ☐30-40 min ☐More than 45 min				
Quantity of liquids: (24 hour day)				
Quantity of food: (24 hour day)				
Frequency: Intervals ☐2 hours ☐3 hours ☐4 hours ☐Other				
Distress/liquids: ☐gag ☐cough ☐choke				
Distress/solids: ☐gag ☐cough ☐choke				
Special feeding techniques:				
Special utensils/nipples:				
Position: ☐Cradled in arms ☐Upright in arms ☐Upright in chair ☐Special seating				
Control of oral secretions: ☐drooling ☐congestion ☐coughing on secretions				
Respiratory disorder: ☐ Oxygen ☐ Aspiration or pneumonia ☐ BPD ☐ Bronchitis or chronic upper respiratory infection ☐ Allergies or asthma ☐ Noisy breathing: ☐ with feeds ☐ Apart from feeds ☐ Gurgly voice quality: ☐during feeds ☐ After feeds ☐ Coughing or choking: ☐ during feeds ☐After feeds ☐ Trouble breathing during feeds				
Other signs of distress: ☐ Fussing during feeding ☐ Head turning to avoid feeding ☐ Falling asleep during feeding ☐ Cyanosis ☐ Postural changes: ☐ stiffening ☐ Hyperextending				
Regurgitation: ☐vomiting ☐nasal regurgitation				
Other Factors: ☐Past medical/surgical history:☐Upper GI				

Figure 5 Clinical feeding evaluation.

(b)

Name:

Clinical Examination	Comments		0 = within normal limits 1 = concern 2 = abnormal	
Face:				
Lips & Cheeks:				
Mandible:				
Tongue:				
Maxilla & Palate:				
Thorax:				
Muscle tone and movement patterns:	☐ Tone normal ☐ Hypertonicity ☐ Hypotonicity ☐ Variable Proximal stability: ☐Adequate ☐ Deficient Distal stability: ☐Adequate ☐ Deficient			

Sucking:	Non-nutritive			Nutritive				
Strength	Strong☐	Moderate☐	Weak ☐	Strong☐	Moderate☐	Weak☐		
Suction	Yes ☐	No ☐		Yes ☐	No ☐			
Compression	Yes ☐	No ☐		Yes ☐	No ☐			
Coordinated	Yes ☐	No ☐		Yes ☐	No ☐			
Breaks in suction	Yes ☐	No ☐		Yes ☐	No ☐			
Initiates suck	Yes ☐	No ☐		Yes ☐	No ☐			
Loss of liquid	Yes ☐	No ☐		Yes ☐	No ☐			
Rhythmic	Yes ☐	No ☐		Yes ☐	No ☐			
COMMENTS:								

Swallowing:	☐ normal ☐ doesn't manage secretions ☐ multiple swallows ☐ noisy breathing (when?)	☐ history of respiratory infections ☐ gulping Comments:			
Respiratory Quality:	☐ normal ☐ increased respiratory effort ☐ apnea ☐ periodic breathing ☐ wheezing	☐ stridor ☐ Chest retraction Comments:			
Communication	☐ Nonverbal ☐ Verbal ☐ Intelligible ☐ Babbles ☐ Vowel vocalizations only ☐ Consonants ☐ Voice Quality normal ☐ Abnormal ☐ Breathy ☐ Shrill ☐ Hypernasal ☐ Gurgly ☐ Weak ☐ Hyponasal ☐ Pitch normal ☐ High ☐ Low ☐ Volume normal ☐ Weak ☐ Overloud Comments:				

Figure 5 Continued.

(c)

Name:

Stage of Infant vocalization	☐Phonation (cry suckling sounds, nasal) 0-1 mos. ☐Cooing (sounds with velar and uvular movements back, throaty sounds, Cooing and laughter emerge) 2-3 mos. /ah/ /uh/ ☐Expansion (Variations in pitch, volume, breath control, and place of articulation. Emergence of squealing, yelling, growling, prolonged vocalizations. 4-6 mos. /o/ /oo/ /m/ b/ /h/ ☐Reduplicated Babbling (strings of identical syllables) 6-10 mos. ☐Variegated Babbling (Each successive syllable sequenced in utterance is not identical to the other syllables) 11-12 mos. ☐Jargon (Contains fully stressed and reduced stress syllables within one utterance.) 12 mos.
Stage of Dysarthria	☐I. Normal (functioning WNL) ☐II. Mild Dysphagia (nourished with special dietary/medical management) ☐III. Moderate Dysphagia (nourished with dietary management and adaptive strategies) ☐IV. Severe Dysphagia (inadequate nourishment and/or airway protection in spite of management.) ☐ V. Profound Dysphagia (non-oral feeding is required)
Summary:	
Recommendations:	

_____
Speech- Language Pathologist

Figure 5   Continued.

it functionally for communication. The therapist assesses the type, rate, and quality of the infant's vocalization to determine whether it is normal, abnormal, or delayed. There are multiple systems affecting the infant's skills in this area (e.g., neuromuscular, language processing, sensory processing). The speech therapist must keep these systems in mind to effectively evaluate and plan for treatment in this area.

4. Communication Function

Communication involves generating an idea or a thought that needs to be transmitted, initiating it, receiving a message, and understanding it. The infant with cerebral palsy may have limited communication abilities secondary to motor, vision, and/or hearing impairments. A complete speech, language and hearing evaluation should be done with children exhibiting impairments in any of these areas. The speech therapist's job during the interdisciplinary assessment is to determine the impact of the infant's impairments on their communication skills. In the infant, some of the areas to be considered are their level of play, receptive and expressive, and language functioning. An excellent scale for measuring the infant's communication and interaction is The Rossetti Infant-Toddler Language Scale (63).

VI. ANALYZING THE DISCIPLINE-SPECIFIC ASSESSMENT DATA

During the interdisciplinary assessment, therapists gather discipline specific assessment data. Together, they combine their clinical reasoning skills to analyze the data and determine which impairments are hindering the infant's functional development. Sound clinical reasoning incorporates the knowledge, experience, judgment, problem solving, and decision making of the practitioners (64). Working together improves the potential to accurately determine which systems are causing those impairments.

In this analysis process, the therapists look first at *how* the infant is moving and interacting. Each therapist will be observing different functional positions or tasks. This requires critical observation skills and it may be helpful to ask some of the following questions:

1. How atypical is the response?
2. How often is the atypical or abnormal response elicited and under what circumstances or conditions?
3. What is going on in other areas of development that may be influencing this behavior?
4. How does the atypical or abnormal movement affect function?
5. Can the responses be managed with specific structuring, environment alterations, or handling by parent, therapist, or caregiver?

Next, and most importantly, the therapists determine what impairments may be causing the abnormal movement patterns and behaviors observed. This is the process of analyzing *why* the impairments may be occurring and which systems are involved. This is a critical process and care must be taken to carefully analyze the possible contributions from each of the systems previously discussed. Working together, the members of the assessment team can share their discipline-specific knowledge and clinical reasoning and experience to insure that each of the systems is thoroughly investigated and the most significant impairments are exposed.

Table 5 is one example of how this information can be organized to assist the therapist in analyzing the assessment data for the eventual development of goals and treatment strategies. In the top half of the table, space is provided to input demographic and diagnostic information. There is an area to note the strengths of the infant and the family. These can often be utilized to enhance treatment strategies and outcomes.

The middle section of the table has three columns. In the left column, Observation of Performance Areas, space is provided to list descriptions of *how* the infant moves. For example, if a 7-month-old infant is placed in a sitting position, the therapist may observe excessive spinal extension, causing the infant to arch backward. While this is a very obvious observation, there may be a number of impairments that cause this motor behavior.

In the next column, Impairments, the therapist must ask *why* the infant may be moving or behaving in a particular way. This may be the most difficult part of the assessment process, requiring the therapist to generate hypotheses regarding all of the possible organ systems that may be contributing to the impairments observed. Table 1 provides a list of the common organ systems to consider. Related to the example above, these may be some of the possible impairments that cause the infant to arch backward.

1. Increased muscle tone in the head, trunk, and extremities—a neuro-muscular system impairment.
2. Inadequate balance of trunk extensors and abdominal—a neuromuscular system impairment.
3. Decreased ability to maintain a sufficient airway without adequate balance of neck extensors and flexor muscles—a respiratory system impairment.
4. Decreased ability to process multisensory input and extends as part of a stress response—a sensory or regulatory system impairment.
5. Feeding or reflux problems that are relieved by extending the neck and back—a respiratory or gastrointestinal system impairment.

Any or all of these impairments may contribute to *why* the infant is arching backward. The clinical experience of the therapist plays a crucial role in his or her ability to select the correct impairments, prioritize them, and develop specific intervention strategies to address each one.

Finally, based on the observations and hypothesized impairments, the therapist makes a list of *what* age-appropriate functions have not yet emerged. This

Table 5 Assessment Worksheet

CHILD:	DATE:
BIRTHDATE:	CHRONOLOGICAL AGE:
DIAGNOSIS:	ADJUSTED AGE:

Strengths (Included in this list are any motor, cognitive, communication, behavioral, attitudinal and/or family-related strength which will assist the child achieve his or her functional goals.)

Organ Systems to access impairments of body structure and function.

Musculoskeletal	Posture & Balance
Sensory	Neuromuscular
Gastrointestinal	Regulatory
Cardiopulmonary	Processing

Observations	Impairments	Functional Limitations/Activity
Description of motor movement and patterns. (How they do it?)	*Loss or abnormality of body structures or physio-logical body function. (Organ Systems)* (Why are they doing it?)	*Restriction of ability to perform functional activities. Secondary to impairments in body structure or function.* (What they can't do?) *Relate the impairments to discipline-specific functional limitations. This will assist you in keeping treatment directed toward function.*

Disability/Participation: *(Restricted participation in typical societal roles.)*

Societal Limitations/Contextual Factors: *(Barriers to full participation imposed by societal attitudes, architectural barriers, social policies, and other external factors.)*

information is placed in the final column, Functional/Activity Limitations. In the example of the 7-month-old infant, the backward arching may interfere with a variety of functional activities including sitting independently, using both hands to play with a toy, or babbling. Working as a team, the therapists and the family can better analyze the most significant contributing factors influencing the behaviors observed. Their collaboration enhances the identification of the impairments that contribute to the functional/activity limitations and allows the team to hypothesize potential disabilities and societal limitations.

VII. CHAPTER SUMMARY

In this chapter, one model for a multidisciplinary assessment of the infant with suspected cerebral palsy has been presented. This model is based on the assumption that all of the physiological systems contribute to motor control. By approaching the assessment as an interdisciplinary team, the expertise of each team member can be utilized to identify the system impairments that interfere with function. The team then writes up the assessment and develops the treatment plan, and functional goals and intervention strategies can be determined. This will be discussed in Chapter 7 and the entire process will be presented in a case study in Chapter 9.

REFERENCES

1. Greenspan S. Infancy and Early Childhood: The Practice of Clinical Assessment and Intervention with Emotional and Developmental Challenges. Madison: International University Press, 1990.
2. Boyle R, Anderson S. Caring for Infants and Toddlers with Disabilities: A Manual for Physicians. Norge, VA: Child Development Resources, 1995.
3. Bayley N. Bayley Scales of Infant Development–II. New York: The Psychological Corporation, 1993.
4. Folio MR, Fewull RR. Peabody Developmental Motor Scales and Activity Cards: A Manual. Allen, TX: DLM Teaching Resources, 1983.
5. Miller L, Roid G. Toddler and Infant Motor Evaluation. San Antonio: The Psychological Corporation, 1993.
6. Piper M, Darrah J. Motor Assessment of the Developing Infant. Philadelphia: Saunders, 1994.
7. World Health Organization. International Classification of Impairments, Disabilities and Handicaps (ICIDH). Beta2 Draft. Website: www.who.org, 1999.
8. National Council for Medical Rehabilitation Research. Research Plan for the National Center for Medical Rehabilitation Research. Washington, DC: National Institutes of Health, 1993, Publication No. 93–3509.

9. Gibbs E, Teti DM. Interdisciplinary Assessment of Infants. Baltimore: Paul H. Brookes Publishing Company, 1990.

10. Meyers P, Youngstrom MJ. Guide to occupational therapy practice. Am J Occup Ther 1999; 5:256.

11. Als H. A synactive model of neonatal behavioral organization. Phys Occ Ther Ped 1986: 6:3–54.

12. Ayres AJ. Sensory Integration and the Child. Los Angeles: Western Psychological Service, 1979.

13. Ayres AJ. Sensory Integration and Praxis Test. Los Angeles: Western Psychological Service, 1991.

14. Fischer A, Murray E, Bundy A. Sensory Integration: Theory and Practice. Philadelphia: Davis, 1991.

15. Williamson GG, Zeitlin S. Assessment of coping and temperament: contributions to adaptive functioning. In: Gibbs EE, Teti DM, eds. Interdisciplinary Assessment of Infants. Baltimore: Paul H. Brookes Publishing Company, 1990:215–226.

16. Degangi G, DiPietro J, Greenspan S, Porges S. Physiological characteristics of the regulatory disordered infant. Infant Behav Dev 1991; 14:37–50.

17. Blanche E. Infants and Toddlers: Understanding the Impact of Sensory Processing. Continuing Education Course. Los Angeles (unpublished), 1996.

18. Stallings S. Sensory integration: Assessment and intervention with infants and young children. In: Case-Smith J, ed. Pediatric Occupational Therapy and Early Intervention. Woburn, MA: Butterworth-Heiemann, 1998:223–254.

19. Ornitz EM. Normal and pathological maturation of vestibular function in the human child. In: Romand R, ed. Development of Auditory and Vestibular System. New York: Academic, 1993: 479–536.

20. Atkinson J. Human visual development over the first six months of life: A review and a hypothesis. Human Neurobiol 1984; 3:61–74.

21. Glass P. Development of visual function in preterm infants: Implications for early intervention. Infants Young Children 1993; 6:11–20.

22. Kranowitz CS. The Out-Of-Sync Child. New York: Berkley Publishing, 1998:112–113.

23. Frick S, Lawton-Shirley N. Auditory Integrative Training from a Sensory Integrative Perspective. Rockville, MD: American Occupational Therapy Association Inc, 1994.

24. Shumway-Cook A, Woollacott M. Motor Control: Theory and Practical Applications. Baltimore: Williams and Wilkins, 1995:223.

25. Olney SJ, Wright S. Cerebral Palsy. In: Campbell SK, ed. Physical Therapy for Children. Philadelphia: WB Saunders Co, 1995:489–523.

26. Shumway-Cook A, Woollacott MH. Motor Control: Theory and Practical Application. Baltimore: Williams and Wilkins, 1995:28–37.

27. Corcos D, Gottlieb GL, Penn RD. Movement deficits caused by hyperexcitable stretch reflexes in spastic humans. Brain 1986; 109:1043–1058.

28. Tardieu G, Tardieu C, Colbeau-Justin P, Lespargot A. Muscle hypoextensibility in children with cerebral palsy: II. Therapeutic implications. Arch Phys Med Rehabil 1982; 63:103–107.

29. O'Sullivan MC, Miller S, Ramesh V, Conway E, Gilfilian K, McDonough S, Eyre

JA. Abnormal development of the biceps brachii phasic stretch reflex and persistence of short latency heteronymous reflexes from the biceps brachii in spastic cerebral palsy. Brain 1998;121:2381–2395.

30. Damiano DL Vaughn C, Abel MF. Muscle response to heavy resistance exercise in children with spastic cerebral palsy. Dev Med Child Neurol 1995; 37:731–739.
31. Sutherland DH. Gait Disorders in Childhood and Adolescence. Baltimore: Williams and Wilkins, 1984.
32. Nashner L, Shumway-Cook A, Martin O. Stance posture and control in a select group of children with cerebral palsy: Deficits in sensory organization and muscular coordination. Exp Brain Res 1983; 49:393–409.
33. Winstein, CJ. Designing Practice for Motor Learning: Clinical Implications. In: Van-Sant AF, ed. Contemporary Management of Motor Control Problems. Washington DC: Foundation for Physical Therapy, 1991:65–76.
34. Bobath B, Bobath K. Motor Development in the Different Types of Cerebral Palsy. London: William Heinemann Medical Books Ltd, 1981.
35. Campbell SK. Central nervous system dysfunction in children. In: Campbell SK, ed. Pediatric Neurologic Physical Therapy. New York: Churchill Livingstone Inc, 1984:1–12.
36. Wolf LS, Glass RP. Feeding and Swallowing Disorders in Infancy. Tucson: Therapy Skill Builders, 1992.
37. Bar-Or O. Role of exercise in the assessment and management of neuromuscular disease in children. Med Sci Sports Exerc 1986; 28:421–427.
38. Damiano DL, Abel MF. Functional outcomes of strength training in spastic cerebral palsy. Arch Phys Med Rehabil 1998; 79:119–125.
39. Stout JL. Physical fitness in childhood and adolescence. In: Campbell SK, ed. Physical Therapy for Children. Philadelphia: W B Saunders Company, 1995:127–154.
40. Lundberg A. Maximal aerobic capacity of young people with spastic cerebral palsy. Dev Med Child Neurol 1978; 20:205–210.
41. Rose J, Gamble J, Burgos A, Medeiros J, Haskell W. Energy expenditure of walking for normal children and for children with cerebral palsy. Dev Med Child Neurol 1990; 32:333–340.
42. Bar-Or O. Pathophysiological factors which limit the exercise capacity of the sick child. Med Sci Sports Exerc 1986; 18:276–282.
43. Darrah J, Fan J, Chen L, Nunweiler J, Watkins B. Review of the effects of progressive resisted muscle strengthening in children with cerebral palsy: A clinical consensus exercise. Pediatr Phys Ther 1997; 9:12–17.
44. Rosenthal SR, Sheppard JJ, Lotze M. Dysphagia and the Child with Developmental Disabilities. San Diego: Singular Publishing Group Inc, 1995.
45. Bradley N. Motor control: Developmental aspects of motor control in skill acquisition. In: Campbell SK, ed. Physical Therapy for Children. Philadelphia: WB Saunders Co, 1995:39–77.
46. Shumway-Cook A, Woollacott MH. Motor Control: Theory and Practical Application. Baltimore: Williams and Wilkins, 1995:119–122.
47. Cordo P, Nashner L. Properties of postural adjustment associated with rapid arm movements. J Neurophysiol 1982; 47:287–302.

48. Horack F, Nashner L. Central programming of postural movements: adaptations to altered support surface configurations. J Neurophysiol 1986; 55:1369–1381.
49. Nashner LM, Shumway-Cook A, Marin O. Stance and posture control in select groups of children with cerebral palsy: Deficits in sensory organization. Exp Brain Res 1983; 49:393–409.
50. Case-Smith J. Assessment. In: Case-Smith J, ed. Pediatric Occupational Therapy and Early Intervention, 2d ed. Boston: Butterworth-Heinemann, 1998:49–82.
51. Köng E. Fróhdiagnose und frótherapie der zerebralen bewegunsstörungen. Kinderärztliche Praxis 1999; 4:222–243.
52. Alexander R, Boehm R, Cupps B. Normal Development of Functional Motor Skills: The First Year of Life. Tucson: Therapy Skill Builders, 1993.
53. Bly, L. Motor Skills Acquisition in the First Year. Tucson: Therapy Skill Builders, 1994.
54. Video: Early Infant Assessment Redefined. Chicago: Pathways Awareness Foundation, 1993.
55. Sutherland DH. Gait Disorders in Childhood and Adolescence. Baltimore: Williams and Wilkins, 1984.
56. Woollacott MH, Shumway-Cook A. Development of Posture and Gait Across the Lifespan. Columbia: University of South Carolina Press, 1990.
57. Boehme R. Improving Upper Body Control: An Approach to Assessment and Treatment of Tonal Dysfunction. Tucson: Communication Skill Builders, 1988.
58. Henderson A, Pehoski C. Hand Function in the Child: A Foundation for Remediation. Boston: Mosby, 1994.
59. Lawrence DG, Kuypers HG. The functional organization of the motor system in the monkey. I. The effects of bilateral pyramidal lesions. Brain 1968; 91:1–14.
60. Exner C. Development of hand functions. In: Case-Smith J, Allen A, Pratt P, eds. Occupational Therapy for Children, 3d ed. St. Louis: Mosby, 1996: 268–306.
61. Fisk J. Sensory and motor integration in the control of reaching to visual targets. In: Bard C, Fleury M, Hay L, eds. Development of Eye-Hand Coordination Across a Lifespan. Columbia: University of South Carolina Press, 1990:75–98.
62. Parham LD, Fazio L. Play in Occupational Therapy for Children. Boston: Mosby, 1997.
63. Rossetti L. The Rossetti Infant-Toddler Language Scale. East Moline: LinguiSystems Inc, 1990.
64. Palisano RJ, Campbell SK, Harris SR. Clinical decision-making in pediatric physical therapy. In: Campbell SK, ed. Physical Therapy for Children. Philadelphia: WB Saunders Co, 1995:183–204.

7
The Written Assessment, Treatment Planning, and Intervention Strategies

Gay L. Girolami
Pathways Center, Glenview, Illinois

Judy M. Gardner and Diane Fritts Ryan
DuPage Easter Seals, Villa Park, Illinois

I. INTRODUCTION

In the previous chapter we presented a model for collecting assessment data and organizing and categorizing the observations gleaned during that assessment process. In this chapter, we will discuss how the information collected and organized in Chapter 6 can be used to create a written document, write functional goals, develop a treatment plan, and create intervention strategies.

II. WRITING THE MULTIDISCIPLINARY ASSESSMENT

After organizing the data collected during the assessment, the therapist must produce a written document to describe and interpret the observations, discuss the correlation between impairments and functional limitations, formulate conclusions, and provide recommendations for intervention. We endorse a format that is simple, concise, and positively written. Whenever possible, the information should be compiled as a single, interdisciplinary document. This provides a more holistic overview of the infant's performance and sets the tone for a team treatment approach. The assessment document should be sent to the family, referring physician, and other professionals identified by the family.

If you are working independently, the same format for documentation can be followed, but, of course, it will be written up from a single point of view. We are aware that in some situations only one discipline is available for assessment or the referring physician may request an assessment in only one therapy discipline.

In this section, we will discuss and describe the information to be documented in the written interdisciplinary assessment. In many centers the format for the assessment is preordained by the facility. However, if you have an opportunity to provide input regarding the organization and content of the document, we recommend the following content areas (Fig. 1):

> Background data (*history, reason for referral, parental information, and concerns or information obtained from other professional reports*)
> Assessment data (*functional abilities and strengths, organ system impairments, functional limitations, and compensations*)
> Analysis and summary of strengths, impairments, and limitations
> Recommendations (*type of treatment, frequency of treatment, and outside referrals*)
> Functional goals. (Chap. 6, Fig. 3)

A. Background Data

Generally the team, or one member of the team, who assumes responsibility for this portion of the written assessment, creates the section on background information. This is often called the history. The history should contain information regarding parental concerns, physical abilities, daily routine, ongoing medical care, and other therapies or interventions that the child may be receiving. Subjective information from other professional reports should be relative to therapy. It can include information from follow-up clinics or other professional assessments such as orthopedics, neurology, or gastroenterology, but only as it relates to physical, occupational, or speech therapy issues. Information available from other medical records, that is not pertinent to the treatment you will provide, need not be included. As a rule of thumb, if it does not impact on your treatment or provide information about the functional level of the infant, it most probably can be eliminated from your report.

B. Assessment Data

In the observation section of the written assessment, the therapists each record and analyze the clinical observations and objective data specific to their discipline. This includes the infant's functional abilities, regulatory abilities, posture

Child's Name: Date of Birth:

Assessment Date:

HISTORY *(Background Data)*
- **Reason for Referral**
- **Medical History**
- **Parent Concerns**
- **Information from other professionals**

OBSERVATIONS *(Assessment Data)*
- **Functional Abilities** *(discipline related information)*

- **System Impairments Related to Function**
  Postural Control and Balance
  Regulatory System *(discipline related information)*
  Postural System *(discipline related information)*
  Neuromuscular System Musculoskeletal System
  Sensory System
  Cardiopulmonary System
  Gastrointestinal System

SUMMARY *(Data Analysis)*
- **Strengths** *(functional, behavioral, physiological system related)*
  Child
  Family
- **Functional Limitations** *(age related)*

- **Impairments** *(by system)*

RECOMMENDATIONS
- **Occupational Therapy**
- **Physical Therapy**
- **Speech and Language Therapy**
- **Other Professional Assessments to Consider**

GOALS
- **Occupational Therapy**
- **Physical Therapy**
- **Speech and Language**

Figure 1 Multidisciplinary assessment.

and movement patterns, and impairments in the various systems, particularly the
regulatory, neuromuscular, sensory, musculoskeletal, gastrointestinal, and cardiopulmonary systems. Results from standardized testing, joint measurements, and
other quantitative data should also be recorded and interpreted. Significant or
predictable disabilities and current or potential societal limitations should be
noted.

C. Data Analysis

In the summary section of the assessment, the interrelationship of these data must be analyzed as it enhances or interferes with the infant's functional abilities. In the process, the infant's strengths and the most critical impairments and functional limitations should be identified. It is essential to write up the information in a way that emphasizes the child's abilities. Assessments often overlook the client's strengths, focusing only on the impairments and functional limitations. We believe that it is important to acknowledge the strengths and build on these when selecting intervention strategies. In addition, this approach may assist the family to see their child in a positive light, even in the face of obvious limitations. In this way, we begin our initial interactions with the family by working from a point of strengths rather than weaknesses.

There are many options for discussing the impact of the various system impairments and how they interfere with the acquisition of functional skills. We do not advocate recounting a litany of the abnormal postures and movement patterns used by the infant. The object is not to present a picture of how the child moves, but rather *why he moves as he does*. To do this, we must identify and/ or hypothesize which system impairments are present and how they interfere with function. Through this process, we begin to build the framework for the treatment plan and identification of goals and treatment strategies that will minimize the identified system impairments.

D. Summary

After presenting your analysis of the objective information, and your hypotheses regarding how the impairments interfere with function, you must summarize the most significant impairments and functional limitations in a precise, clearly written paragraph. This will allow anyone to pick up your report and, from the summary, gain a clear picture of the main, discipline-specific issues.

E. Recommendations

Recommendations regarding the need for intervention, referral for additional testing, or other professional consultation should be presented next. When developing recommendations, therapists should consider the family situation, financial resources, and time constraints. Recommendations should be developed as a team and presented to the family as options. Alternative recommendations should be offered, which will allow the family to select the program that works best for their individual situation (1).

F. Functional Goals

The family and all involved therapy disciplines should write the functional goals. Functional goals are based on the identified functional limitations. There is a logical progression between what is interfering with function and what must be accomplished to insure improved functional performance. The treatment goals should identify the expected functional outcomes and provide the foundation for treatment planning and selection of intervention strategies (2).

Goals allow the therapist to verify the efficacy of the selected intervention strategies by documenting measurable changes in functional performance. These objective, measurable changes can then be used to illustrate the effectiveness of intervention and assist the family and clinician in obtaining payment for treatment.

If functional changes cannot be documented, the therapist must reassess the identified impairments, and determine how to revise or modify the goals, treatment plan, and intervention strategies to achieve the desired outcomes. Well-written, measurable goals can prevent the loss of valuable treatment time by assisting the clinician in pinpointing the desired functional outcomes and in planning appropriate intervention protocols that impact on impairments that interfere with function.

Writing functional goals also provides an opportunity for objective communication between the family and the therapists. It is important to schedule regular meetings with the family to discuss the expectations that they have for their child. This discussion may reveal expectations that are developmentally on target, or expectations that are too advanced for the infant's developmental age. The therapist may need to educate the family and to assist them in accepting and writing more developmentally appropriate goals. This process can be delicate.

The clinician has the significant responsibility of educating the family without shattering their dreams for their child. For example, the family may express a desire for their infant to sit independently and play with toys, but developmentally the child cannot yet push up onto extended arms and reach for objects. The therapist can use this opportunity to provide the family with suggestions for positioning that allows the infant to spend some time in a well-aligned sitting position. This can also be used as an opportunity for the therapist to educate the family about precursor activities for learning to sit and play independently. The therapist can explain some of the neuromuscular, musculoskeletal, and sensory benefits of pushing up in prone or playing in supine, and how experiences in these positions form the foundation for sitting and playing. In this manner, the therapist can assist the family in selecting more developmentally appropriate goals without diminishing the importance of the family's aspirations for their child.

In an interdisciplinary clinical setting, we advocate that goals be written as a team. Recall that, at a minimum, the team includes the family and members from all the evaluating disciplines. Goals written in this manner insure that each member of the team is aware of the other's concerns and has a good understanding of where and how each member of the team is directing their treatment intervention. This team approach insures better continuity of treatment, as each team member can try to incorporate aspects of other disciplines' goals into the interventions.

III. WRITING FUNCTIONAL GOAL

A good functional goal should contain the following: *subject, action verb, observable functional performance, conditions of performance*, and *criteria for performance* (2,3). The functional goal should assist to demonstrate measurable, functional outcomes of a treatment intervention. While it is not the main object of this chapter to teach goal writing, we will provide definitions for these terms and some examples.

The *subject* is the client, who will be demonstrating success of the goal. The family or a caregiver may also be included in this category, if it is felt that their ability to perform a specific task or skill will be beneficial to the infant and enhance functional progress.

The *action verb* should be selected to show some posture or movement that is consistent with the desired function. Some examples are walking, standing, reaching, and cup drinking. Verbs that do not allow measurement of the outcome function should not be used. Verbs such as "increase" or "will improve" are often used by therapists and should be replaced with verbs that truly denote movement or action.

Observable function performance is the movement skill that is directly related to the action verb. The movement or function selected should be consistent with the child's age, developmental status, and family concerns. Generally it is important to write a beginning and an end for each movement; for example, Jack will move from long sit to side sit, or Jenny will push up onto extended arms. Constructing goals in this manner will make it easy for anyone to assess performance with certainty.

The next element of the goal should define the *conditions of the performance*; that is, the circumstances and environment under which the goals will be evaluated. Use of specific performance conditions allows objective assessment of the goals by you or another individual. Additionally, performance conditions allow the therapist to adapt the goal to demonstrate progress, for example:

Initial PT Goal: In a play setting, Jenny will push up on extended arms in prone to view a toy as her therapist provides assistance and support at the trunk.

Follow-Up PT Goal: In a play setting, Jenny will independently push up on extended arms in prone to view a toy.

Initial OT Goal: In supported sitting, Jenny will bang a toy on a surface using a gross radial grasp.

Follow-Up OT Goal: Sitting in a high chair, Jenny will bang a toy on a surface using a gross radial grasp.

Initial Speech Goal: Sitting in a high chair, Jenny will drink thickened liquids from a cup as her mother or therapist provides assistance at the jaw.

Follow-Up Speech Goal: Sitting in a high chair, Jenny will drink thickened liquids from a cup without assistance.

The last component of the goal is *measurable or qualitative criteria* to assess the achievement of the performance. Accuracy, distance, and speed can all be used to measure how well the performance is executed. The criteria can also demonstrate changed or improved performance, for example:

Initial Speech Goal: Sitting in a high chair, Jenny will drink thickened liquids from a cup as her mother or therapist provides assistance at the jaw.

Follow-Up Speech Goal: Sitting in a high chair, Jenny will drink nonthickened liquids from a cup as her mother or therapist provides assistance at the jaw.

The therapist must determine whether to alter the conditions of performance or the criteria of performance to demonstrate progress. In some cases, when the infant is making rapid progress, it may be necessary to alter the condition of performance. When the infant is making slower progress, it may be necessary to alter the performance criteria. In either case, you have two choices, which allows you to customize the goals for each infant.

After sitting with the family to write functional goals, therapists will use these goals to create the therapy treatment plan and treatment strategies, which will be presented in the next sections. The goals will also be used to develop the multidisciplinary intervention plan and to document progress during treatment. The creation of the multidisciplinary intervention plan and documentation procedures will be presented in Chapter 8.

IV. TREATMENT PLANNING

Following the written assessment and development of functional goals, treatment planning and development of individual treatment strategies are the logical next steps. Treatment planning is the creation of the road map the therapist follows to assist the client in achieving the functional outcomes identified by the goals. It is the *thought process* used by the therapist to prioritize impairments related to a specific goal and to develop treatment strategies to address each impairment. Treatment planning is used to identify and prioritize the most significant system impairments, and to select strategies to address each of those impairments. However, the challenge for the therapist goes beyond merely selecting treatment strategies; it is also to determine the most efficacious sequence for the strategies (Fig. 2).

The data gathered during the assessment provide the foundation for the treatment planning process. Earlier in this chapter we discussed the importance of listing the infant's strengths and identifying and hypothesizing which impairments interfere with age-appropriate function. Additionally, we wrote functional goals to serve as a baseline for assessing change over a specified period of time.

For novice therapists, it may be helpful to use a form to organize this information. A treatment plan worksheet has been provided to assist therapists in this process (Table 1). Over time, the therapist will be able to process this information cognitively without using this written format.

A. Filling-In the Treatment Planning Worksheet

The worksheet can be used to assist the therapist in planning treatment for each identified functional goal. This insures the development of specific treatment strategies to address the various system impairments interfering with the acquisition of each goal.

This treatment planning worksheet provides an outline that directs the therapist to:

>   Select an identified goal from the written assessment
>   List and prioritize the impairments that interfere with the acquisition of
>   each goal
>   Identify and sequence treatment strategies to minimize the effect of the
>   impairments
>   Assess the effectiveness of each strategy and reflect on how to adapt or
>   modify the strategy.

1. Select an Identified Goal

Well-written functional goals are the key to good treatment planning. As stated earlier in this chapter, the goals should be meaningful to the family and important to the child's current developmental stage. The therapist will need to develop a treatment plan for each of the identified goals.

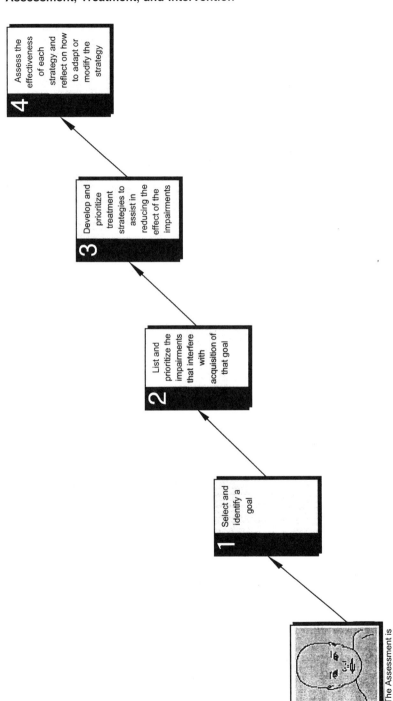

Figure 2 Steps in treatment planning.

Table 1   Treatment Planning Worksheet

Name of Patient and Diagnosis _____ Date: _____

Functional Goal–*Taken from assessment or progress note*	Impairment List–*Prioritize impairments relative to functional limitations*

Treatment Strategies

Sequence strategies relative to prioritized impairments	Expected Outcome–*For each intervention*	Effectiveness–(*Do you need to modify or eliminate the strategy?*)

2. List and Prioritize System Impairments

Next, the therapist must list the system impairments that interfere with the acquisition of that goal. It is sometimes useful to break the goal down into component parts and determine which impairments must be addressed to allow improved performance of the functional task associated with that goal. It is important to note that working on component parts of a goal can be an effective way to treat, but only if those parts are eventually reincorporated and the functional task is practiced in its entirety (4,5).

In either case, simply listing the impairments is not enough. The therapist must next prioritize and sequence these impairments, determining which should be addressed first to achieve the best outcome during each treatment session. Consistent success during treatment will improve the probability of achieving the desired functional goals. Prioritizing and sequencing the impairments is both an art and a science. The therapist must rely on an in-depth understanding of the involved systems, clinical reasoning, and intuition.

3. Identify and Prioritize Treatment Strategies

After prioritizing the impairments, the therapist will develop treatment strategies designed to minimize each of the identified system impairments. Often, with experience, it is possible to develop treatment strategies that pertain to multiple impairments simultaneously. This allows the therapist to address the most crucial impairments throughout the session in a variety of activities and positions, and permits the infant to experience and practice new ways of stabilizing and transitioning within the environment.

Each treatment strategy can be broken down into many components, each of which must be considered. Clinical judgments must insure that the strategy truly addresses the identified impairment, thus leading to the optimal functional outcome. This process will be discussed in greater detail later in the chapter, and a template is provided to help organize each strategy.

Embrey and Hylton (6) have demonstrated that experienced physical therapists have more available treatment scripts and intervention strategies than novice therapists do. In addition, experienced therapists were able to select and alter these strategies with greater speed and variety than novice therapists. This would indicate that treatment planning is an art that can be learned and improved over time.

4. Assess Outcomes of Treatment Session and Strategy

Finally, following the treatment, the therapist should assess the effectiveness of the session, and the effectiveness of each treatment strategy. The therapist should review the outcome of the treatment session related to the goals or components of the goals. It is important to objectively analyze the performance of the infant at the end of the session, and to compare this to the infant's performance at the beginning of the session. Asking some of the following questions may be helpful in evaluating the success of the intervention:

> Did the infant/toddler perform any part of the functional skill with improved posture or alignment?
>
> Did the infant/toddler demonstrate an ability to perform the task with less guidance?
>
> Did the infant/toddler perform some component of the task with greater ease, more speed, less verbal cueing, or greater motivation?

These questions may be helpful in modifying aspects of the treatment session to improve the effectiveness of treatment. This may include identifying additional impairments not observed during the initial assessment, revising or creating new treatment strategies, or even adjusting the environment to produce more effective outcomes (7,8).

The importance of treatment planning cannot be overlooked. It provides an organized, individualized approach to intervention. It allows the therapist to direct the therapy session more effectively, insuring that the following guidelines for treatment planning are incorporated into each session. The end result will be more effective intervention and greater gains for the client.

B. Guidelines for Treatment Planning

It is helpful to observe a number of guidelines when planning treatment:

1. *Communicate with the family on a regular basis.* The family is an important part of the team, and they should be included in goal writing, treatment planning, and regular conferences to discuss any changes in the intervention protocol.

2. *Start from a position of strength.* List the child's strengths and discuss these with the family. This provides an opportunity for you to acknowledge that you recognize each child as an individual. The family will appreciate this affirmation, and you can employ these strengths as you plan treatment strategies.

3. *Goals should be functional.* We cannot stress this enough. If you do not work on functional activities, you will not see the infant incorporate these skills into his daily life. Try to incorporate the remediation of the primary system impairments into goals that highlight the functional tasks the family must address daily. This approach insures greater compliance and directly addresses the immediate needs of the infant and the family.

4. *Goals should be meaningful to the family.* The family will embrace the goals with greater enthusiasm if you include them in the development process. The goals should be directed toward functions that are age appropriate for the

child or assist the family in caring for their child. Parents often select goals that are too advanced for their child. There is often a need to educate the family about development to allow them to embrace goals that form the foundation for the long-term functional outcomes that they desire.

5. *Address the regulatory issues first.* If the infant has difficulty with regulation, find ways to calm and maintain state balance first. Use this information to assist the infant in reorganizing himself as you introduce activities that challenge him. Use these calming and organizing strategies as you introduce sensorimotor input. You should introduce new movements slowly and always be aware of the infant's signals of distress, so you can assist in more adaptive responses (9).

6. *Take time to build a relationship based on trust.* Be playful and engaging in your interactions. Learn the infant's communication style and pay attention to what elicits playfulness in the child. It is comforting and builds trust when the parents see their infant enjoying the treatment session. It will also produce a positive experience that can have an important effect on future treatments.

7. *Create a motivating environment.* Motivation is said to alert and arouse the brain. The conditions of the internal and external environment need to be appropriate to produce motivated behavior. The internal environment needs to be receptive to incoming stimuli (i.e., adequate self-regulation in the infant). The external environment should provide reasonable opportunities for the infant to act on and form relationships with objects and people (10).

In addition, the stimuli must be meaningful to be motivating and engaging. Infants are typically motivated by novelty, increased sensory properties of objects, and positive interactions. The interactions or objects must also be developmentally appropriate, easily initiated, and provide a challenge (11).

Therefore, knowledge of age-appropriate toys and ways of interacting are important. Children with cerebral palsy generally have preferences related to their motor and sensory abilities (12). Incorporating assessment information regarding the infant's preferences for specific sensory input is critical and will aid in the selection of motivating stimuli.

8. *Preparation is not a BAD word.* With the emphasis on function, therapists have come to see preparation as something that should be excluded from treatment plans. However, one might view preparation as those activities that allow the child to more effectively produce the desired functional outcome. Activities that increase mobility improve alignment and sensorimotor knowledge of the movement (i.e., passive movement to allow the child a sensory experience of the movement) can all be beneficial treatment strategies. For example, if a child has very tight hamstrings, it is important to stretch these muscles before introducing functional activities in long sitting.

9. *Integrate sensory input to enhance motor output.* The first year of life is predominately a sensorimotor stage of development (13). Sensory feedback is

important in learning new motor skills; sensory systems contribute to the production of movement (14). All handling has inherent sensory input; this applies to direct input from the therapist as well as input from the environment, including equipment, toys, lighting, and ambient sound. Be aware of your handling speed, tactile input, direction of movement, voice, arrangement of the environment, and combinations of input. How and where you place your hands to provide control, direction, and sensory input must be carefully predetermined and changed to assist, guide, and direct the infant's movement (15). All sensory input can be facilitatory or inhibitory depending on the infant's perception, state of his central nervous system, and how the input is introduced. Be purposeful in the sensory input created by handling, the activities structured, and the interactions presented. Modify input to maximize adaptive responses from the infant.

10.   *Integrate play activities into treatment.* Play, whether structured or spontaneous, can provide motivation, direction, and reinforcement of optimal movement patterns and function. The therapist who can integrate play and creativity into the treatment session will likely see better cooperation and motivation in their client (16). On the other hand, the therapist must realize that highly structured play may inhibit motivation and prevent problem solving and the initiation of new motor behaviors.

11.   *Allow the child to plan and initiate motor behaviors.* Both the task and environment determine how the child will organize his postural system to perform the function (17). During each treatment session, it is important to set up situations that require the child to plan and initiate a variety of motor behaviors. The skills must be practiced in diverse environments to insure the child can effectively alter the postural organization necessary for control.

12.   *Allow the child adequate time to problem solve.* It may take time for the child to problem solve in novel situations. The therapist must step back and permit the child to assess the situation and attempt a variety of movement plans to achieve the desired goal. Knowledge of results is an integral part of learning new skills (18,19). Knowledge of results can be provided through various forms of visual, auditory and kinesthetic feedback (20). Children who have increased processing requirements must be allowed the time to work out the answer before the therapist steps in to assist or guide his movements.

13.   *Practice and repetition are essential.* It is extremely important for the therapist to allow adequate time for practice and repetition when the infant is learning new skills. The therapist should provide an environment that motivates the infant to repeat new motor plans and skills that have been worked on during the treatment session (7). It is also important for the therapist to know what type of practice will effect the most optimal outcome. For example, distributed practice is more effective than massed practice to facilitate learning of new skills (21). Distributed practice requires rest periods that equal or exceed the time it

takes to perform the task. This prevents excessive fatigue and keeps the task challenging rather than boring. Practice should also be scheduled in a variety of environments. These environments should mimic those which are representative of the infant's day. The therapist might use different surfaces or locations to allow the infant to perform the task in a variety of environmental situations.

14. *Therapist handling should decrease as the infant acquires skill*. The therapist must continually assess the infant's ability to perform a task and withdraw guidance to provide an opportunity for the infant to practice unaided. Schmidt (5) has found that guidance is more effective when used in the early practice of an unfamiliar task. Guidance should be used judiciously, allowing a balance between handling and practice.

V. DEVELOPING EFFECTIVE TREATMENT STRATEGIES

During the treatment planning process, the therapist has identified functional limitations, and one or more written goals that address each of the functional concerns. As part of this process, impairments that interfere with acquisition of each goal are prioritized and listed, and general interventions are generated for each of the identified impairments. In this section, we will provide a model for developing treatment strategies for each of the identified interventions that specifically address all of the impairments, thus maximizing the functional performance of the infant.

We have developed a worksheet to assist the therapist in designing treatment strategies that address the identified goals (Table 2). It is important to remember that each of the goals may have numerous intervention strategies because there may be multiple system impairments that interfere with the acquisition of each goal.

A. General Considerations

At the top of each treatment strategy template, a specific goal is identified. Following this, the impairment or impairments to be addressed are listed. Each of the impairments must have a specific treatment strategy to minimize the effect on the infant's function. In some cases, several impairments may be addressed by a single intervention strategy, but, in other cases, the impairment may be so specific that it will require a single intervention or several intervention strategies. Regardless of the impairment being addressed, motivation, mobility, alignment, base of support, sensory input, and environment are key components of every intervention strategy.

Table 2 Treatment Strategy Worksheet

Goal: specific, measurable outcome desired: _____

Element	Description	Rationale/Explanation
Impairment: Specific impairment being addressed		
Anticipated results of this strategy		
Patient: Starting position, including center of gravity (COG) and base of support (BOS), WB/NWB areas, as well as other critical aspects		
Equipment/supplies Position of equipment		
Desired response: parts of the body involved in the activity direction/plane/axis/speed of the movement mobile/stable segments desired muscle activity		
Therapist: Starting position, including COG and BOS		
Movement of the therapist: anticipated direction and plane of motion		
Handling: Keypoints of control; direction and firmness of pressure; timing and other aspects of input Tactile/proprioceptive modalities (e.g., pressure, tapping traction, approximation, vibration, use of temperature)		
Other sensory input (e.g., auditory, verbal cues, visual, vestibular, as well as taste and smell)		

Expected outcome	Modifications	Potential problems/additional considerations
		Acutal results/outcome obtained from use of this strategy:
		Possible adaptation/modification/progression:

B.   Infant Considerations

In each treatment strategy, there are two major players: some aspects of the strategy are specific to the infant and some aspects are specific to the therapist. Each of these considerations has specific areas that must be addressed. With regard to the infant, the therapist must determine the *starting position*; for example, sitting, prone, or standing. Some considerations include the infant's *base of support* and what parts of the body will be weight bearing or non-weight bearing. This can be influenced by a variety of factors: the functional goal, the age of the infant, the ability of the infant, and motivation. The *equipment* used to achieve the desired outcome must also be selected, as well as the size and positioning of that equipment. There are definite reasons to work with a child on your lap, on a ball, or over a roll, which may be related to the activity, the infant's sensory issues, or the need for a stable versus a mobile surface. Finally, the therapist must be keenly aware of the desired outcome of the treatment strategy. In what *direction* do I want the child to move? What *muscle groups* am I trying to activate? What *sensory information* or experience am I trying to provide for this infant? These are just a few of the questions that must be considered.

C.   Therapist Considerations

Therapist considerations are also an important aspect of the treatment strategy. We must decide how to *best position* ourselves to optimize the desired response from the child. There are specific reasons to be in front of the infant, behind the child, or adjacent to the infant. These reasons may be related to the equipment, the anticipated movement of the infant, or the sensory requirements of the infant. *Movement or stability* of the therapist must also be planned. The therapist must also determine whether they will move with the infant or remain stable during the intervention. This can mean movement around the environment or intrinsic weight shifting and movement of the therapist as she provides treatment. With regard to *handling*, the therapist must determine which sensory modalities to employ, how to provide guidance, and when to withdraw assistance and handling. Another aspect of handling is selection of appropriate *key points of control*. The Bobaths (22) first used the phrase describe the choice and modification of hand placement to guide and assist the infant's movement.

Embrey and Adams (15) have studied the ability of novice and expert clinicians to select and modify procedures and key points of control contingent on the responses of the child. Experienced therapists changed their procedures and therefore key points of control every 46 s compared to novice therapists, who altered their handling every 86 s. They also noted that the therapists changed their posture in harmony with the infant. The changes were smooth while those of the novice therapists were abrupt.

With experience, the therapist can more easily and intuitively change the therapy strategy, responding almost instantly to the postural changes, movements, or motivation of the child. This may mean increased or decreased handling, less facilitation, and more guidance or even altering the play activity.

Structuring the environment is another important aspect of the intervention strategy. The therapist must consider the amount of visual, auditory, tactile, and proprioceptive stimuli to offer. Additionally, thought must be given to *where the session will occur* and whether it will be *individual or group treatment*. Each of these decisions is as critical as the selection of the strategy itself. Finally, and perhaps most importantly, each treatment strategy must be motivating and lead to a functional outcome that will be practiced during the treatment session. Although all these considerations may seem overwhelming, especially to the novice therapist, with experience they become more automatic and easier to incorporate in the treatment plan.

During each treatment session, the therapist must determine how long to apply each strategy, and when to adapt or change strategies, based on the response of the child. Evaluation and revision of the treatment strategies should also occur at the end of each session, in preparation for the next treatment. Additionally, evaluation and revision of the treatment plan and intervention strategies should take place each time a progress note is written. Answering the following questions may be helpful in evaluating the success of your treatment strategies and making necessary modifications.

Did this strategy produce the expected effect?
Did I have to modify the strategy significantly?
Did I use this strategy only briefly, perceiving that it was ineffective?
Was the strategy ineffective or do I only need to change some aspect of the strategy (e.g., the equipment, the position, the play activity)?

This analysis will also prevent the application of ineffective treatment strategies, which may be detrimental to the infant over time.

VI. CHAPTER SUMMARY

In this chapter we have presented models for documenting assessment data, goal setting, treatment planning, as well as developing treatment strategies. This planning is critical and must be completed before treatment begins. Without careful data analysis, well thought out functional goals, attention to treatment planning, and development of impairment-related intervention strategies, the efficacy of your treatment will be severely compromised. This impacts not only on clinical performance and self-esteem, but also, more importantly, on the developmental and functional outcomes for infant and the well being of his family.

Yes, the process can be labor intensive. However, as aptitude at analyzing the data improves and the depth of clinical reasoning becomes more sophisticated, the therapist will find it less time-consuming to complete this process, increasing the benefits for the client and personal and professional satisfaction.

Chapter 8 discusses alternative options for treatment implementation and methods to document progress, evaluate and revise functional goals, and alter intervention strategies based on client outcomes. Chapter 9 shows how the processes outlined in Chapters 6 to 8 can be effectively applied to assess and plan treatment for a 10-month-old infant with a diagnosis of cerebral palsy.

REFERENCES

1. Kolobe THA. Working with families of children with disabilities. Pediatr Phys Ther 1992:57–63.
2. Stamer MH. Functional Documentation. San Antonio: The Psychological Corporation, 1998.
3. Vargas JS. Writing Worthwhile Behavioral Objectives. New York: Harper & Row, 1972.
4. Gentile A. The nature of skill acquisition: Therapeutic implications for children with movement disorders. In: Forssbeg H, Hirschfeld H, eds. Movement Disorders in Children. Basel, Switzerland: Karger, 1992:31–40.
5. Schmidt RA, Lee TD. Motor Control and Learning: A Behavioral Emphasis. Champaign, IL: Human Kinetics, 1999:Chap. 10.
6. Embrey DG, Hylton N. Clinical applications of movement scripts by experienced and novice pediatric physical therapists. Pediatr Phys Ther 1996; 8:3–14.
7. Larin HM. Motor learning: Theories and strategies for the practitioner. In: Campbell SK, ed. Physical Therapy for Children. Philadelphia: WB Saunders, 1995; 9:157–181.
8. Embrey DG, Yates, L, Nirider B, Hylton N, Adams L. Recommendations for pediatric physical therapists: Making clinical decisions for children with cerebral palsy. Pediatr Phys Ther 1996; 8:165–170.
9. DeGangi GA, DiPietro JA, Greenspan SI, Porges SW. Psychophysiological characteristics of the regulatory disordered infant. Infant Behavior Devel 1991;14:37-50.
10. Dunn W. Motivation. In: Royeen C, ed. AOTA self study series: Neuroscience Foundations of Human Performance. Rockville, MD: American Occupational Therapy Association, Inc, 1991.
11. Pierce D. The power of object play for infants and toddlers at risk for developmental delays. In: Parham LD, Fazio L, eds. Play in Occupational Therapy for Children. St. Louis: Mosby, 1997:88–111.
12. Blanche E. Doing with—not doing to: Play and the child with cerebral palsy. In: Parham, LD, Fazio, L, eds. Play in Occupational Therapy for Children. St. Louis: Mosby, 1997:202–218
13. Piaget J. The Origins of Intelligence. New York: Norton, 1952.

14. Blanche EI. Intervention for motor control and movement organization disorders. In: Case-Smith J, ed. Pediatric Occupational Therapy and Early Intervention, 2d ed. Boston: Butterworth-Heinemann, 1998:Chap. 11.
15. Embrey DG, Adams LS. Clinical applications of procedural changes by experienced and novice pediatric physical therapists. Pediatr Phys Ther 1996; 8:122–132.
16. Campbell SK. The infant at risk for developmental disability. In: Campbell SK, ed. Decisions in Pediatric Neurologic Physical Therapy. New York: Churchill Livingstone, 1999; 7:260–332.
17. Shumway-Cook A, Woollacott MH. Motor Control:Theory and Practical Application. Baltimore: Williams and Wilkins, 1995:28–37.
18. Gentile AM. Skill acquisition: Action, movement, and neuromotor processes. In: Carr JH, Shepherd RB, eds. Movement Science. Rockville, MD: An Apsen Publication, 1987:93–154.
19. Schmidt RA. Motor learning principles for physical therapy. In: Van Sant AF ed. Contemporary Management of Motor Control Problems. Washington, DC: Foundation for Physical Therapy, 1991:49–64.
20. Higgins S. Motor Skill Acquisition. Phys Ther 1991; 71:123–139
21. Schmidt RA. Motor learning and performance. Champaign, IL: Human Kinetics, 1991.
22. Bobath K, Bobath B. The neurodevelopmental treatment. In: Scrutton D, ed. Management of the Motor Disorders of Cerebral Palsy. Clinics in Developmental Medicine, No. 90. London: William Heinemann Medical Books Ltd, 1984.

8

Treatment Implementation, Reassessment, and Documentation

Gay L. Girolami
Pathways Center, Glenview, Illinois

Diane Fritts Ryan and Judy M. Gardner
DuPage Easter Seals, Villa Park, Illinois

I. INTRODUCTION

After performing the initial assessment, writing up the assessment and goals, and planning treatment, the therapist is now ready to intervene. Figure 1 details the entire intervention process: the clinical assessment (Chapter 6), the written assessment, treatment plan, and intervention strategies (Chapter 7), and the service delivery format, documentation, and reassessment (this chapter).

There are a variety of models to select from when implementing therapy services. Interventions may be provided using the traditional direct therapy model, consultation, or group treatment. The format selected will strongly depend on the individual needs of the infant and constraints of the family. Therapy can be provided in a clinic, at home, or as part of a 0 to 3 program. This chapter provides descriptions of each of the service delivery models, as well as a discussion of various adjunct therapy services.

Regardless of which therapy model is employed, written documentation must be produced to validate the treatment plan and assess progress and functional outcomes. In this chapter, the various types of documentation will be discussed and sample forms provided to assist the therapist in this process.

Finally, consideration must be given to the reassessment process. This process is used to assist therapists and families to redefine the impairments that

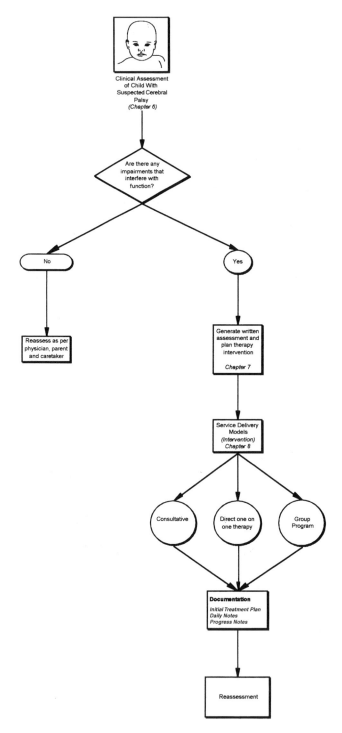

Figure 1 Intervention process.

continue to interfere with function, and to revise the recommendations and goals to reflect the infant's current functional status.

II. CONSIDERATIONS THAT INFLUENCE THE FAMILY'S SELECTION OF TREATMENT SERVICES

Following the clinical assessment, the multidisciplinary team summarizes the findings and makes recommendations for intervention including the types of therapy and the frequency of treatment. It is important to design accessible service delivery systems that are culturally competent and responsive to family identified needs (1). The following are principles to guide the family and therapist when determining the format, frequency, and sequencing of treatment:

> The family's need or concern exists only if the family perceives that the need or concern exists.
> The identification of family priorities and concerns is based on an individual family's determination of which aspects of family life are relevant to the child's development.
> The identification of family resources, including emotional, financial, and environmental constraints (2).

A. Family Concerns

During the assessment, it is important for the multidisciplinary team to be aware of the family's concerns. This information can provide a framework for the presentation of the assessment data and recommendations for intervention. When the family's concerns are not acknowledged, the therapists' recommendations may seem irrelevant or unsympathetic to the family's perception of their child.

A family may come to an assessment with specific concerns regarding their infant. Following the discussion of the assessment data and recommendations, unexpected issues can be revealed, and the family may need time to process this information. In some cases, the information may not only be unexpected, but difficult for the family to accept. The ultimate decision to accept or modify the recommendations belongs to the family. By recognizing and respecting the family's strengths and methods of coping, the team is better able to assist them in understanding the assessment data and the rationale for the recommendations.

In another scenario, a family may be concerned about whether their infant is able to tolerate the amount of intervention recommended. The medical fragility, significance of regulatory issues, or young age of the infant may initially require treatment recommendations to be altered. For example, one discipline may initiate regular direct therapy with consultative intervention from the other disciplines.

In another situation, a family may be apprehensive about the treatment recommendations because they may not be familiar with the different therapies, particularly as they relate to the immediate concerns they have for their infant. Educating the parents about the specific role of each discipline and its function in the assessment and intervention process is critical to the family's understanding and acceptance of the intervention recommendations.

B. Family Priorities

It is important for the team to recognize that the family's priorities for their infant may be different than that of the team. For example, a family who has an infant with a history of poor weight gain may not be able to relate to other identified impairments that affect gross and fine motor function. The team may need to modify the focus of their recommendations and interventions, and relate them more specifically to the family's immediate priorities. When high-priority goals are targeted first, family members are more likely to be incentivised to participate in the treatment plan. If these priorities are adequately managed, the family may be more open to work on other therapy goals initially viewed as less important (3). Acknowledging the family's priorities will also engender trust in the therapy team and build the foundation for open communication and empowerment of the family.

C. Family Resources

The family resources are the strengths, abilities, and supports that can be mobilized to meet the family's concerns and needs (2). The therapist must be able to recognize and respect the family needs and concerns regarding their resources. Some of the variables that can impact on the family's decisions regarding therapy recommendations may include financial resources, transportation, distance to travel, time schedules, and the health and well-being of the family. Therapy is seen as a dynamic process in which therapists and parents work together as partners to define and prioritize the needs of the infant with cerebral palsy (CP) (4).

III. SERVICE DELIVERY MODELS

The intervention model selected should be individualized, flexible, and accessible for the infant and his family. Some of the most common models include direct one on one, consultative, and group therapies. When possible, the child's natural environment is the preferred location.

A. Direct Therapy Model

Direct one-on-one intervention is often the initial model. This allows the therapist to work directly with the parent and infant. The therapist is able to address the concerns, frustrations, and changes that often occur more frequently in infants. In addition, the more frequent direct contact increases the comfort level and trust between the infant and therapist as well as the therapist and parents. In the direct treatment model, the therapist can more accurately gauge the input they are providing, address parental concerns, and modify intervention strategies and home programs. As progress is made, the therapist can alter the frequency of the treatment sessions based on the immediate needs of the infant and the comfort level of the family.

During each treatment session, time should be allotted to discuss how the session goals relate to the desired functional outcomes. Throughout the session, the parent should be encouraged to participate in the handling strategies by playing and interacting with their infant. The therapist should also teach and provide an opportunity for the parent to practice handling strategies and home-programming activities. This may include positioning with the use of equipment or suggestions for holding, carrying, diapering, bathing, feeding, or other activities of daily living. The parent's participation in the therapy program increases their understanding of the treatment goals and their comfort level in caring for their infant. At each subsequent treatment session, the therapist should begin by addressing questions or concerns the parents may have regarding their infant's progress, goals, or home-programming activities.

B. Consultative Model

In some situations, the therapist will take on a consultant's role to the parents or other facilitators working with the infant. This is often the model of choice for an infant who is unable to be brought to the clinic because of medical or family reasons. The consultative model can also be used for those infants whose functional goals can be addressed by providing the parents with a home program. In either case, the home program provides the family with suggestions and strategies that can be implemented as part of the daily routine. The intervention strategies should incorporate the infant's emerging skills, including those that can be elicited by positioning changes, equipment adaptations, or environmental adjustments. Follow-up sessions are scheduled to modify the home program, respond to parental concerns, and to make recommendations for other services.

C. Group Model

In this model, infants with similar functional goals can be treated together with one or more therapists providing handling suggestions to the parents or caregivers. The therapists structure the sessions to provide opportunities for handling practice and suggestions for home program activities. The group model provides advantages for both the parent and infant. The group setting enables parents with similar concerns to communicate and to offer support to one another. The infants may benefit from the opportunity to be treated in an environment that fosters motivation and interaction with their peers. For the infant with sensory or regulatory issues, a group environment may be less stressful, and therefore a more effective delivery model.

In some cases, the group model can be used to facilitate infants as they transition from direct services into day care or community-based programs. Alternatively, both the direct therapy and consultative models can be employed to provide intervention in playgroups, day care, or infant stimulation programs. These settings provide an excellent forum for the carryover of intervention strategies, positioning, and activities of daily living designed to achieve the desired functional outcomes. Often these environments provide the opportunity for infants to learn and model their nondisabled peers in both motor as well as social behavior.

D. Summary of Models

There are many creative and innovative ways of implementing these service delivery models. The model providing the most comprehensive and collaborative intervention that integrates the infant's therapy needs and the family's priorities and resources should be selected.

The following questions may be helpful to the therapist when determining which of the above models is most appropriate for each individual infant and family:

Is this the best service delivery model to meet infant's identified goals?
Does the model selected meet the families identified goals, priorities and resources?
Is the service being provided in the most family centered way?
Will this model contribute to the most optimal treatment outcomes?

Regardless of the model chosen for intervention, communication between the family and all team members is essential.

IV. ADJUNCTS TO THERAPY

In addition to therapy, and regardless of the model selected, adjunctive interventions should be considered when planning and implementing treatment. The infant's daily activities offer opportunity to incorporate the home programming into natural routines. How the infant is positioned, carried, and handled, and how the infant moves independently contributes to the development of body image and acquisition of functional skills. It is critical for the infant to incorporate these daily experiences using the most normal movement patterns possible as he learns how his body functions with greater independence and coordination. The therapist can be instrumental in recommending assistive technology, splinting, and orthotics that make daily functions easier and more efficient.

A. Assistive Technology and Equipment

Assistive technology (AT) is the use of equipment, tools, and service animals to allow persons with disabilities to actively direct the performance of tasks that would otherwise be prevented or made difficult (5). Virtually anything that makes a task easier to complete qualifies as AT. AT can include almost any useful device, from high-tech computer-generated augmentative communication devices, to seating and positioning equipment for the infant. Every day people with and without disabilities use technology to function more fully in society.

Technology has become a powerful force in the lives of individuals with disabilities. It has allowed people greater control over their own lives. They can participate in and contribute more fully to activities in their home, school, work environment, and community. In addition, AT enhances their ability to interact with individuals who do not have disabilities (6). The use of assistive technological devices and services by individuals with disabilities can reduce the costs of the expenditures associated with early intervention, education, rehabilitation, and health disabilities (6).

Even in its seminal stage, AT has enhanced the delivery of therapy services and the acquisition of functional outcomes. For the young infant with cerebral palsy, AT is an essential element of treatment implementation. This might include a variety of commercially available infant seats to custom-made seating devices that allow the infant to experience age-appropriate posture and activities before he has the postural control to achieve them independently. It may also include the use of more technology-advanced devices such as switches and communication devices. Through AT, the infant is able to accomplish a variety of motor tasks and achieve more functional independence.

B. Splinting and Orthotics

Infants with cerebral palsy may develop muscle contractures and structural deformities that impact on functional skills (7). The use of splinting and orthotics to address these issues has been shown to improve postural control, hand function, and to facilitate standing balance and gait. The use of splinting and orthotics is preventative and conservative interventions should be applied early to enhance functional outcomes (8).

Children with cerebral palsy move in restricted ranges of motion and develop little variety in their movement patterns. In the upper extremities, wrist flexion and hand fisting can interfere with functional reach and grasp. In the lower extremities, knee extension with ankle plantar flexion is a common pattern that may develop as early as 4 to 6 months in children with spastic CP. If this position is not modified, this pattern will eventually result in the development of foot and ankle deformities including equinus or equinovalgus (9).

The decision to use splinting and/or orthotics should be made as a team. The orthopedist and therapist should discuss with the family the structural and functional rationale underlying the use of a splint or orthotic device. However, the professionals must respect the family's ability to acknowledge and accept the recommendation. The therapist may need to assist the family in understanding how these devices may improve functional outcomes and prevent potential contractures or deformities (10).

V. DOCUMENTATION

Once the model and frequency for therapy have been established with the family, intervention can be initiated. Regardless of how the therapy is provided, documentation procedures must be implemented. Written documentation will be necessary for a variety of reasons, including assessing progress and revising the goals, treatment plan, and treatment strategies. Additionally, documentation is essential to obtain payment from insurance or other funding sources.

Figure 2 is a schematic of the relationship between the treatment planning process discussed in Chapter 7 and the documentation required to support the treatment plan and goals. In this section, the various types of documentation, including an initial treatment plan, daily notes, and progress notes, will be discussed.

If the infants assessed are enrolled in federally funded programs, the model for the documentation may be predetermined. For infants enrolled in such programs, the Individualized Family Service Plan (IFSP) must be used (11). However, if the infants treated are not enrolled in a federally funded program, then the following documentation formats may be helpful.

A. Initial Treatment Plan

The initial treatment plan will provide information regarding the starting date and type or types of therapy to be administered, as well as the location and fre-

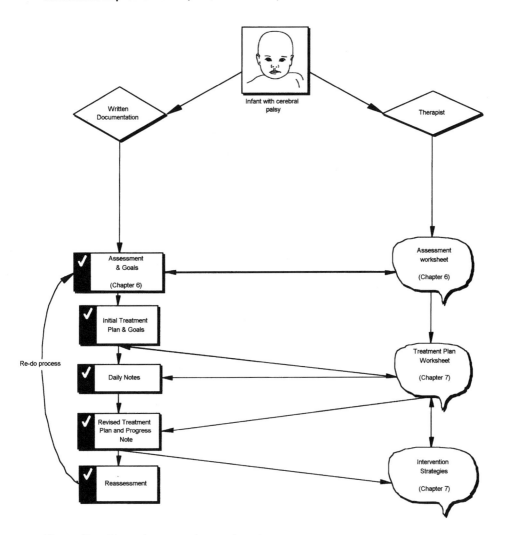

Figure 2   Written documentation vs. therapist process.

quency of each therapy. Figure 3 provides an example of how an initial treatment plan can be organized.

The functional goals, which have been developed with the family and used by the therapists for treatment planning, serve as baseline outcome measures. For each functional goal, the therapist should create a list of components that are needed to achieve the goal. These are based on the impairments identified during

Patient Name:	Start Date:
DOB:	Location of treatment: ☐home ☐Clinic
Diagnosis/ICD:	OT: ☐ X per ___ Name:
Referring Physician:	PT: ☐ X per ___ Name:
	ST: ☐ X per ___ Name:
	Other ☐

Functional Goals & Components	
1. Kaitlyn will pull to stand & play at a small table.	☐ OT ☒ PT ☐ ST ☐ Other
a. Ability to kneel with fully extended hips	
b. Ability to dissociate the lower extremities for half kneeling.	
c. Ability to actively dorsiflex the ankle joint.	
d. Ability to shift weight forward over the weight bearing foot.	
e. Ability to generate adequate muscle force to attain standing.	
2.	☐ OT ☐ PT ☐ ST ☐ Other
3.	☐ OT ☐ PT ☐ ST ☐ Other
4.	☐ OT ☐ PT ☐ ST ☐ Other
5.	☐ OT ☐ PT ☐ ST ☐ Other
6.	☐ OT ☐ PT ☐ ST ☐ Other
7.	☐ OT ☐ PT ☐ ST ☐ Other

Referrals/Other
☐ Clinic Visits

☐ Equipment   ☐ Additional Services _____

☐ Consultation by _____   Expected Date of Review _____

Date: _____   Parent Signature _____

Date: _____   Therapist Signature _____

Figure 3 Initial treatment plan.

the initial assessment. For example, for a therapy goal such as *Kaitlyn will independently pull to stand to play at a small table*, the components that Kaitlyn must acquire to achieve this goal may include:

1. Ability to kneel with fully extended hips.
2. Ability to dissociate the lower extremities for half kneeling.
3. Ability to actively dorsiflex the ankle joint.
4. Ability to shift weight forward over the weight-bearing foot.
5. Ability to generate adequate muscle force to attain standing.

At the end of the initial treatment plan, space is provided to document information regarding referrals to other professionals, consultations, or equipment suggestions the family may want to consider.

B. Daily Documentation

Daily notes are an important part of treatment documentation; they provide a means of chronicling the interventions, relating them to the functional goals, assessing the effectiveness of the intervention strategies, and analyzing the outcome of each session. The notes also provide a framework for communication. Any member of the team, including the family and the infant's physician, can read these notes and clearly see the direction and emphasis of the treatment. In addition, third-party payment strongly hinges on this documentation.

Figures 4 to 6 are examples of daily note formats that can be concisely and quickly completed. The daily note can be generated monthly to document all of the treatment sessions provided during that period of time. The note should include identifying information, specifically the name and age of the infant, and the name, discipline, and license number of the treating therapist. Following that information, the discipline-specific goals and components are listed.

As a means of documenting each session, a series of treatment intervention categories are listed on a grid followed by a space to document progress toward the goals. The therapist places the number and letter of the goal and component next to the applicable treatment intervention categories used during the session. This format is used to indicate the relationship between the goals and components, and each applicable treatment intervention category. Using the sample goal and components from the initial treatment plan in Figure 3, if the therapist worked on lower extremity dissociation to improve half kneeling, the letter 1b would be inserted next to the *range of motion*, *postural control*, and *strengthening* treatment intervention categories. In the space following the grid, a brief narrative can be written describing the specific treatment interventions or the infant's responses to those interventions. This permits the therapist to document changes in behavioral performance and areas of continued concern.

Month/Year:		Therapist:	
Patient:		License #:	
Date of Birth:		Page	of
Treatment Recommendation	x-week/X-mos		

Goals

1. *(Taken from Table 1)*
   - a.
   - b.
   - c.

2.
   - a.
   - b.
   - c.

Date of Session   **Treatment Interventions** (Place goal number next to method.)

	Range of Motion/Flex		Strengthening		Endurance		Balance
	Coordination		Gait Training		Mobility Skills/Transfer		Splinted/Casting
	Postural Control		Neuromuscular Re-education		Manual Therapy		Consultation
	Gross Motor Skills						

Progress Toward Goals:

Signature: _____

Date of Session   **Treatment Interventions** (Place goal number next to method.)

	Range of Motion/Flex		Strengthening		Endurance		Balance
	Coordination		Gait Training		Mobility Skills Transfer		Splinted/Casting
	Postural Control		Neuromuscular Re-education		Manual Therapy		Consultation
	Gross Motor Skills						

Progress Toward Goals:

Signature: _____

Figure 4   Physical therapy daily progress notes and treatment plan.

Documentation about each treatment session allows the therapist to assess the effectiveness of the interventions and, if necessary, to revise treatment strategies. The daily notes insure that the treatment interventions are truly in sync with the infant's needs and address identified impairments and functional goals.

C.   Progress Notes

Progress notes are written to review the infant's current status and areas of continued concern, assess functional outcomes, and revise the goals, recommendations,

Month/Year:	Therapist:
Patient:	License #:
Date of Birth:	Page of
Treatment x-week/ x-mos. Recommendation	

Goals
1. *(Taken from Table 1)*
   a.
   b.
   c.

2.
   a.
   b.
   c.

Date of Session   Treatment Interventions (Place goal number next to method.)

	Range of Motion		Strengthening		Endurance		Coordination
	Postural control		Functional Reach		Weight Bearing		Bilateral Skills
	Hand Skills		Daily Living Skills		Visual Skills		Visual Motor Skills
	Sensory Modulation		Sensory Discrimination		Praxis & sequencing		Play Skills
	Splinted/Casting:		Equipment		Consultation		Other

Progress Toward Goals:

Signature: _____

Date of Session   Treatment Interventions (Place goal number next to method.)

	Range of Motion		Strengthening		Endurance		Coordination
	Postural control		Functional Reach		Weight Bearing		Bilateral Skills
	Hand Skills		Daily Living Skills		Visual Skills		Visual Motor Skills
	Sensory Modulation		Sensory Discrimination		Praxis & sequencing		Play Skills
	Splinted/Casting:		Equipment		Consultation		Other

Progress Toward Goals:

Signature: _____

Figure 5 Occupational therapy daily progress notes and treatment plan.

and treatment plan. It is important to reassess the infant more frequently than you might assess an older child. The developmental changes seen in the first year of life are significant and demand vigilant attention to insure that the treatment plan and goals reflect the immediate needs of the infant.

In Figure 7, we have provided a progress note format. Figure 7a includes pertinent data related to the infant and the therapist. This is followed by an update of the infant's current status and areas of continued concern. Frequency of ther-

Month/Year:	Therapist:	
Patient:	License #:	
Date of Birth:	Page	of
Treatment Recommendation	x-week/x-mos.	

Goals

1. *(Taken from Table 1)*
   - a.
   - b.
   - c.

2.
   - a.
   - b.
   - c.

Date of Session   Treatment Interventions (Place goal number next to method.)

	Strength /Oral-Motor		Sensory Modulation		Respiration/Phonation		Augmentative Communication (AAC)
	Range of Motion-Oral Motor		Language processing/Comprehen.		Swallowing/Oral - Motor		Consultation
	Praxis & Sequencing		Expressive Language/ Comm. Verbal & Non-verbal		Food Transitioning		Saliva Control
	Motor Coordination for Speech		Sound sequencing		Feeding Skills		Postural Control
	Parent Education				Equipment		Other

Progress Toward Goals:

Signature: _____

Date of Session   Treatment Interventions (Place goal number next to method.)

	Strength /Oral-Motor		Sensory Modulation		Respiration/Phonation		Augmentative Communication (AAC)
	Range of Motion-Oral		Language Processing/Comprehen.		Swallowing/Oral - Motor		Consultation
	Praxis & Sequencing		Expressive Language/ Comm. Verbal & Non-verbal		Food Transitioning		Saliva Control
	Motor Coordination for Speech		Sound sequencing		Feeding Skills		Postural Control
	Parent Education				Equipment		Other

Progress Toward Goals:

Signature: _____

Figure 6 Speech therapy daily progress notes and treatment plan.

apy, attendance, home programs, equipment, surgeries, or orthotics are examples of information related to the infant's current status. Parental, medical, or environmental concerns, as well as a review of the impairments that continue to interfere with the acquisition of functional abilities, should also be included in this section. This is followed by a discipline-specific summary of the infant's progress, changes in frequency or treatment, and recommendations for additional services or other interventions that may benefit the infant.

In the first column of Figure 7b, the goals from the initial treatment plan or previous progress note are listed. In the second column, the therapist should comment on progress made toward achievement of each goal or impairments that continue to interfere with achievement of the goal. There are check boxes to indicate whether the goal has been achieved or will be continued, revised, or replaced with a new goal. The goals are revised or rewritten to reflect the influence of the impairments, continued functional limitations, and the most pressing concerns of the family. The new or revised goals are written in the third column and become the baseline for assessing outcomes in the subsequent progress note. As part of this process, the therapist must also review the treatment planning worksheet and revise or create intervention strategies that are consistent with the new goals.

VI. THE REASSESSMENT PROCESS

After 9 to 12 months of treatment, the infant should be reassessed using the same initial assessment format detailed in Chapter 6. Following reassessment, therapists should meet with the family to review the infant's progress, update the functional goals, and revise the treatment plan (see Fig. 8).

Following this meeting, a written reassessment should be generated. Pertinent subjective information from the previous year should be written in the current status section in lieu of a medical history. The objective information will require reassessment of each of the physiological systems to determine which impairments continue to interfere with function (see Fig. 9).

In the summary, a list of new strengths, impairments, and functional limitations should be generated. The functional limitations will reflect the discipline-specific developmental issues that impede progress and interfere with acquisition of the identified goals. Recommendations for therapy and/or further referral should be provided, and the revised goals should be listed. As always, the treatment planning worksheet and treatment strategies will also be revised based on the new assessment information.

(a)

☐Physical Therapy ☐Occupational Therapy ☐Speech Therapy

Patient Name:
DOB:
Diagnosis/ICD:
Referring Physician:
Date Of Note:

Therapy Dates:
Location of treatment: ☐Home ☐Clinic
Physical Therapy: ___ X per ___
Occupational Therapy: ___ X per ___
Speech Therapy: ___ X per ___

System Impairments:
☐Neuromuscular
☐Regulatory
☐Musculoskeletal

☐Gastrointestinal
☐Cardiopulmonary
☐Posture & Balance
☐Sensory/Processing

Status & Areas of Concern:

Summary:

Revised Treatment Plan:
☐Physical therapy ___ X per wk.
☐Occupational therapy ___ X per wk.
☐Speech therapy ___ X per wk
☐Other ___
☐Re-evaluate ☐PT ☐OT ☐ST

Recommendations:
☐Clinic Visits
☐Home Visits
☐Equipment Changes
☐Consultation by ___
☐Additional Services

Progress reviewed with:
☐Patient
☐Family
☐Physician
☐Other

Date: _____ Therapist Signature _____ License #
Date: _____ Therapist Signature _____ License #
Date: _____ Therapist Signature _____ License #

(DISCIPLINE SPECIFIC PROGRESS & GOALS ATTACHED)

(b)

Patient Name: _____

Date of Note: _____

Functional Goals & Components	Comments	Future Goal

1. Kaitlyn will pull to stand & play at a small table
  a. Ability to kneel with fully extended hips.
  b. Ability to dissociate the lower extremities for half kneeling.
  c. Ability to actively dorsiflex the ankle joint.
  d. Ability to shift weight forward over the weight-bearing foot.
  e. Ability to generate adequate muscle force to attain standing.
	☐Achieved ☐Continue ☐Revise ☐Discontinue	

Functional Goals & Components	Comments	Future Goal
2.	☐Achieved ☐Continue ☐Revise ☐Discontinue	

Functional Goals & Components	Comments	Future Goal
3.	☐Achieved ☐Continue ☐Revise ☐Discontinue	

Date: _____ _____ Therapist Signature _____ License # _____

Figure 7 Progress note and treatment plan.

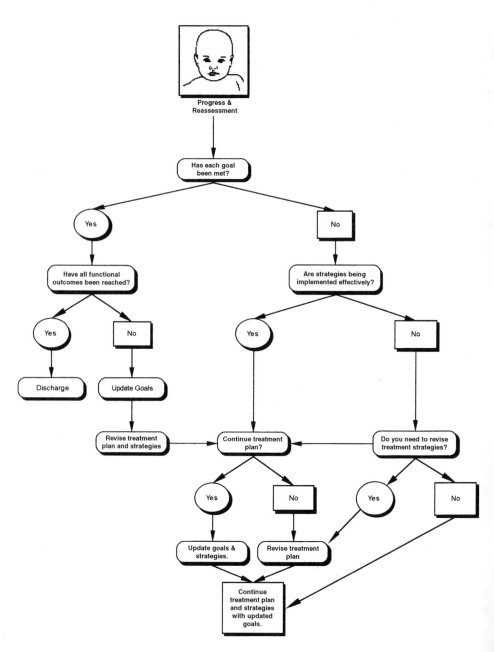

Figure 8 Reassessment.

Child's Name: **Date of Birth:**

Reassessment Date:

Current Status *(Background Data)*
- **Treatment type and frequency**
- **Parent concerns**
- **Information from other professionals**
- **Surgical interventions**
- **Assistive technology/equipment**
- **Orthotics/splints**

OBSERVATIONS *(Assessment Data)*
- **Functional abilities *(discipline-related information)***

- **System impairments related to function**
  Postural Control and Balance
  Regulatory System *(discipline related information)*
  Postural System *(discipline related information)*
  Neuromuscular System Musculoskeletal System
  Sensory System
  Cardiopulmonary System
  Gastrointestinal System

SUMMARY *(Data Analysis)*
- **Strengths** *(functional, behavioral, physiological system-related)*
  Child
  Family
- **Functional limitations** *(age related)*

- **Impairments** *(by system)*

RECOMMENDATIONS
- **Occupational therapy**
- **Physical therapy**
- **Speech and language therapy**
- **Other professional assessments to consider**

GOALS
- **Occupational therapy**
- **Physical therapy**
- **Speech and language**

Figure 9   Multidisciplinary reassessment.

VII. SUMMARY

This chapter has addressed options for treatment and family considerations that may affect the implementation of those options. The importance of written documentation was discussed and examples of an initial treatment plan, daily notes, and progress notes were provided. Finally, the importance of reassessment was presented along with a format for writing up the reassessment information.

The implementation of therapy for the infant with cerebral palsy focuses on function and attempts to optimize the infant's ability to respond to daily physical needs and activities. In order to accomplish this objective, therapy must be a continuum of assessment–treatment planning–intervention–and reassessment until the identified functional outcomes have been achieved. A guide to this process has been detailed in Chapters 6 to 8. An example of this continuum is outlined in Chapter 9 in a case study of a 10-month-old with cerebral palsy.

REFERENCES

1. Smith B. The Division for Early Childhood Position Statements and Recommendations Relating To P.L. 99–457 and Other Federal and State Early Intervention Policies. Washington, DC: Division for Early Childhood of the Council for Exceptional Children, 1987.
2. Kaufmann RK, McGonigel MJ. Identifying family concerns, priorities, and resources. In: McGonigel MJ, Kaufmann RK, Johnson MK, eds. Guidelines and Recommended Practices for the Individualized Family Service Plan, 2d ed. Bethesda: Association for the Care of Children's Health, 1991:47–56.
3. Case-Smith J. Defining the early intervention process. In: Case-Smith J, ed. Pediatric Occupational Therapy and Early Intervention. Boston: Butterworth-Heinemann, 1998:27–48.
4. Law M, Darrah J, Pollock N. Family-centered functional therapy for children with cerebral palsy: an emerging practice model. In: Law M, ed. Family-Centered Assessment and Intervention in Pediatric Rehabilitation. New York: Hawthorne Press, 1998:83–102.
5. Seelman KD. What Is Assistive Technology? National Institute on Disability and Rehabilitation Research. Washington D.C.: U.S. Department of Education, 1999.
6. Technology-Related Assistance for Individuals with Disabilities Act of 1988. Assistance for Individuals with Disabilities Act of 1988. Public Law 100–407. August 19, 1988:1383.
7. LeVeau BF, Bernhardt DB. Developmental biomechanics: effects of forces on the growth, development and maintenance of the human body. Phys Ther 1984; 64: 1874–1882.
8. Cusick BD. Splints and casts: managing foot deformity in children with neuromotor disorders. Phys Ther 1988; 68:1903–1912.
9. Hainsworth F, Harrison MJ, Sheldon TA, Roussounis SH. A preliminary evaluation

of ankle orthoses in the management of children with cerebral palsy. Dev Med Child Neurol 1997; 39:243–247.

10. Olney SJ, Wright S. Cerebral palsy. In: Campbell SK, ed. Physical Therapy for Children. Philadelphia: WB Saunders Co, 1995:489–523.

11. Dunst CJ. Implementation of the individualized family service plan. In: McGonigel MJ, Kaufman RK, Johnson BH, eds. Guidelines and Recommended Practices for the Individualized Family Service Plan, 2d ed. Bethesda: Association for the Care of Children's Health, 1991:67–77.

9

Assessment and Treatment Planning
A Case Study

Gay L. Girolami
Pathways Center, Glenview, Illinois

Diane Fritts Ryan and Judy M. Gardner
DuPage Easter Seals, Villa Park, Illinois

I. CASE STUDY: MICHELLE

A. Introduction

In Chapters 6–8, principles for executing an interdisciplinary assessment, as well as planning and implementing treatment, have been described. Templates to assist the team in organizing information and developing strategies have also been discussed. This chapter presents a case study of Michelle, a 12-month-old infant with cerebral palsy. The assessment principles and forms discussed in the previous three chapters will be used to provide an actual example of how the information gathered during a multidisciplinary assessment can be organized and treatment planning and intervention can be planned and executed.

B. Assessment

The assessment is performed to gather data regarding the family's concerns and the infant's strengths, impairments, and functional limitations. After analysis of these data, the assessment is written, goals are developed, and the treatment plan is finalized. This section presents this process for the infant in the case study.

Child's Name: Michelle   **Assessment Date:** 11-99

Birthdate: 12-98   **Diagnosis:** Cerebral Palsy

Adjusted Age: 9 months   **Chronological Age:** 12 months

Strengths

- Age appropriate
    Regulatory skills
    Play & social interests
    Receptive language
- Emotionally supportive family interested, participates in all aspects of therapy, but some time limitations because of family size
- Excellent endurance for therapy
- Hand function on left in supported positions
- Some ability to explore body parts in supported positions
- Some ability to produce reciprocal lower extremity movement
- Vision and hearing appears within normal limits

Observations In All Performance Areas	Impairments That Impact Function	Functional Limitations/Activity
Upper Body	**Musculoskeletal System**	
• Neck hyperextension in all positions	• ROM restrictions in cervical, pecs, lats, shoulder elevator, internal rotator, pronator, wrist, hand and finger flexor muscles	Michelle is unable to drink from an open cup.
• Increased shoulder elevation in all positions		
• Shoulder internal rotation in all positions		Michelle is inefficient in accepting food from a spoon.
• Scapular winging during reaching	• Decreased strength in scapular depressor, upward rotator, humeral flexor and abductor, elbow extensor, forearm supinator and wrist/finger extensor and thumb abductor muscles	
• Forearm pronation & wrist flexion		
• Hand fisting in all positions right > left		Michelle is unable to use an age appropriate biting and chewing pattern.
• Poor UE weight bearing in all positions	• Decreased range of movements and strength of tongue, lips, and jaw	
• Decreased forward shoulder flexion in all positions		Michelle is limited in her ability to use expressive language.
• Decreased isolated movement in UEs	**Neuromuscular System**	
• Poor protective extension	• Poor timing and initiation of shoulder girdle muscles	Michelle uses limited pitch, range and volume in her speech production.
• Increased stiffness in extremities with vocalization	• Poor ability to initiate and sustain muscle activity in scapular depressors, upward rotators, humeral flexors and abductors, elbow extensors, forearm supinators and wrist/finger extensors and thumb abductors	
• Frequent open-mouth posturing		Michelle is unable to speak without increasing the muscle stiffness in her extremities.
• Hard glottal attack when initiating vocalization		
• Poor timing of breathing, sucking and swallowing during feeding	• Decreased isolated movement in face, lips and tongue	
• Aversive to tactile input around face and mouth	• Poor timing and sequencing of respiratory and phonatory muscles	
	Sensory System	
	• Inadequate UE and oral motor sensory experiences secondary to decrease ability to explore the environment	

(a)

Areas	Impairments That Impact Function	Functional Limitations/Activity
Trunk • Decrease ability to generate adequate muscle tone in the neck and trunk musculature • Increased thoracic rounding and posterior pelvic tilting in sitting • Poor ability to initiate trunk rotation in all positions • Poor pelvic mobility for postural alignment and transitions • Decreased weight shifting in prone, sitting and four point, and standing • Shallow respiratory pattern • Difficulty transitioning into and out of prone, sitting, four point and standing • Poor ability to align head, trunk, upper and lower body for functional movements and with respect to gravity and base of support • Poor head and body righting reactions • Inadequate equilibrium responses • Inability to reach for objects placed outside her base of support • Restricted movement of the respiratory musculature in all postures • Noisy breathing during inspiration	**Musculoskeletal System** • Decreased strength in back extensor and abdominal muscles • Decreased ROM (see Upper Body section) **Neuromuscular System** • Decreased ability to initiate muscle activity in the back extensors and abdominals more pronounced in antigravity positions • Decreased ability to sustain muscle activity in back extensors and abdominals more pronounced in antigravity positions • Poor timing, sequencing and concentric and eccentric control of trunk flexors and extensors **Posture and Balance** • Limited ability to maintain the appropriate relationship between all body segments for postural responses and transitions • Limited ability to maintain center of mass over base of support transitions, mobility and functional tasks • Decreased ability to anticipate the postural organization necessary for transitions and functional tasks secondary to decreased sensory and motor experience **Cardiopulmonary** • Secondary effect of the cardiopulmonary complications resulting from prematurity	• Michelle is limited in the ability to vary patterns of grasp and release. • Michelle is unable to engage in bilateral upper extremity play. • Michelle is delayed in age appropriate play independently. • Michelle is deficient in object play. • Michelle is unable to reach for toys or objects placed overhead. • Michelle is unable to support on her upper extremities for transitions. • Michelle is delayed in her visual motor development. • Michelle is unable to maintain her posture while visually scanning the environment. • Michelle is limited in her ability to independently explore her environment.
Lower Body • Increased muscle stiffness and resistance to hip, knee and ankle flexion • Increased extensor muscle activity at the hip, knee and ankle in all positions • Increased ankle eversion and toe clawing in all positions • Poor ability to initiate and isolate unilateral LE movements in all positions • Inadequate LE disassociation • Poor participation of LEs for transitions • Decreased variability and frequency of LE movements for stability and transitions	**Musculoskeletal System** • ROM restrictions in hip flexors, adductors and internal rotators, hamstrings gastrocsoleus, and toe flexors • Decreased LE strength in hip extensors, abductors, external rotators, quads, hamstrings, tibialis anterior, gastrocsoleus and toe extensors **Neuromuscular System** • Decreased ability to initiate activity in the muscles of the LE, more pronounced in antigravity positions • Decreased ability to sustain activity in the muscles of the LE, more pronounced in antigravity positions • Poor timing, sequencing and concentric and eccentric control of LE muscles **Sensory System** • Inadequate LE sensory experiences secondary to decreased ability to explore the environment	• Michelle is unable to independently sit on a small bench and reach for or play with toys. • Michelle is unable to maintain four-point position and reach for a toy. • Michelle is unable to use creeping to explore her environment. • Michelle cannot maintain a half kneel position for playing. • Michelle is unable to stand and play at a small table. • Michelle is unable to maintain a foot flat position in weight bearing positions.

(b)

Figure 1 Assessment worksheet.

1. Assessment Worksheet

Before writing the assessment, it is important for the team to fill out the Assessment Worksheet (see Fig. 1). This form is designed to assist the therapist in identifying the infant's strengths and sorting and analyzing the data collected during the assessment.

In column 1, observations about the infant's alignment, muscle activity, and movement capabilities in the various performance areas are listed. Reviewing the Assessment Worksheet for this case study (Fig. 1), the reader will note that the observations are divided by areas: upper body, trunk, and lower body. Organizing observations by areas of the body seems to be a more efficient means of organizing data. Observations can also be listed by performance areas, but, eventually, impairments will recur in each performance area.

After listing the various observations concerning *how* the infant moves, the team must hypothesize *why*; that is, which systems may be impaired. It is important to consider how each system may contribute to the postures and movements observed. These hypotheses are listed in the impairment column on the Assessment Worksheet.

Finally, discipline-specific, age-appropriate, functional limitations are listed in column 3. These functional limitations will form the foundation for the construction of the functional goals, in addition to other goals that the family may have for their infant.

2. Written Assessment

The format for the written assessment for this case study was outlined in Chapter 7. This begins with history or background data and may include the reasons for referral, medical history, parent concerns, and pertinent information from other professionals who have evaluated the infant.

This is followed by the observations or assessment data and includes information about the infant's functional abilities and impairments in the various systems. Filling in the Assessment Worksheet will be very beneficial and assist the therapist in creating the written information related to the assessment data.

Finally, a summary of the infant's strengths, age-related functional limitations, and impairments is written. Then recommendations for the type and frequency of interventions are specified, along with a list of general discipline-specific goals. These goals will be presented to and discussed with and finalized with the family. The final goals will be recorded in the Initial Treatment Plan (see Fig. 2) and become the baseline outcomes for measuring progress.

For this case study, the background data and summary information are provided in a narrative format. The content for the assessment data can be found in the Assessment Worksheet (Fig. 1) and will not be written in narrative form. The

Patient Name: Michelle	Start Date:	☒ OT: 2 X per Week
DOB: 12-98	Location of treatment: ☐ Home ☒ Clinic	☒ PT: 2 X per Week
Diagnosis/ICD: Cerebral Palsy		☒ ST: 1 X per Week
Referring Physician:		

Functional Goals				
1. Michelle will drink from an open cup held by another person.	☐ OT	☐ PT	☒ ST	☐ Other
2. Michelle will eat when being spoon-fed in 15 minutes while maintaining proper postural alignment, while positioned in a high chair.	☐ OT	☐ PT	☒ ST	☐ Other
3. Michelle will use 2-3 word phrases to spontaneously express her needs, without associated reactions.	☐ OT	☐ PT	☒ ST	☐ Other
4. Michelle will independently bite off and rotary chew solid foods appropriate for her age, without associated reactions.	☐ OT	☐ PT	☒ ST	☐ Other
5. Michelle will reach overhead for an object with either upper extremity while independently floor sitting.	☒ OT	☐ PT	☐ ST	☐ Other
6. Michelle will visually explore her environment using 180 degree while maintaining upright sitting position.	☒ OT	☐ PT	☐ ST	☐ Other
7. Michelle will shape her hands and maintain grasp around various size objects, to allow for independent exploration of toys.	☒ OT	☐ PT	☐ ST	☐ Other
8. Michelle will hold a hand size container with one hand while putting small objects in with the other (bilateral).	☒ OT	☐ PT	☐ ST	☐ Other
9. Michelle will support her weight on one extremity in a sitting position, while reaching for a toy with the other extremity.	☒ OT	☐ PT	☐ ST	☐ Other
10. Michelle will demonstrate age appropriate visual-motor skills in an adapted sitting position.	☒ OT	☐ PT	☐ ST	☐ Other
11. Michelle will independently sit on a small bench and reach for toys.	☒ OT	☒ PT	☐ ST	☐ Other
12. Michelle will maintain a four-point position when reaching for a toy.	☒ OT	☐ PT	☐ ST	☐ Other
13. Michelle will use creeping to explore her environment.	☐ OT	☒ PT	☐ ST	☐ Other
14. Michelle will maintain a half-kneeling position to play at a low table.	☐ OT	☒ PT	☐ ST	☐ Other
15. Michelle will independently stand to play at a small table.	☐ OT	☒ PT	☐ ST	☐ Other
16. Michelle will maintain her feet flat on the floor, with no toe clawing, in all weight bearing positions.	☐ OT	☒ PT	☐ ST	☐ Other

Referrals/Other
☒ Clinic Visits
☒ Orthopedic clinic for baseline consult and discussion regarding prescription for orthotics   ☐ Additional Services _____
☒ Equipment
    Adaptations to high chair, floor sitter with tray, insert for stroller
☐ Consultation by _____   Expected Date of Review _____
        Date: _____   **Parent Signature**
        Date: _____   **Therapist Signature**

Figure 2 Initial treatment plan.

recommendations for therapy and the functional goals can be found in the Initial
Treatment Plan (Fig. 2).

(a) Background Data.   Michelle is 12 months old, with an adjusted age
of 10 months. She was the first of triplets born by C-section at 29 weeks gestational age. Her birth weight was it 1.9 kg, and she was hospitalized for the first
7 weeks of life with the following complications:

> Twin-to-twin transfusion syndrome (multiple blood transfusions)
> Severe cardiomyopathy (treated and gradually resolved)
> Ventilator dependent with meds for first 10 days
> Grade II retinopathy (no treatment recommended)
> Mild apnea of prematurity (treated with theophylline and weaned by 1
>   month)
> Mild pulmonic stenosis and bronchiolitis (treated with albuterol)
> Left corioplexis hemmorrage (resolved)

Both the physician and parents were concerned about her slow motor development. She was referred at 7 months adjusted age for a multidisciplinary evaluation. Her parents became concerned because, when compared to her siblings,
Michelle's motor development was delayed and her extremities were stiff and
difficult to bend.

(b) Observations.   The strengths, observations, impairments and functional limitations are documented on the Assessment Worksheet in Figure 1.

(c) Summary.   Michelle, one of triplets, whose adjusted age is 10
months, was seen by physical, occupational, and speech therapists as part of a
multidisciplinary assessment (see Fig. 3–16). She was easily engaged and appeared to enjoy the movement and interaction possibilities provided by the therapists. Her parents were present during the assessment and provided information
about Michelle's daily schedule, as well as their concerns regarding their infant's
development.

Michelle exhibits decreased muscle tone in her neck and trunk. Increased
muscle tone is evident in all extremities and is more pronounced in the lower
limbs and throughout the right side. This atypical distribution of muscle tone
interferes with Michelle's ability to isolate, initiate, sustain, and grade muscle
activity for the performance of age-appropriate gross, fine, and oral motor skills.
Secondary to the reduced muscle activity and paucity of active movement, Michelle demonstrates mild range-of-motion restrictions in the spine, shoulder girdle, and upper and lower limbs, which also impacts on the development of independent motor skills.

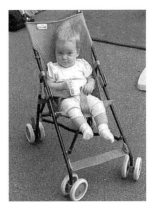

Figure 3 *Stroller*: Michelle was brought to the assessment by her parents and arrived in this stroller, which allows a position of posterior pelvic tilting, thoracic spine flexion, and cervical spine hyperextension. Her legs are extended and feet plantarflexed.

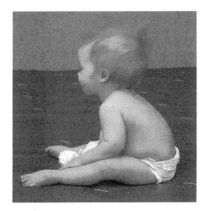

Figure 4 *Long sit*: Placed in long sitting, Michelle sits with a posterior pelvic tilt, which results in thoracic flexion and cervical hyperextension. Michelle has scapular abduction and shoulder internal rotation that may be a result of the position of the pelvis and spine position and may also be indicative of possible tightness in the muscle groups around the shoulder girdle. Her legs are abducted and flexed, allowing a wide base of support to sustain sitting balance. Her knees are somewhat flexed, which may indicate decreased hamstring range of motion. Plantarflexion and eversion are visible at the ankle joint and may be indicative of gastrocsoleus and peroneal muscle tightness.

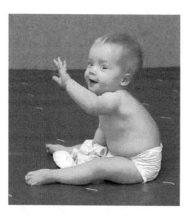

Figure 5 *Sit with reach*: Posture is similar to that in Figure 2, but, with overhead reaching, increased shoulder elevation, shoulder internal rotation, and poor scapulo-humeral dissociation are apparent. These postures limit the range and variability of her reach. The trunk muscles are inactive, and this muscle inactivity contributes to poor ribcage mobility. Michelle shows little variety in her facial expressions and consistently maintains an open-mouth posture.

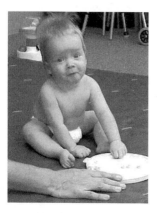

Figure 6 *Sit/grasp*: The base of support is widened by increasing hip abduction and knee flexion; this base is used to maintain sitting balance for fine motor tasks. This wide base of support increases the posterior pelvic tilting to balance the forward movement of the upper trunk for reaching tasks. The fisting in the right hand, seen in other positions, increases with use of the left hand for fine motor grasping tasks. The left hand shows an immature gross grasp when reaching for a small piece of cereal. Michelle's poor ability to grade her facial musculature is evident in the change of facial expression seen in this figure. Her previously low-tone affect (Fig. 2) changes dramatically to a more high-tone grimacing expression. This impacts on her ability to develop oral facial muscle strength and interferes with her ability to develop rotary chewing.

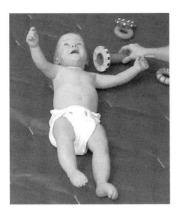

Figure 7 *Supine/extended legs*: Supine is Michelle's preferred position for play. She pushes back into the support surface with cervical hyperextension and strong lower extremity extension and toe clawing. This posture interferes with downward visual gaze and Michelle's ability to bring her hands to midline. Belly breathing, although appropriate for age, is shallow and irregular.

(d) Recommendations. Physical therapy—twice weekly, to address limitations that interfere with mobility and the acquisition of age-appropriate gross motor skills; occupational therapy—twice weekly to address limitations in ability to reach and grasp objects and use upper extremities for weight bearing and transitions; and speech therapy—once weekly to address feeding, respiration, and phonation concerns.

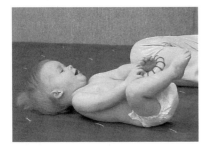

Figure 8 *Supine/flexed legs*: Michelle demonstrates the ability to alter her upper and lower extremity posture, but lacks variety in her movements and alternates between flexion and extension postures. Regardless of her ability to bring her arms to midline, she remains unable to achieve eye hand/foot integration.

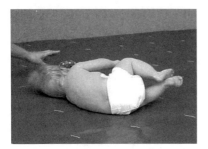

Figure 9 *Rolling to side:* Michelle is able to independently roll to either side, but uses neck, trunk, and hip flexion to initiate the transition. She is unable to dissociate lower extremities and exhibits no lateral head or trunk righting.

(e) Goals. The recommendations for frequency of treatment and the discipline-specific functional goals are recorded on the Initial Treatment Plan (see Fig. 2).

C. Initial Treatment Plan

The information regarding the frequency of therapy, as well information about the providing therapists, is recorded in the initial treatment plan. The discipline-

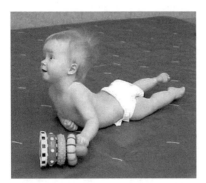

Figure 10 *Prone/flexed elbow*: Michelle can independently achieve prone on forearms. She uses excessive neck, trunk, and LE extension to sustain this posture. This interferes with weight shifting and the development of trunk and shoulder girdle strength and control, as well as lower extremity dissociation. It also limits scapulo-humeral range of motion, lower arm and hand development, and eye–hand coordination.

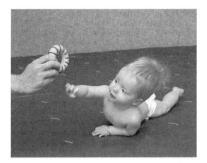

Figure 11 *Prone/reach*: Michelle uses increased cervical and lumbar extension to initiate weight shifting. This interferes with elongation of the dorsal spinal musculature, activation of the abdominal muscles, and pelvic mobility. Trunk and shoulder girdle weakness causes inefficient weight shifting for reaching, and Michelle collapses onto the weight-bearing arm. This inability to sustain weight and to push up onto extended arms impacts on the development of supination and elbow, wrist, and finger control.

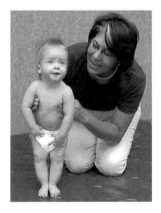

Figure 12 *Standing/front view*: When placed in standing, Michelle uses strong extension in the hips, knees, and ankles to sustain weight bearing. Her arms are held close to the body to assist with antigravity postural control. The strong activation of antigravity muscles limits the initiation of movement and interferes with the ability to develop concentric and eccentric muscle control.

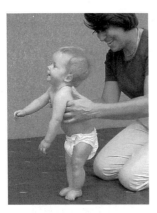

Figure 13 *Standing/side view*: From the side, the effect of the strong lower extremity extension can be better observed. This posture forces Michelle's center of mass behind her base of support and interferes with the development of independent standing balance. Cervical spine hyperextension contributes to tongue protrusion and jaw instability.

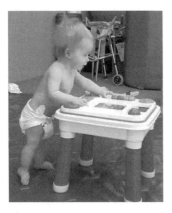

Figure 14 *Standing/table*: The anterior support provided by the activity table allows Michelle to achieve improved LE weight bearing. On the left side she is able to maintain her foot under her center of mass and demonstrates some ability to balance knee flexion/ extension. The right foot remains strongly extended at the knee and ankle, with no ability to initiate movement.

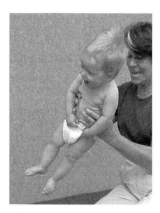

Figure 15 *Vertical suspension*: When held vertical and tilted, Michelle is unable to integrate lateral head and trunk righting and hip abduction to sustain antigravity postural stability. Instead, extensor muscle activity is greatly exaggerated and she uses neck flexion, shoulder elevation, and protraction. Michelle uses her hands to grasp her diaper, another attempt to stabilize her body in space.

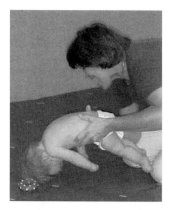

Figure 16 *Protective extension*: When tipped forward to elicit protective extension, Michelle again reverts to the exaggerated lower extremity extensor muscle activity, along with neck flexion, shoulder elevation, and protraction. She is unable to dissociate her arms from her upper body to achieve a protective response.

Name of Patient: ___Michelle___   **Date:** ___   **Therapist:** ___Judy Gardner___

Functional Goal – *one goal taken from Assessment or Progress Note*	Impairment List - *Prioritize Impairments Relative to Functional Limitation*
Michelle will be spoon-fed in 15 minutes, while maintaining proper postural alignment.	• ROM restrictions in cervical, pecs, lats, shoulder elevator, internal rotator, and pronators.
	• Decreased strength in scapular depressor, upward rotator, humeral flexor and abductor.
	• Decreased range of movements and strength of tongue, lips and jaw.
	• Decreased isolated movement in face, lips and tongue.
	• Poor timing and sequencing of respiratory and oral-motor muscles.
	• Inadequate UE and oral motor sensory experiences secondary to decrease ability to explore the environment.
	• Limited ability to maintain the appropriate relationship between all body segments for postural responses and transitions.
	• Decreased ability to anticipate the postural organization necessary for transitions and functional tasks secondary to decreased sensory and motor experience.

Treatment

Interventions - *Sequence strategies relative to prioritized impairments*	Expected Outcome - *for each intervention*	Effectiveness *(Do you need to adapt, revise or eliminate the strategy?)*
• Activities to promote symmetry of the head, shoulders, and trunk for feeding.	• Michelle will sit in good alignment of head and trunk during spoon-feeding.	
	• Michelle will eat the required amount of food by spoon in 15 minutes or less.	
• Activities to improve timing of suck, swallow and breathing patterns.		
• Activities to increase activation of respiratory mechanism for feeding and phonation.	• Michelle will maintain a regular and normal breathing pattern during feeding.	
• Activities to promote head and jaw stability.	• Michelle will use stable jaw to allow her upper lip to retrieve food, and her tongue to activate the swallow.	
• Activities to encourage Michelle to initiate transitions into high levels of chewing and cup drinking.	• Michelle will use the above movement patterns to transition into chewing and cup drinking.	

Figure 17 Speech treatment planning worksheet.

Name of Patient: Michelle   **Date:**   **Therapist:**   Diane Fritts Ryan

Functional Goal – *taken from Assessment or Progress Note*	Impairment List - *Prioritize Impairments Relative to Functional Limitation*
Michelle will reach overhead for a toy with either hand while independently floor sitting.	• UE and LE ROM Limitations (scapula-humeral, trunk lateral and rotational muscles, hip extensors) • Decreased mobility of thoracic spine • Decreased activity in abdominals • Decreased pelvic-femoral disassociation and stability • Decreased scapula depression/upward rotation with humeral flexion with trunk extension • Decreased active trunk extension with humeral flexion

Treatment

Interventions - *Sequence strategies relative to prioritized impairments*	Expected Outcome - *for each intervention*	Effectiveness *(Do you need to adapt, revise or eliminate the strategy?)*
• Activities to promote ROM and mobility to UEs, Trunk and LEs • Activities to improve trunk extension with UEs free for reach in prone, sidelying, sitting while inhibiting LE extension • Activities to improve trunk extension with scapula depression shoulder flexion and external rotation using WS and WS with reach in prone, plantigrade, and sitting • Activities to encourage exploration of toys using both hands while posture is supported • Assistive device to encourage UE and hand development while supporting upright sitting posture until independent sitting is achieved	• Full passive range of motion in lateral spine scapula- humeral, shoulder, elbow and wrist muscles • Reach with assisted trunk extension • Weight bearing and reach with assisted trunk extension • Both upper extremities/hands engaging in play with neck flexion and downward visual gaze, shoulder girdle depression and neutral rotation	

Figure 18 Occupational treatment planning worksheet.

Name of Patient: **Michelle** Date: _____ Therapist: **Gay L. Girolami**

Functional Goal – *taken from Assessment or Progress Note*

Michelle will independently stand to play at a small table.

Impairment List - *Prioritize Impairments Relative to Functional Limitation*

- UE and LE ROM Limitations
- Decreased strength of Trunk and U & LE muscle groups
- Increased muscle tone in all extremities
- Decreased spinal and pelvic mobility
- Decreased ability to initiate, sustain, and control muscle activity for unilateral forward shoulder flexion, elbow extension, and wrist ext.
- Decreased ability to initiate, sustain, and control muscle activity for unilateral hip flexion, knee flexion and ankle dorsiflexion

Treatment

Interventions - *Sequence strategies relative to prioritized impairments*

- Activities to promote ROM and mobility in the UEs, Trunk and LEs
- Activities to improve trunk stability and rotation in prone, sitting, modified four point and standing
- Combine improved ROM and rotation with weight bearing and reaching activities in prone, sitting, modified four point, and standing
- Activities to increase activation and agonist/antagonist control of upper and lower extremities in prone, sitting, modified four point and standing
- Weight shifting activities in prone, sitting, modified four point, and standing to improve ability to initiate and sustain muscle activity for weight bearing, reaching and rotation activities
- Activities to encourage Michelle to initiate weight shifting, reaching in prone, sitting, modified four point and standing
- Activities to encourage Michelle to initiate transitions into and out of prone, sitting, modified four point, and standing.

Expected Outcome - *for each intervention*

- Increased joint mobility and muscle length in trunk, upper/lower extremities
- Increased ability to sustain muscle activity in the upper extremities and trunk in all postures
- Improved ability to reach in all planes of movement while sustaining postures in sitting, four point and standing
- Improved ability to initiate movement in the upper and lower extremities for transitions, reaching, and lower extremity weight bearing
- Improved ability to initiate upper and lower extremity movements for weight shifting outside the base of support without losing balance
- Improved lower extremity disassociation for crawling, half-kneeling and standing

Effectiveness (*Do you need to adapt, revise or eliminate the strategy?*)

Figure 19 Physical therapy treatment planning worksheet.

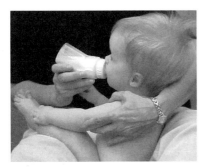

Figure 20 Michelle is placed in a flexed sitting position, inhibiting abnormal extension of the body. Symmetrical head and neck elongation is maintained. The therapist inhibits shoulder elevation and internal rotation, humeral extension. This promotes expansion of upper chest. An "upright" bottle is used to maintain a forward gravity posture of the tongue for sucking and effective swallowing pattern.

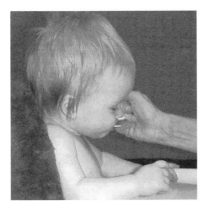

Figure 21 Michelle is placed in a high chair seat with an abductor between her legs to encourage an upright sitting position. Two small rolls are placed behind her shoulders to inhibit retraction and extension of the shoulders. Once Michelle is actively using a "chin tuck" head posture with a stable jaw, the spoon is placed on the lower lip in a horizontal position. Michelle is encouraged to suck the food off the spoon with her upper lip. The therapist continues to integrate lip closure skills and jaw stability.

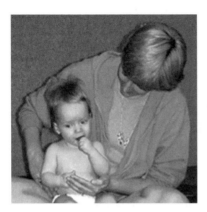

Figure 22 In order to promote full integration of skills previously discussed, Michelle is placed in her mother's lap. Mother is inhibiting external rotation of shoulders, while Michelle is independently placing small pieces of cereal in the lateral portion of the bucal area of the mouth. Michelle is demonstrating a dynamic use of capital head flexion, jaw stability, lip closure, and little overflow of spasticity in extremities. She is also maintaining regular respiratory pattern during eating.

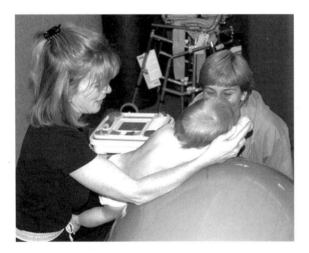

Figure 23 This position focuses on elongation of scapulo-humeral and lateral trunk muscles. The ball provides a mobile surface to use the infant's body weight shifting over laterally and back to midline. Gentle traction through the upper extremity is applied. This gradually increases humeral external rotation and flexion, elbow extension, and supination, elongating muscles throughout the upper extremity. The therapist uses her other hand to dissociate the lower extremities and inhibit the hip extension/adduction pattern to allow for greater elongation and activation through the trunk.

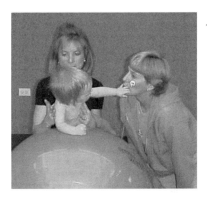

Figure 24 From the elongation of muscles in Figure 23, we now progress to increase activation of trunk and shoulder girdle in this sidelying position with forward reach. The therapist's hands assist to maintain alignment and elongation through the trunk and shoulder girdle, while also assisting with weight shifting in the frontal plane. The therapist watches for Michelle to activate lateral head lifting and reaching with the opposite upper extremity. Again, the therapist's front hand is also positioned to dissociate the lower extremities and inhibit increased muscle tone. Mom is an ideal "sticker board" to entice Michelle to reach and weight shift forward toward midline.

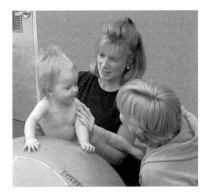

Figure 25 Michelle pushes onto extended arm weight bearing, requiring increased elongation on the weight-bearing side as well as increased humeral extension. Activation of wrist and finger extensors is possible. Depression of the less-weighted humerus assists Michelle in midline orientation of her head and beginning activation of shoulder depressors, giving her "more neck." This series shown in Figures 23–25 should be repeated to both sides.

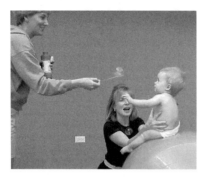

Figure 26 Michelle is now sitting on the ball with the therapist's hand assisting in alignment and weight shifting of the trunk over the pelvis in the frontal plane. The therapist uses her forearms to maintain abduction and neutral rotation of the lower extremities to enhance trunk activity. Michelle reaches up and out with one arm as the therapist uses her index finger to inhibit excessive scapula movement. The other extremity is inhibited by the therapist in a position of humeral external rotation and depression. This assists in trunk alignment and stability as well as upper extremity dissociation. Michelle begins to experience an erect trunk with arms free to reach out in space. This should be repeated on both sides.

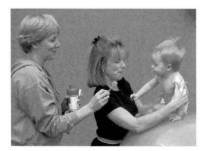

Figure 27 Michelle is combining trunk extension with forward reach of right hand, while also beginning to weigh bear on left arm. The therapist controls the left humeral alignment in neutral rotation and elbow extension as well as trunk extension. This requires a subtle lateral weight shift toward the left hip. The weight shift and reaching activity from Michelle also activates scapula depression and scapula trunk musculature as well as elbow, wrist, and finger extension. This should be repeated to both sides.

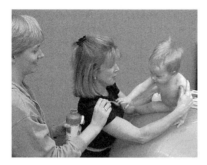

Figure 28 With further weight shift to the left side, Michelle is now reaching out of her base of support, which is preparatory for transitions. This activity also increases the demands throughout the muscles of the left scapula, shoulder, and lower arm and hand. Mom is directing Michelle's vision and reach of the right arm forward and across midline with her head in a neutral position. This placement assists in actively lengthening the cervical extensors and shoulder elevators.

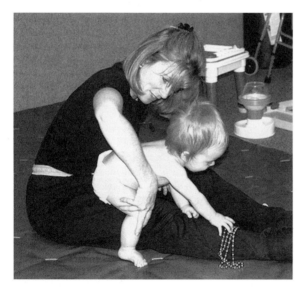

Figure 29 Here is another position to combine trunk extension with active shoulder flexion and elbow extension in the arms. This time Michelle is reaching bilaterally to the therapist's leg, which serves as a surface that encourages wrist extension. Michelle is moving her extended trunk over the pelvis anteriorly with beginning weight through the lower extremities and feet.

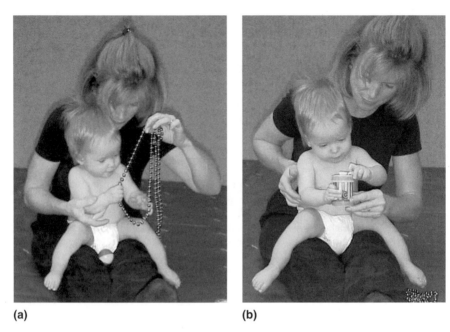

(a)   (b)

Figure 30 These two photos demonstrate Michelle freeing both hands in midline while supported in sitting on the therapist's lap. It is important for Michelle to experience more upright positioning while using both hands to reach and explore objects. The therapist's hands encourage alignment of the humerus in neutral rotation and depression from Michelle's lower arm using slight downward traction. The therapist is also assisting forearm rotation to maximize visual motor exploration of the object (a). In (b), the therapist uses even less assist to align upper trunk and arm by minimally adducting Michelle's shoulder. Michelle is able to control her alignment and activate appropriate head, trunk, and shoulder muscles on her own. The therapist assists in stabilizing the toy in Michelle's hand for increased wrist extension, as Michelle is not able to shape her right hand around this object independently yet. The pelvis is slightly posteriorly tilted in these activities because Michelle is still unable to incorporate full trunk extension with bilateral fine motor tasks. However, visual motor and upper body control are improved. Future sessions should continue to link bilateral hand and visual motor function with erect floor or bench sitting.

specific goals are also included on the form and these goals will provide a baseline to measure progress and achievement of the identified functional outcomes.

The initial treatment plan should be developed and discussed with the family. The plan may need to be modified to accommodate the family's priorities and resources. The Initial Treatment Plan created for Michelle can be found in Figure 2.

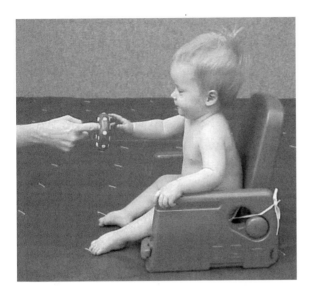

Figure 31 This photo illustrates a possibility for Michelle to experience both arms free for play in a stable, upright sitting position. Here, gravity will assist Michelle in shoulder depression, as well as support to the trunk and pelvis. The tray provides a surface for Michelle to get experience with age-appropriate tabletop visual motor tasks. This will assist in the development of reach with a more erect trunk, but also further the development of hand function and independent play. As independent sitting and reaching improve, the chair would no longer be necessary.

1. Treatment Planning Worksheet

After developing the Initial Treatment Plan, each therapist must then develop a discipline-specific intervention protocol. The Treatment Planning Worksheet is a tool for the therapist to use in completing this aspect of the intervention process. Ideally, a separate Treatment Planning Worksheet is filled in for each goal. The therapist then identifies and prioritizes the impairments associated with each goal and develops a sequence of treatment strategies to address the impairments. These strategies are intended to assist the infant to eventually achieve the identified functional goals.

Next to each treatment strategy is a space to describe the intended outcome of each intervention. After each session, the therapist can also use this worksheet to document effectiveness of the strategies or revisions that should be made prior to the next treatment session. Figure 17 to 19 provide examples of this process using one of the speech (Fig. 17), occupational (Fig. 18), and physical (Fig. 19) therapy goals written for Michelle. In addition, Figures 20–46 show discipline-

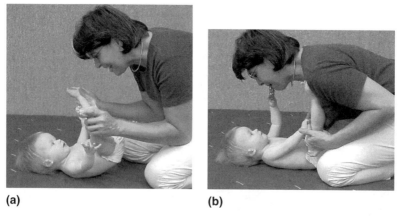

(a)   **(b)**

Figure 32 Therapy begins with two activities to alter Michelle's extended lower extremity posture and to lengthen the hip adductors, internal rotators, and hamstrings. These supine activities also encourage elongation of the cervical extensors, and with side-to-side weight shifting improve activation of the muscles around the trunk. Michelle enjoys this position and begins to interact with the therapist, reaching out to grasp a toy.

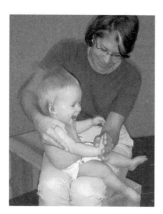

Figure 33 With increased mobility, activities in sitting are used to continue anterior-posterior pelvic mobility and add lateral weight shifting to increase activation of muscles in the trunk and pelvis. These sitting activities are combined with preparation of the right upper extremity for weight bearing. While maintaining the infant's shoulder and arm in a position of shoulder depression, forward flexion, and external rotation, along with elbow and wrist extension, this activity uses joint compression and deep pressure to improve sensory awareness and increase muscle length and muscle activity in the upper extremities.

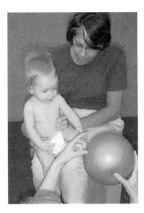

Figure 34 Following preparation of the trunk and upper extremities, we observe improved trunk and pelvic mobility and decreased shoulder elevation. The lower extremity extensor pattern has also decreased with the improved trunk and pelvic position and increased muscle activity in the trunk. Play activities are introduced to elicit active trunk rotation and forward reaching.

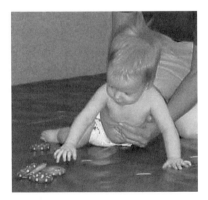

Figure 35 To build on previous trunk mobility and upper extremity preparation for weight bearing, a side sitting position is used to add the additional component of lower extremity dissociation. Here, we see interest in reaching with the more involved right upper extremity, while maintaining a position of good left upper extremity weight bearing and lower extremity dissociation.

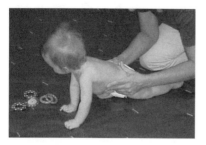

Figure 36 By assisting Michelle to shift her weight forward, the transition to bilateral upper extremity weight bearing can be made. This increases muscle activity in the shoulder girdle, trunk, and pelvis by encouraging weight shifting and reaching in various planes. This position can also be used to improve range of motion of the hip flexors.

specific treatment sequences for the goals identified on the three Treatment Planning Worksheets.

2. Treatment Strategies

Once the sequence of treatment strategies for each goal has been identified, a Treatment Strategy Worksheet should be developed for each strategy. This worksheet is designed to assist the therapist in considering all the elements necessary to produce treatment strategy. These elements reflect considerations relevant to the infant, the therapist, and the environment. Using this worksheet permits the

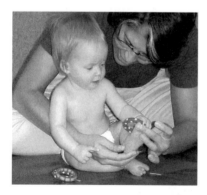

Figure 37 In this sequence (see Figs. 38 and 39), we are ready to challenge the motor activity achieved earlier in treatment in a more antigravity position. First, improved hip external rotation and ankle dorsiflexion range of motion must be achieved.

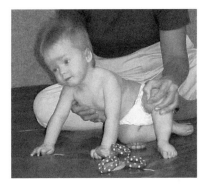

Figure 38 Michelle is assisted into a position of upper extremity weight bearing with increased hip external rotation and ankle dorsiflexion. Improved range of motion and muscle activity in the hip and ankle are facilitated by guiding weight shifting in various planes. Joint compression is applied to enhance proprioceptive awareness and increased weight bearing in the lower limb and foot.

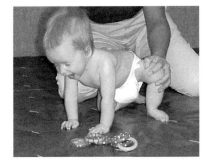

Figure 39 Using play to motivate a forward weight shift, Michelle is able to achieve a position of bilateral upper extremity weight bearing and lower extremity hip dissociation and weight bearing on the left foot. To enhance muscle activity, Michelle should be guided through and encouraged to initiate weight shifting. Side-to-side weight shifting will improve muscle activity around the shoulder girdle and increase hip abduction in both hips, as well as hip external rotation and ankle dorsiflexion in the leg that is weight bearing through the foot.

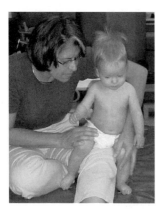

Figure 40 Moving to a sitting position, it is possible to continue to provide weight bearing and improve range of motion in the lower extremities. It is easier to control the weight bearing when one foot is prepared at a time. We also see decreased shoulder elevation and improved spinal extension, secondary to the modified four-point activities practiced earlier.

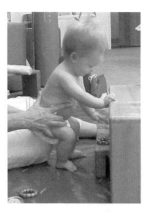

Figure 41 After weight bearing and range of motion have been prepared in the feet and ankles, it is combined with activities to improve pelvic mobility and forward weight shifting in preparation for standing. Here, Michelle's pelvis is maintained in forward flexion, but a toy is used to motivate her to shift her weight forward. This enhances activation of the lower extremity muscles in a more flexed pattern that will allow Michelle to eventually achieve a standing posture without pushing back into extension, her pattern of choice.

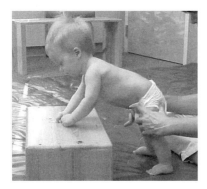

Figure 42 With this motivation to weight shift forward, Michelle is able to achieve a bear-standing posture. This reinforces the upper extremity weight bearing and combines this with work in the shoulder girdle, trunk, and lower extremities. You will note that her feet are strongly "pushing" (increased plantarflexor activity) into the support surface for stability. Since her range of motion has been prepared, this posturing is indicative of her instability in this position. This demonstrates a common strategy, which we all may use in novel situations (i.e., stiffening joints to decrease the amount of available movement). For treatment purposes, this posture can be used as a benchmark. As Michelle's lower extremity strength and ability to control and activate lower extremity muscle groups improves the toe clawing and overactivity of the plantarflexors will decrease.

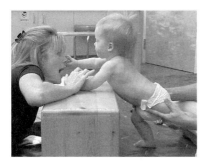

Figure 43 To decrease the overactivity in the plantarflexors, Michelle must be provided with other means to achieve and sustain her postural stability. This can often be achieved by facilitating movement. As Michelle reaches forward, the weight shift requires more activation of muscle activity in the shoulder girdle, trunk, and lower extremities. For the treating therapist, it is often easier insure optimal weight bearing and to guide the eccentric/concentric muscle activity at the hip, knee, and ankle by working with one lower extremity at a time. This also reinforces the hip dissociation and assists Michelle in realizing that her lower extremities can work independently of each other.

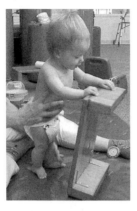

Figure 44 Moving into standing and using a mobile support surface, Michelle must continue to anticipate and plan new strategies to sustain the antigravity posture. She appears relaxed and enjoys rocking the bench while standing. Again you will note the tendency to revert to the increased plantarflexor activity indicative of the need for continued practice in this position.

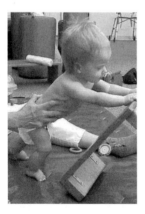

Figure 45 Once again, the treatment strategy of lower extremity dissociation is employed. This increases Michelle's awareness that her lower extremities can initiate and sustain different muscle activities and must not always function as a unit. Additionally, this posture can be used to increase hip flexor and plantarflexor range of motion in the extended (left) lower extremity, while encouraging muscle grading and control in the forward, flexed lower extremity.

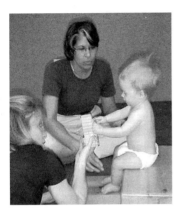

Figure 46 In this last photo, Michelle is given the opportunity to practice the skills that have been worked on in speech, occupational, and physical therapy. Following her therapy, Michelle is able to sit independently while playing with a toy. We observe improved sitting posture with good cervical flexion, mouth closure, decreased shoulder elevation, and the ability to sustain a position of lower extremity hip and knee flexion while using the upper extremities to reach forward for the toy. It is extremely important to provide these play opportunities to allow Michelle to practice and incorporate new skills and improve her body awareness.

therapist to analyze the success of each strategy and systematically determine which aspects to alter in order to improve the intervention and achieve the desired functional outcomes.

Figures 47–49 are examples of three discipline-specific treatment strategies. Each figure illustrates this process for one of the identified strategies listed on the Treatment Planning Worksheets.

Over time, the novice therapist will develop a repertoire of intervention strategies that can be applied with some modifications for infants with similar impairments and identified functional outcomes. Eventually, with experience, the therapist will be able to perform this process with minimal effort.

D. Charting Progress

The daily and progress note templates in Chapter 8 could be used to chart information related to Michelle's daily treatments and progress over time. Since this case study represents a single multidisciplinary assessment and one treatment session, these forms are not included in this chapter.

Goal: Michelle will be spoon-fed in 15 minutes, while maintaining proper postural alignment

ELEMENT	DESCRIPTION	RATIONALE/EXPLANATION
Impairment: Specific Impairment being addressed	Poor timing and sequencing of respiratory and oral-motor skills.	Michelle has difficulty timing her suck swallow with her respiratory pattern, which results in feeding taking a long time.
Anticipated results of this strategy	Michelle will sit in good alignment of head and trunk during spoon-feeding. She will eat the required amount of food by spoon in 15 minutes or less.	Michelle will lean how to use capital flexion or a "chin tuck" to swallow more effectively. This should inhibit the neck extension and shoulder elevation.
Patient: Starting position, including Center of Gravity (COG) and Base of Support (BOS), WB/NWB areas, as well as other critical aspects.	Michelle will be in a flexed position in the therapist's lap. Then moved to an adapted high chair. Then sitting on mom's legs on the floor.	Varying the location of this strategy from lap, in very inhibiting position, to supported high chair and then back to mom's lap with lighter inhibition. This will show Michelle that she can carry over the strategy in a variety of places and people. Then she won't get stuck with only one feeder, and one way to be fed.
Equipment/supplies Position of equipment.	Shallow bowl spoon with correct diameter for Michelle size of mouth. Adapted high chair that fits Michelle well. Stage 2 food, and cheerios.	"Sit Right" insert is placed in base of the chair with two small rolls placed in the sides of the chair.
Desired response: • parts of the body involved in the activity • direction/plane/axis/speed of the movement • mobile/stable segments • desired muscle activity	Michelle will use her head movement independent of the rest of her body. She will be able to use her tongue and lips off her jaw, which will serve as the base of stability.	As jaw stability is taken over by Michelle, place the spoon on the lower lip to make her use more isolated lip movement to remove food.
Therapist: Starting position, including COG and BOS	The therapist will sit Michelle in her lap with Michelle facing her mother.	Start in the most controlled position to learn new movement pattern and gradually reduce control to Michelle to use.
Movement of the therapist: • anticipated direction and plane of motion	The therapist begins with strong inhibition and gradually reduces tactile input to cueing and Michelle takes over the movement. Food is presented at a regular rate to allow for the swallow. Gradually increasing the rate to improve timing of suck-swallow response with the food.	Teach Michelle to use a normal oral-motor pattern synchronized with a regular breathing pattern.
Handling: • Keypoints of control; direction and firmness of pressure; timing and other aspects of input. • Tactile/proprioceptive modalities *(e.g.) pressure, tapping traction, approximation, vibration, use of temperature*	• Michelle will be placed in the therapist's lap or adapted seating position. Make sure that Michelle is in a position to prevent abnormal extension of the body and facilitate flexion in the knees, hips, trunk and head. Center her head and maintain neck elongation.	Show Michelle how to use a "chin tuck" movement with only slight head flexion to swallow more effectively.

• Use a shallow bowled spoon. Place the bowl of the spoon on the tongue and push inward gently. Partially close the jaw with inward pressure on the chin. Allow for a closed mouth. Wait for slight flexion of the head. Then withdraw the spoon with slight downward movement of the spoon. (With bilateral lip closure.) When Michelle starts using the "chin tuck" on her own, place the spoon horizontal to her lips (This is only done after jaw stability has been established.) Place the spoon on the lower lip and allow Michelle to suck the food off with her upper lip. Continue to integrate lip closure skills and jaw stability with rapid feeding rate.	Use spoon to stabilize the jaw, and inhibit extensor patterns through Michelle's neck to allow normal lip and tongue movement to move food to the swallow.
• Give Michelle independent practice using finger foods (small dissolvable piece of cereal). Use the positioning techniques discussed and allow her to put small pieces in the side of her mouth. Use jaw stability to munch on foods. Wait for lip closure. Place the food in the buccal area of the mouth to encourage lateral tongue mobility, and independent jaw stability.	As jaw stability is taken over by Michelle, place spoon on the lower lip to make her use more isolated lip movement to remove the food. Allow Michelle to repeat the strategy with other food, to improve carry-over of motor planning. Also it will prepare her for goals in cup drinking and finger feeding.
Other sensory input *(E.g. auditory, verbal cues, visual, vestibular, as well as taste and smell.)*	Auditory reinforcement of "good job." Feed Michelle foods that taste and smell good, at temperatures she likes.	Things that taste good to her easily motivate Michelle. Sometimes distractibility is a good thing when working on timing of the swallow.

Figure 47 Speech therapy treatment strategy worksheet. Goal: Michelle will be spoonfed in 15 mins, while maintaining proper postural alignment.

ELEMENT	DESCRIPTION	RATIONALE/EXPLANATION
Impairment: _Specific Impairment being addressed_	-Decreased activity in abdominals -Decreased active trunk extension with humeral flexion	
Anticipated results of this strategy	Improved ability to sit erect and reach forward	Infant compensates with UE position as part of the postural system. UE have not developed ROM or motor control for reaching.
Patient: Starting position, including COG and BOS, WB/NWB areas, as well as other critical aspects.	Sitting on the ball with LEs abducted and E.R.	This position assists in inhibiting increased muscle tone and maintaining alignment in LE which assists in trunk alignment over the pelvis.
Equipment/supplies Position of equipment.	Large therapy ball, firm	Easy to impose WS in many directions and give the infant the feeling of the movement through the pelvis.
Desired response: • parts of the body involved in the activity • direction/plane/axis/speed of the movement • mobile/stable segments desired muscle activity	Reach forward 90° while being shifted slightly to lateral hip (this is done to both sides)	Needed for beginning ability to reach overhead while maintaining independent sitting.
Therapist: Starting position, including COG and BOS	In front of infant on tall knees with one hand on the infant's non-reaching humerus; the other hand widely spread along the infant's ribs to pelvis of the infant's reaching hand with firm pressure down stabilizing the infant symmetrically on the ball.	Visual contact with the infant while discouraging neck hyperextension as well as being a good biomechanical position to impose handling strategies.
Movement of the therapist: • anticipated direction and plane of motion	Lateral WS over the pelvis and hip with traction down through both of therapist's hands into infant's pelvis.	
Handling: • Keypoints of control; direction and firmness of pressure; timing and other aspects of input. • Tactile/proprioceptive modalities _(e.g.) pressure, tapping traction, approximation, vibration, use of temperature_	- One hand externally rotating and depressing non-reaching shoulder; other hand widely spread along the infant's ribs to pelvis of the infant's reaching hand with firm pressure downward to stabilize the infant on the ball. - Time the lateral WS on the ball with the presentation of the bubbles (guiding mom to hold the wand slightly lateral, up and where infant's hand would contact when elbow is straight. Therapist uses the non-reaching hand of the infant in the amount of E.R. necessary to assist with trunk extension and alignment to be maintained in primarily the frontal plane as the infant is laterally shifted to the pelvis of the reaching hand. - Then the infant is brought back to midline. This is repeated a few times to each side.	-Maintains alignment before initiating movement and during the movement as well. -Proper timing allows the infant's reach to assist in initiating WS through the pelvis as well as functionally pairing the movement with the infant's play intention. -This will assist with trunk extension and alignment being maintained in primarily the frontal plane.
Other sensory input _(e.g. auditory, verbal cues, visual, vestibular, as well as taste and smell.)_	Visual and auditory cue from mom with the bubbles to direct reach, head and trunk and WS. Placement and timing as discussed prior.	Infant is easy to motivate with age appropriate play/interaction but timing and placement is important for success with treatment strategy and building movement into body scheme.

Figure 48 Occupational therapy treatment strategy worksheet. Goal: Michelle will reach overhead for a toy with either hand while independently floor sitting.

ELEMENT	DESCRIPTION	RATIONALE/EXPLANATION
Impairment: *Specific impairment being addressed* 60%	Over activity of the extensor muscles of knees and ankles causes decreased ability to initiate and control agonist/antagonist muscle activity around the hip, knee and ankle joints. This over activity also contributes to joint range limitations and decreased range of motion of the hips flexors, hamstrings and gastrocsoleus muscle groups.	The over activity of the extensor muscle groups of the lower extremity causes Michelle's center of mass to be shifted backward. To sustain a standing position, Michelle compensates by flexing forward at the hips. This compromises her standing balance and interferes with the development of independent standing.
Anticipated results of this strategy:	In standing, Michelle will demonstrate improved alignment of the trunk, hip and knees and weight bear symmetrically on both feet.	For Michelle to develop standing balance, she needs to independently sustain adequate postural alignment and maintain an improved base of support including feet flat on the floor.
Patient: Starting position, including COG and BOS, WB/NWB areas, as well as other critical aspects.	Michelle will be encouraged to play at a bench that requires her to use upper extremity support and to stand with mild hip and knee flexion and ankle dorsiflexion. Her base of support will be her upper extremities and her feet. Her center of mass should be over her feet with the knees flexed in from the COM and the hips behind.	When knee extension and ankle plantarflexion are strong and cause balance to be compromised, it is easier to treat in a semi-flexed position rather than upright standing. The flexed position requires concentric/eccentric muscle activity at the hips, knees and ankles. The height of the bench must be carefully selected to insure that hip and knee flexion is adequate to make activation of the extensor muscles difficult, but not too low to cause over activity of the flexor muscles.

Figure 49 Physical therapy treatment strategy worksheet. Goal: Michelle will independently stand to play at a small table.

ELEMENT	DESCRIPTION	RATIONALE/EXPLANATION
Equipment/supplies Position of equipment.	A small bench to provide upper extremity support and a play surface. Toys to engage Michelle and increase the time spent playing at the bench. Toy should be large enough to easily manipulate. Perhaps bean bags for tossing or cars for rolling. If the play tasks are too difficult, this may affect the ability to play and control lower extremity muscle activity.	The bench is used to create an optimal starting posture for the treatment strategy (see above) and also to provide a support surface for the upper extremities and toys. When part of the weight is distributed to the upper extremities, the weight on the lower extremities is decreased. This makes it easier to activate the LE muscles in more optimal patterns of eccentric and concentric control.
Desired response: • parts of the body involved in the activity • direction/plane/axis/speed of the movement • mobile/stable segments • desired muscle activity	Facilitate and guide A/P and side to side weight shifting in supported standing with feet symmetrical and in a reciprocal position. This activity is directed toward increasing joint flexibility at the hip, knee and ankle. It will also improve Michelle's ability to grade hip, knee, ankle flexion and extension. The speed of the movement and the amount of flexion and extension should be guided by the therapist in response to the child's ability.	This weight shifting will result in reciprocal activation of the muscles at the hip, knees and ankle. The weight shifting and reciprocal foot placement will increase the range of the hip flexors, hamstrings and plantarflexors on the leg that is extended backward. Additionally, this activity will result in activation of shoulder girdle and trunk muscles to sustain the upper body posture. The lower extremities will be most actively involved, but the trunk and shoulder girdle must also be active.
Therapist: Starting position, including COG and BOS	Behind Michelle kneeling or sitting. The therapist's COM should be over the BOS to allow weight shifting in any direction without loss of balance.	Sitting on the knees offers the therapist more opportunity to move in any direction, but it is often difficult to sustain this posture for long periods. If the therapist sits, it is important to choose a sitting position that allows mobility. Long sitting is very difficult because of the therapist's own range limitations.

Figure 49　Continued.

ELEMENT	DESCRIPTION	RATIONALE/EXPLANATION
Movement of the therapist: • anticipated direction and plane of motion	Therapist should be in a position to easily initiate both anterior/posterior and side to side weight shifts as these movements are facilitated and guided in the child.	When the therapist moves in tandem with the child it is easier to guide and facilitate the child's movement. This tandem movement creates a harmony between the therapist and child.
Handling: • Key points of control; direction and firmness of pressure; timing and other aspects of input. • Tactile/proprioceptive modalities *(e.g. pressure, tapping traction, approximation, vibration, use of temperature)*	When employing this strategy with the lower extremities in a reciprocal position, handling might be directed through the pelvis and one lower extremity. This allows the therapist to provide input and guidance to maintain pelvic alignment in all planes and to provide proprioceptive input into the base of support. The extended lower leg is used to direct weight shifting and maintain alignment of the lower extremity joints.	Using the pelvis and lower extremity as key points allows the therapist to assist the child to learn how to maintain the COM over the BOS and sustain balance and postural control. Additionally these two key points provide the optimal hand placement to maintain proper spine and pelvic alignment, as well as lower extremity alignment and weight-bearing. The child can be guided to experience and respond to movement in all planes.
Other sensory input: *(e.g. auditory/verbal cues, visual, vestibular, as well as taste and smell)*	Sensory input might include auditory cues that indicate the desired direction of the movement rather than how to move an extremity or body part. For example "Get the car on the floor," rather than "Bend your knees." The visual system can be accessed by strategically placing the toys to cue the child regarding the direction of weight shift.	By using auditory cues that provide goal directed suggestions, the therapist can optimize handling by providing the child with suggestions for movement without directly telling her to bend or straighten or weight shift. Children with neurological conditions often have difficulty isolating and initiating specific movements, but can more easily respond to a play-related goal. The verbal cues can be enhanced by visual cues that emphasize the direction or goal of the movement. That is, where you place the play activity can enhance the functional outcome of your treatment strategy.

Figure 49 Continued.

E. Summary

This case study demonstrates the assessment and treatment planning process detailed in Chapters 6 to 8. Templates have been provided to guide the therapist through the thought process of organizing and analyzing the assessment data and developing a sequence of intervention strategies based on the identified impairments and goals.

Michelle continues to receive physical and occupational therapy twice a week and speech therapy once a week. She has made progress toward all of her identified goals and her treating therapists continue to use this assessment and treatment planning process to chart progress and update goals and intervention strategies. Michelle is an excellent example of the effectiveness of early identification and intervention, and of how careful assessment and treatment planning can improve the functional outcome for children with cerebral palsy.

10

Research in Cerebral Palsy
Yesterday and Today

Charlene Butler
Health and Special Education Consultant, Seattle, Washington

As we learned in the first chapter of this book, only 50 years ago there was little understanding of, or attention to, cerebral palsy in the United States. It was in 1947 that a group of six physicians met in Chicago to promote academic and scientific discourse on cerebral palsy by forming the organization that eventually became the American Academy for Cerebral Palsy and Developmental Medicine (AACPDM). These six men from different medical backgrounds—neurology, neurosurgery, pediatrics, orthopedic surgery, and physical medicine—recognized the importance of pooling resources and ideas from their respective fields. With that far-reaching mindset, they laid the groundwork for an important model of interdisciplinary collaboration that eventually expanded to include physical, occupational and speech therapy, special education, psychology, and bioengineering—and grew to include a significant international membership.

Almost immediately, the formation of the AACPDM led to an on going emergence of new ideas about treatment. These ideas arose from the increasing involvement of clinicians in the many disciplines who became interested in moving the field forward by exploring new methods that might enhance the quality of life for children with cerebral palsy. Applying their evolving understanding of physiological and developmental processes, they formulated innovative approaches to the treatment and management of this complex disorder.

I. EVOLUTION OF TREATMENTS

A wide variety of approaches were proposed and pursued by the different specialists without validation by scientific investigation. In the rush to be helpful, there was a tendency to want to believe in and adopt recent treatments. These new ideas were promoted by well-intentioned practitioners and often appeared to make a lot of sense, based on the current understanding of physiology and developmental theory. Many of these ideas were based on medical treatments that had been successful in other conditions, such as polio. Some were new approaches, often named for their originators (e.g., Bobath, Rood, Vojta, Doman-Delacato), whose charismatic personalities were instrumental in widespread acceptance of unproven therapies. Other approaches employed adaptive equipment and, later, assistive technology.

The thrust of intervention changed as time went by. Late diagnosis and intervention of a predominantly orthopedic nature (i.e., surgery and bracing) gave way to early identification and early intervention programs of a multidisciplinary nature but with an educational orientation.

By the 1960s, the neuromaturational theory of development was guiding assumptions made about motor development and control, as well as proposed interventions (1). Neurodevelopmental therapy (also known as NDT and the Bobath method) derived from this neuromaturational perspective and has dominated physical, occupational, and speech therapies (2). Other predominant approaches, based on this perspective, include Rood's sensorimotor approach, proprioceptive neuromuscular facilitation (PNF), and Ayres' sensory integration (SI) therapy. These interventions attempted to promote typical developmental progressions and to inhibit abnormal reflexes, tone, and movement patterns.

More recently, neuromaturational principles are being reexamined in the light of contemporary systems theories (3). Dynamic systems theory, for example, is being advanced as an alternative way to explain and describe child development and has begun to influence therapeutic evaluation and treatment. Instead of viewing motor development as the unfolding of prescribed patterns in the central nervous system, the central nervous system is seen as only one component of motor development and control. Organization of motor control depends on the interactive relationships among child, task, and environmental variables. Assessments of tasks and environments, therefore, are as important as assessments of the child. Interventions occur within the context of functional activities and may focus on the child, task, or environment. Treatment principles emphasize age-appropriate, goal-directed tasks; practice; transfer of learning; and timing of feedback.

II. ABSENCE OF SCIENTIFIC VALIDATION

Attention turned increasingly toward research; but circumstances led to relatively little pursuit of treatment outcome studies. One obstacle was a general reluctance to withhold any treatment that might help. This reluctance was coupled with little demand from parents, third-party payers, or practitioners for hard evidence of efficacy. Moreover, the rigorously controlled studies that are necessary to establish efficacy of an intervention are especially difficult to accomplish in this population. As a consequence, researchers focused on other important questions about the causes and incidence of cerebral palsy, prognosis, and diagnosis. These questions could be answered appropriately with analytical, correlational and other types of studies that are more easily accomplished than controlled trials needed for definitive answers about treatment outcomes. The efficacy studies that were conducted tended to be anecdotal or descriptive in nature, without control groups, and composed of small numbers of children. The larger group studies were hampered by lack of clear definition of subjects within the general diagnosis of cerebral palsy and by the heterogeneity of subjects within the samples. Subjects with varying degrees of severity and type of abnormal movement, other impairments commonly associated with cerebral palsy, a range of cognitive ability, and age span from infant to adult often comprise the sample of "cerebral palsy." There were also mechanical limitations of sorting and analyzing data in the years before computer capability was widely available.

As a result of the reluctance to withhold treatment, the lack of demand for scientific evidence of efficacy, and the relative difficulty of doing efficacy studies, the value of treatment approaches in cerebral palsy through the years has been more extolled than proven. Despite convincing scientific evidence of their effectiveness—or lack thereof—some interventions became the standard of care while others came to be regarded as "alternative" or "controversial." Still others disappeared altogether. Therefore, the issue of which treatments should be pursued has been contentious between specialists who held opposing views, tempered with varying degrees of skepticism. Parents, faced with conflicting recommendations, have had to pursue appropriate intervention through faith in their child's doctors, therapists, or teachers, rather than on the basis of scientific validation of efficacy.

III. INCREASING INTEREST IN TREATMENT OUTCOMES RESEARCH

By the mid-1980s, however, increased interest and focus on the importance of scientific research about treatment outcomes began to be apparent. Clinicians interested in moving the field forward pursued postgraduate training in research methodology. The AACPDM began offering instructional courses in research methodology to help clinicians understand the issues and problems in conducting research and how to interpret the results of research studies. Papers selected for presentation at the meetings of the academy were also required to reflect research rather than "show and tell" about treatments being explored.

A scientifically cautious approach to the adoption of new treatments appeared in meetings and publications. Practitioners were urged to temper their enthusiasm for new theories or treatments until their efficacy could be subjected to scientific scrutiny. For example, when selective dorsal rhizotomy, a new treatment for reducing spasticity was reported in 1982, there was a sense of urgency in the clinical and research community that it be validated before it became an accepted practice (4). Investigation of selective dorsal rhizotomy was organized and undertaken by a variety of different investigators as quickly as possible.

IV. EVIDENCE-BASED HEALTH CARE MOVEMENT

Health care, in general, has been undergoing a paradigm shift in recent years. Coincident with this shift, research in the field of cerebral palsy has increasingly focused on investigations of treatment outcomes. In the past, medical practice has been primarily based on expert opinion supported by an understanding of basic mechanisms of disease or physiology and on extensive, but uncontrolled, clinical observations (5). The new paradigm is evidence-based practice. This is the integration of clinical expertise with the best available clinical evidence from systematic research (6). It is characterized by knowledge of treatment outcomes based on research and on involving individual patient's rights and preferences in making clinical decisions about their health care.

Adults with disabilities and parents of children with disabilities, through political advocacy, have transformed the potential of lives of people with disabilities by bringing them into the mainstream of family and community life. People with disabilities, therefore, need treatment programs that improve their ability to participate in activities in normal settings. They have been increasingly vocal that their medical care should target improved function.

Fiscal pressures are also fueling this paradigm shift in developmental medicine. The abundance of resources in the United States and the western industrial nations has created the circumstance that all interventions that might possibly benefit a child have been implemented. Now, however, there is increasing demand from politicians, economists, and payers to provide the ''best'' treatment for the least amount of money. At the same time, developing countries, where resources are extremely limited, are experiencing an increasing survival rate of children with disabilities. Fledgling intervention programs for children with cerebral palsy are steadily emerging in all the developing countries. These programs must judiciously allocate their meager resources to treatments that have been shown to be the most effective in giving children with cerebral palsy an improved quality of life.

V. PROBLEMS IN APPRAISAL OF THE TREATMENT OUTCOMES LITERATURE

In response to the worldwide need for a critical and useful appraisal of the existing scientific literature, the American Academy for Cerebral Palsy and Developmental Medicine began efforts in 1995 to develop summaries of evidence about interventions in developmental medicine (7). Immediately, however, stumbling blocks appeared.

The multidisciplinary nature of developmental disabilities, in general, and cerebral palsy, in particular, poses a challenge when it comes to evaluating outcomes research. A simple review of the literature yields a hodgepodge of information from the multiple disciplines that publish research in a wide variety of specialty journals. In addition, there is little consistency in what has been measured and how it was measured. Physiologically concerned specialists have focused on outcomes such as spasticity; therapeutically concerned specialists have investigated outcomes related to gait, hand use, and speech; and developmentalists have concentrated on outcomes such as social interactions, learning, or emotional well being. These circumstances make it difficult to identify all the relevant studies, to assess the efficacy of individual treatments, and to compare the outcomes of one intervention with those of another.

Outcome measures, to date, have been determined almost exclusively by health care professionals, not by the people who live with the treatments and face the reality of the outcomes. Groups, such as the Advisory Board to the National Center for Medical Rehabilitation Research, have made it clear that people living with disabilities are concerned with outcomes that reduce their functional limitations. They want to be able to perform more activities and increase their participation in the normal societal roles. It is in these dimensions that people experience their medical condition. Take, for example, the sometimes controversial issue about whether the treatment of youngsters with cerebral palsy should focus exclusively on interventions to develop eventual ambulation or whether it should also allow the use of wheelchairs. A treatment plan that prioritizes eventual ambulation with interventions to reduce spasticity and facilitate normal movement patterns offers an unknown potential to walk at some future time. In the meantime, restricted mobility affects every aspect of the child's life and development. Alternatively, a treatment plan that involves a wheelchair makes it possible to perform more of the roles of childhood that depend on mobility immediately. A wheelchair can provide a self-controlled, easy, and timely means of mobility to keep up with peers in various kinds of gross motor play, perform household chores, and explore the neighborhood community. Only the people who must live with the treatment decisions can evaluate whether the cost of eventual ambulation of unknown quality or quantity may be worth while. These costs must be counted in dollars, pain, time in intensive therapy in lieu of time in other activities, orthotic use, and perhaps years of literally lagging behind peers in participation of normal roles at home, school, and in the community due to restricted mobility.

The lack of rigor in the efficacy studies that have been done poses another challenge to evaluating outcomes research. Interventions supported only by biological theory, testimony, or common sense and uncontrolled observations have been the norm in the treatment of cerebral palsy, as in medicine, in general. The fact that a treatment idea is sensible, based on our current and imperfect understanding of the physiology or epidemiology of cerebral palsy, is no guarantee that the approach will make a clinical difference. It is important to know whether decisions can be based on the results of rigorously controlled investigations or to know whether to be much more circumspect because a decision may rest only on the results of uncontrolled observations—or even weaker evidence.

VI. A CONCEPTUAL FRAMEWORK FOR REVIEWING TREATMENT OUTCOMES

To overcome these hurdles, review of outcomes research required a conceptual framework for considering treatment outcomes. The framework needed to accommodate data from multiple disciplines, to make sense of the existing disparate scientific findings, and to promote consensus about which treatments work (i.e., are efficacious) and which treatments matter to children and their families. After deliberation of the merits of classification systems to accomplish this, the AACPDM endorsed and implemented a two-part framework that makes it possible to (1) classify and consolidate diverse treatment outcomes in a meaningful way and (2) indicate the strength of the evidence so readers can know with what degree of confidence it can be used (8). This framework will structure the development of evidence tables that are a convenient way to summarize what is known, what is not yet known, and what it would be helpful to know about various interventions.

The AACPDM framework will be used in the next chapter to explore the existing evidence for several interventions for infants and young children with cerebral palsy. An understanding of the basic concepts and definitions of the framework is essential background for following the structure of the evidence tables and the analyses they make possible. Readers who are already familiar with this framework may want to skip the rest of this chapter. Readers who are interested in detailed information about the framework, and how to use it, will want to supplement the following information by reading the AACPDM *Method-*

ology for Developing Evidence Tables and Reviewing Treatment Outcomes Research, which can be found on the Internet at www.aacpdm.org (9).

A. What Kind of Evidence Do We Have?

The first part of the AACPDM framework is a classification system of disablement that was used in Chapter 5 to discuss considerations in providing therapy services. The NCMRR and the World Health Organization have identified five dimensions of human functioning in which congenital abnormalities, developmental disorders, genetic conditions, injury, or disease and its consequences may create medical and social disablement. This classification of disablement was used again in Chapter 6 to discuss comprehensive clinical evaluation and treatment planning. As we will see in Chapter 11, the classification can also be used to aggregate research findings and to demonstrate the gaps in our knowledge about outcomes. Even widely varying data can be consolidated and analyzed in an evidence table constructed from these five dimensions. Table 1 summarizes the five dimensions and Table 2 demonstrates how selected effects of cerebral palsy may manifest in these dimensions.

An evidence table organized by these dimensions has an additional benefit beyond accommodating diverse data. It lends itself to an examination of interactions across dimensions that may occur as a result of an intervention. This is important because there has been an underlying, but untested, assumption in treatment of cerebral palsy that these are five "levels" of a hierarchical causal pathway. In a hierarchical perspective, periventricular leukomalacia causes spasticity, which is responsible for awkward gait, which leads to restricted participation in community activities. While this may be true, the corollary, that successful treat-

Table 1 Five Dimensions of Human Functioning

Dimensions	Description
Pathophysiology	Interruption or interference of normal physiology and developmental processes or structures
Impairment	Loss or abnormality of body structure or physiological body function
Functional limitation/ activity	Restriction of ability to perform functional activities
Disability/participation	Restricted participation in typical societal roles
Societal limitation/ contextual factors	Barriers to full participation imposed by societal attitudes, architectural barriers, and social policies and other external factors

Table 2 Examples of Variety of Effects of Cerebral Palsy on Dimensions of Human
Functioning

Dimension	Examples
Pathophysiology	Cystic lesions and white matter loss as a result of periventric- ular leukomalacia of the premature infant's brain
Impairment	Spasticity, contractures, low endurance, perceptual dysfunc- tion
Functional Limitation/ activity	Awkward walking with fatigue; difficulty dressing; poor con- centrating and sustained listening; reading problems
Disability/participation	Education in restricted environment, limited sports access, lack of dating opportunity, lack of contribution to family by doing fair share of chores, not able to attend commu- nion at church, unable to achieve independent living
Societal limitation/ contextual factors	Exclusion from school/city team sports, denial of medical treatment or equipment by insurer, government apathy to- ward the provision of low-income independent living units for people with disabilities, failure of voters to support transportation bond for wheelchair lifts on public buses

ment at one "level" (i.e., the impairment dimension) will automatically and positively affect another "level" (i.e., functional limitation) has not been confirmed
by scientific observation.

The assumption of a hierarchy has had two effects on research efforts.
For example, in the area of spasticity management, the assumption that reducing
spasticity will automatically yield positive outcomes in function and social roles
has prioritized our interventions toward those that alter spasticity. In addition,
investigators have generally not measured treatment effects on function and disability, but have restricted their measures to effects on spasticity.

These five dimensions may prove to be multidirectional, not hierarchical,
with complex interactions; in other words, effects may be top-down, bottom-up,
or lateral. For example, antispasticity drugs may intervene in the pathophysiological dimension by affecting neurotransmitters; orthopedic surgery may act in the
impairment dimension by changing range of motion. There may be positive, negative, or no effects of these drug or surgical interventions in the dimensions of
functional limitation and disability. Assistive technology, such as powered mobility, may compensate for functional limitations by providing an alternative means
of efficient locomotion. It may decrease disability by allowing a student to be
independent and to move about school faster and with less effort. Its use may
or may not have positive or negative effects in the impairment dimension, such
as improved head control (positive), skin breakdown (negative), or increased knee

contractures (negative).Use of assistive technology may have effects in the functional limitation dimension, through loss of ability for independent transfers, or conversely, increase of transfer ability due to high motivation and effort to access public transportation. Training for the Wheelchair Olympics may increase ability. It may or may not also decrease emotional impairment for a person with depression or low self-esteem. The relationships among the five dimensions of functioning have not been, but need to be, systematically investigated.

B. How Credible Is the Evidence We Have?

It is important to know whether health care decisions (especially those involving high risk to people) can be based on the results of rigorously controlled investigations or that they can rest only on the results of uncontrolled clinical observations—or even lesser evidence. Potentially useful interventions in health care originate with a common sense idea, or with expectations that are based on knowledge of the pathophysiology of a medical condition and the mechanism of action of an intervention. Sometimes they are based on beliefs arising from unsubstantiated theories of physiology or from analogies to other conditions. These forms of evidence may constitute the sole basis for an intervention that is being offered. Usually, however, these types of evidence serve only in a preliminary way, until the intervention has been submitted to systematic observation and evaluation.While the foregoing types of evidence can have a compelling logic, the actual effectiveness of an intervention can only be established by external evidence derived through empirical research.

1. AACPDM Classification of Levels of Evidence

Table 3 shows the AACPDM levels of evidence, which classify empirical and nonempirical evidence on the basis of its internal validity or credibility.

As a rule of thumb, level I designs are well-controlled experiments that must also include random allocation and manipulation of the intervention. Level II designs do not include randomization, but are otherwise well controlled experiments or comparison studies. Level III designs are comparison studies, but one (or both) of the comparisons is retrospective. Levels I to III all include some control group or condition, the purpose of which is to establish an expectancy about the outcome in people in the absence of intervention. Level IV designs have no comparison group or condition. If there is a firm base of expectancy (i.e., all people with a certain condition previously died within 1 year of diagnosis), then a control is not needed to demonstrate convincing evidence for an intervention. For most conditions, however, we lack good descriptive information (natural history of conditions) or baseline information, so an expectancy about outcome is necessary to establish convincing evidence about an intervention.

Table 3 AACPDM Classification of Levels of Evidence

Level	Nonempirical	Group research	Outcomes research	Single subject research
I		Randomized controlled trial All or none case series		N-of-1 randomized controlled trial
II		Nonrandomized controlled trial Cohort study with concurrent control group	Outcomes research analytic survey	ABABA design Alternating treatments Multiple baseline across subjects ABA design
III		Case-control study Cohort study with historical control group		
IV		Case series without control group		AB design
V	Case reports Anecdotes Expert opinion without explicit critical appraisal (or testimony) Theory based on physiology, bench, animal research Common sense/first principles			

Any study which is not well controlled is downgraded to the next lower level.

Level V evidence is nonempirical evidence—or level IV case series with high potential for bias reducing the information more to the equivalency of case reports at level V. Level V evidence can only hint at possible relationships between intervention and outcome. Any research design that is not well controlled is downgraded to the next lower level.

2. Definitions of Research Types

Because there is no standard taxonomy for discussion of research concepts and designs, even within the field of medicine, the following definitions are given for the terms used in the classification. Some variations of these designs are included; others may be encountered in the literature.

(a) Randomized Controlled Trials. The distinguishing feature of the randomized controlled trial (RCT), in group research, is that people are randomly allocated to a group that is offered the intervention or a group that is offered nothing, "usual care," a placebo, or some other intervention. When groups are relatively small, strategies in addition to random allocation may be used to increase the similarity of the groups. Strategies such as matching and stratification by age or disability, for example, will precede random allocation; statistical strategies such as analysis of covariance will follow completion of data collection.

Variations of the RCT include the randomized crossover trial. This is a RCT with the added feature of internal comparison of people against themselves as well as external comparison of the groups. People are randomly allocated to an intervention and control group and receive the intervention or control condition for a specified period of time, as in the RCT. Then the groups cross over (i.e., the group that received the treatment initially now receives the control condition and vice versa).

(b) All or None Case Series. Not all certain knowledge is obtained through controlled experiments. Experiments are necessary only when our expectation of an outcome is not certain. If an outcome is essentially certain, such as a uniformly fatal disease, a case series in which one or more people survive after receiving an intervention provides very convincing evidence. Criteria for the all or none case series are met when all people died before the treatment became available, but some now survive on it; or when some people died before the treatment became available, but none now die on it. Another example of an all or none case series are outcomes that can only occur as a result of the intervention such as operative mortality and perioperative risks.

(c) N-of-1 Randomized Controlled Trials. In single subject research, treatment versus control conditions are manipulated within a single person; the order of these exposures is randomly allocated. There are several variations of the N-of-1 RCT, sometimes called a randomized crossover trial; these include

the blind crossover trial or double-blind crossover trial. A person frequently undergoes pairs of periods in which one period applies an experimental treatment (B) and the other applies a placebo or baseline (A)—in other words, an ABABA type of design.

The order of these two periods within each pair is randomly selected so that the conduct of the trial may be, for example, ABBAAB. Treatment outcomes are monitored to document the effect of the treatment currently being applied. Pairs of treatments are *repeatedly* measured until the person being treated and the investigator are convinced that the treatment period is clearly different, or clearly not different. In a blind trial, the person making the outcome assessments is blind to the treatment condition; in a double-blind trial, both the subject and the assessor are unaware of the treatment condition. Although this method can also provide a group comparison when more than one subject has been studied, the focus of the published report is the individual comparisons. Alternatively, when multiple N-of-1 randomized controlled trials conducted under the same protocol have been summed and a group comparison is provided, this is called a multiple crossover trial.

Another variation of the N-of-1 RCT is the alternating treatment design in which the subject is exposed to the treatment condition and control condition(s) in close temporal proximity. For example, a subject is assessed during a 20-minute exposure to a control condition followed by a 20-minute exposure to the treatment condition; these exposures are determined by random allocation. Yet another variation is the multiple baseline across subjects design; several subjects are assessed for differing periods of exposure to the nontreatment condition (called baseline) and then assessed during treatment exposure. The order in which subjects change from the control condition to the treatment condition is established through random allocation.

(d) Nonrandomized Controlled Trials. This is like a RCT with one exception: subjects are not randomly allocated to groups. Instead, the groups are convened on the basis of factors such as convenience (e.g., a comparison of people in two regional hospitals), availability (children who attend the investigator's clinic), or voluntary behavior of the subjects. A variation is the crossover design without randomization. Similarly, the absence of random allocation of treatment and control conditions to a single subject makes the alternating treatment design and multiple baseline across subjects design the single subject research equivalent of this experimental design, as does the ABABA design. Multiple observations of potential change between treatment and control phases are possible.

(e) Cohort Study with Concurrent Control Group. This study is essentially the same as the nonrandomized controlled trial.

(f) Outcomes Research Analytic Survey. This is not a direct study of people. Instead, "groups" are created from retrospective review of information obtained from a database. This is sometimes called a correlational study. De-

pending on the criteria used for inclusion in a database, the observations might be controlled and calibrated. The database can be on a large scale (e.g., national surveillance registry for spina bifida) or a small scale (e.g., the spina bifida clinic of a hospital). In outcomes research, the investigator starts with an intervention of interest, sorting all the people in the database in rows, according to whether they received the intervention or not, and then sorting them in columns, according to whether they had the outcome of interest or not. As an example, the investigator uses a database that was created by a hospital's neuromuscular clinic to follow up its patients with cerebral palsy. Data can be extracted that allow the following question to be answered: Are children with spastic diplegia cerebral palsy who received selective posterior rhizotomy (SPR) surgery more likely to walk unaided at age 10 than children who did not? The investigator organizes the numbers obtained as indicated in Table 4.

The numbers in cells a,b,c, and d are analyzed for differences in rates of outcomes. A major value of this design is that it demonstrates whether the outcomes we might expect to observe (or have observed) in controlled experiments are also being observed in the real world of clinical care.

(g) Case-Control Study. Like the outcomes research analytic survey, this, too, is a correlational study of ''groups'' created by retrospective review of information for analysis. In this correlational analysis, not all people who receive an intervention are tracked, only those with a particular outcome. Similarity of people with an outcome of interest (cases) to people without the outcome (controls) can only be established retrospectively; and their previous exposure to an intervention of interest can only be verified retrospectively. In the most common form of this design (called a 2 × 2 case-control study), the investigator starts by identifying a group of people who already have an outcome of interest (called cases) and another group of similar people who do not have the outcome of interest (called controls). The investigator then retrospectively examines the histories of both groups to determine current or previous exposure to the intervention. This design is useful for establishing the relationship between low-frequency outcomes that may be important (i.e., serious adverse outcomes) and an interven-

Table 4 Outcomes Research Analytic Survey (example)

	Outcome of interest (unaided walking)	
	Present	Absent
Exposed to intervention (SPR)		
Yes	a	b
No	c	d

tion. Using the same example as that used in defining outcomes research (i.e., spastic diplegia, selective posterior rhizotomy, and unaided walking), the matrix that is created for the analysis looks exactly the same; the numbers in the cells of course, differ.

A variation of this design is sometimes called a matched case-control study, which begins by identifying the cases; then, for each case, a specified number of controls (typically two to five) that match the case with respect to several important characteristics (e.g., gender, age) are identified. Another variation is used when the intervention can occur in degrees or categories of intensity, such as the dose of a drug or exposure to varying degrees of asbestos; this is called a $2 \times k$ case-control study, with the k referring to the number of degrees or categories of intensity of the intervention.

(h) ABA Design. In this study, baseline is established for the outcome of interest through multiple measures made over a period of time. A treatment period follows and the level or trend of the outcome is established. Finally, the treatment is withdrawn with multiple measurements made again to observe whether the outcome reverses. It allows two comparisons of change between treatment and control phases.

(i) Cohort Study with Historical Control Group. This is a cohort study that compares two groups of people, but only one group is currently studied by the investigator. Rates of outcomes for the studied group are compared with those of a control group of people who were studied at an earlier time when, or in a place where, treatment policy (or availability) differed from that being investigated. Alternatively, the rates are compared with rates of outcomes published for a similar group who received a different intervention (literature control). Because the comparison studies were not conducted under the same protocol, it is almost certain that the people and the way their outcomes were measured is not the same, posing significant threats to the validity of results under this research design.

(j) Case Series Without Control Group. A case series typically consists of a single group of people who receive an intervention and are followed for a time to observe their outcomes. The outcome is measured before and after the intervention, but any rate of change is not compared directly with the rates that occurred in people who were not receiving the intervention but were otherwise comparable. In the absence of a firm base of expectancy or a control group to establish an expectancy, a rate of change in a single group has little credibility. The observed rate of change may have been influenced by some factor other than the intervention or may have even happened without the intervention. The single subject research equivalent of this group design is the AB design. In the AB study, the investigator makes repeated measures during a baseline phase followed

by measures during an intervention phase. Only one comparison of change between treatment and control phases is possible.

(k)   Case Reports.   These describe small collections of cases that usually involve a careful review of records. Their main value is in documenting the occurrence of events that otherwise are known to be exceedingly rare.

(l)   Anecdotes.   Anecdotes are uncontrolled observations reported in a study. They do not establish causality, but they are useful to document that an outcome has, at least, been observed to occur in association with the intervention. Anecdotal reports of outcomes may also be useful for the formation of hypotheses for subsequent study. Anecdotal evidence includes comments reported by the author with or without any quantification. If the information is formalized and/ or quantified (e.g., subjects' responses in an interview or questionnaire at the conclusion of a study), but not compared to responses to similar questions elicited prior to treatment, this is regarded as anecdotal evidence.

(m)   Expert Opinion Without Explicit Critical Appraisal (Testimonial Evidence).   This is defined as a statement of belief by an individual or a group about the effect of an intervention on an outcome without description of supporting evidence or rationale.

(n)   Theory Based on Physiology, Bench, or Animal Research.   Evidence about an intervention is said to be theoretical, if (1) no empirical observations exist about the effect of the intervention on outcomes, but (2) there is an appeal to a set of beliefs, based on knowledge of the pathophysiology of the disease and the mechanism of action of the intervention. This can be based on basic science (bench) research, animal research, or an analogy (i.e., screening for breast cancer may rest on the evidence—(or belief)—that screening for another type of cancer is effective in reducing mortality).

(o)   Common Sense or First Principles.   Occasionally there will be virtually unanimous agreement about the merits of an intervention, despite the fact that there is no external evidence pertaining to the intervention and no obvious biological theory that directly supports it. In developmental disabilities, an example of a common sense intervention is the multidisciplinary approach to care of children with complex developmental disabilities. An example of a first principles or common sense intervention that went wrong, however, is the CAST study. Controlling blood pressure in people with aortic dissection is based on the principle that lowering blood pressure will reduce ventricular output and so decrease the risk of further extension of the dissection. First principles suggest that prophylactic treatment with antiarrhythmics that reduce these arrhythmias must also reduce mortality. The CAST study randomized people with these post-MI ar-

rhythmias to flecainide/encainide or placebo, but found that more people on an antiarrhythmic died than those on placebo.

VII. SUMMARY

Research about the treatments for cerebral palsy has a relatively short history. In the 50 years since academic and scientific discourse formally originated, the field has moved through and beyond a fertile period of exploring innovative treatments that might improve the quality of life of people with cerebral palsy. In the rush to be helpful, treatments proliferated and were adopted or discarded with little concern for systematic scientific evaluation. Instead of evaluating treatment outcomes, research efforts focused on issues of etiology, diagnosis, prognosis, and the development of measurement tools.

With maturation, the field has evolved to the understanding that even though a treatment idea based on current knowledge or theory of physiology is sensible, this does not guarantee that the approach will work. Moreover, there is a need to know in which dimensions of disablement an approach does work so that those who live with cerebral palsy can decide which outcomes matter most to them. Coincident with this evolution has been the generalized paradigm shift in medicine to evidence-based practice. The result has been the recognition that, until there is a firmer grasp on the efficacy and relevance of our treatments in cerebral palsy, responsible clinicians must temper their enthusiasm for established, or new, treatments with a sober and scientifically cautious approach to their continuation or adoption.

The American Academy for Cerebral Palsy and Developmental Medicine has assumed leadership in describing a conceptual framework in which evidence-based efficacy of various treatments in use, and new options that appear, can be evaluated. With this tool, the field has the potential for moving forward in several ways with regard to treatment outcomes. Consensus can be reached about the levels for which there is evidence of efficacy. Meaningful comparisons between interventions can be made. Use of the model should prompt the research community to include multiple outcome measures in study protocols to establish whether effects of an intervention in one dimension can be linked to effects in other dimensions. Research agendas will be guided because the dimensions where adequate information is lacking, as well as the need for more definitive types of research designs, can be visualized and future research encouraged to address these gaps in our knowledge.

REFERENCES

1. Adams R, Snyder P. Treatments for cerebral palsy: Making choices of intervention from an expanding menu of options. Infants *and* Young Children 1998; 10:1–22.

2. Campbell SK. The child's development of functional movement. In: Campbell S, VanderLinden D, Palisano R, eds. Physical Therapy for Children. Philadelphia: W.B. Saunders, 1994:1–7.

3. Bly L. A historical and current view of the basis of NDT. Pediatr Phys Ther 1991; 3:131–135.

4. Peacock WJ, Arens LJ. Selective posterior rhizotomy for the relief of spasticity in cerebral palsy. S Afr Med J 1982; 62:119–24.

5. Sackett D, Rosenberg W, Muir Gray J, Haynes R, Richardson W. Evidence-based medicine: what it is and what it isn't. Br Med J 1996; 312:71–72.

6. Sackett DL, Richardson WS, Rosenberg W, Haynes RB. Evidence-based Medicine: How to Practice and Teach EBM. New York: Churchill Livingstone, 1997.

7. Butler C. Outcomes that matter. Devel Med Child Neurology 1995; 37:753–754.

8. Butler C, Goldstein M, Chambers H, S Harris, R Adams, J Darrah, J Leach. Evaluating research in developmental disabilities: a conceptual framework for reviewing treatment outcomes. Devel Med Child Neurol 1999; 41:55–59.

9. Butler C. AACPDM Methodology for Developing Evidence Tables and Reviewing Treatment Outcome Research. Internet at www.aacpdm.org: American Academy for Cerebral Palsy and Developmental Medicine, 1998 (Last Update: August 1, 1999).

11

Evidence Tables and Reviews of Treatment Outcomes

Charlene Butler
Health and Special Education Consultant, Seattle, Washington

> I have no hesitation in advising you to experiment in support of your views
> because, whether you confirm them or refute them, good must come from
> your exertions—*Michael Faraday, 1834.*

The pursuit of answers about treatment outcomes may create tensions within
us—between our belief in unbiased empirical examination of the issues and our
concern that the possible revelation of inadequate evidence will result in medical
care being withheld from these children. Without objective observations, however, we cannot know which interventions work, for whom, and under what conditions. Without this knowledge we cannot know whether we need to search
further for interventions that do work or that work better.

The goal of this chapter is to explore a way of thinking about the evidence
gleaned from "our experiments" or studies of various treatments and to expand
our thinking about the effects of what we do in our clinical practices. Using the
conceptual framework described in Chapter 10, results of studies can be consolidated in evidence tables that will lead us toward being able to confirm or refute
the efficacy of treatments in use or new treatments as they appear.

A selective review of three types of treatments or interventions for very
young children with cerebral palsy will demonstrate how outcomes data may be
organized and analyzed to determine the current state of the evidence about any
intervention. As we will see from the reviews of treatments that have been selected for analysis, this framework lends itself to evaluating (1) a very specific
type of intervention (e.g., feeding via gastrostomy tube): (2) an intervention that
may vary from one clinician to another in precisely how it is practiced (e.g.,
neurodevelopmental therapy or NDT); and (3) an intervention that may be com-

posed of other interventions (e.g., early intervention with physical therapy for infants considered to be at risk for developing cerebral palsy includes a variety of motor therapies).

I. METHOD FOR CONDUCTING REVIEWS OF INTERVENTIONS

A. Subjects

Given the paucity of treatment outcome studies conducted only with children diagnosed with cerebral palsy under the age of 3, these reviews include studies that contained at least some infants or preschoolers. When results are given for the youngest subgroup of subjects within a larger study, just the results for these youngest children are included in the evidence tables.

B. Literature Search

Each of the reviews includes published studies for which full text is available in English and is accessible through the U.S. university library system, and studies for which published abstracts are available. Searches were conducted through the electronic, bibliographic MEDLINE data base of the National Library of Medicine (1966 to spring of 1999) using two search programs (Clinical Query of PubMed and EndNote) and the exploded terms *cerebral palsy, infants,* and *preschool children* as well as types of studies (e.g., *clinical trials, cohort studies*). Reference lists in studies and review articles and researchers knowledgeable about this intervention were consulted.

C. Organization of Summary and Evidence Tables

The first table in each review summarizes the studies. Section 1 of this table describes the intervention and the subjects. Section 2 describes the research methodology and indicates whether specific results were available for the subjects with cerebral palsy. Each study is classified to indicate the relative strength of the credibility (i.e., internal validity) of the outcomes it produced; these levels of evidence were described in detail in Chapter 10. AACDPM guidelines are followed for determining the level of evidence each study represents (1). Where studies of subjects with mixed diagnoses provide separate results, only those results for the subjects with cerebral palsy are shown in the subsequent evidence tables. When studies are conducted in two parts or when there are two or more subgroups for whom outcomes are reported, the evidence tables show outcomes as such.

The second table in each review summarizes the results for each study. Some studies report a group result, usually a mean score, that reflects the difference between treatment and another condition. This may be the difference between a treated group and a control group. In a case series that has no control group, the group result is the assessed difference between the group before treatment compared to after treatment. Alternatively, some studies report the uniformity of effect within the treated group (i.e., the number who improved, the number who worsened, and the number who were unchanged). Some studies report both types of results.

Each result is classified according to the dimension of disablement in which it had an effect. These five dimensions were described in detail in Chapter 10. AACDPM guidelines are also followed to determine the dimension of disablement represented by each result (1). Greater confidence can be placed in any results that were subjected to statistical evaluation and that were from studies with higher internal validity (i.e., levels of evidence); this information is also contained in the second summary table. Section 1 of this summary table shows results of treatment when compared to another condition. When uniformity of results within a treated group is reported, these results are shown in Section 2 of the table.

Evidence tables are a convenient way to consolidate evidence. The third table in each review aggregates all the research results and demonstrates the current state of our knowledge about the intervention. Section 1 of the evidence table aggregates the outcomes of treatment when it has been compared to another condition; Section 2 aggregates what is known about the uniformity of effects within treated groups. Finally, evidence about adverse effects or medical complications is reported in a fourth table.

D. Analysis of Evidence

The reviews of research seek to evaluate not only the effect of an intervention based on its anticipated mechanism of action in the expected dimension, but also to evaluate possible effects in other dimensions of disablement. Evidence tables will be analyzed to answer the following questions for each intervention:

1. What evidence exists about the effects of the intervention in the dimension in which there is an anticipated mechanism of action and how uniform are those effects?
2. What evidence is there about its effects in the other dimensions?
3. What linkages exist for treatment effects within and between these dimensions of disablement and in which directions?
4. Are there subgroups for whom the intervention may be more or less effective?

    5.   What kinds and magnitude of complications have been documented?

    6.   What is the strength of the evidence for the intervention?

E. Caution About Drawing Conclusions

In science, in general, we can never be *sure* of anything; we can only be 95% sure or 99% sure. In the absence of certainty, we must always retain at least the willingness to accept an alternative hypothesis. Moreover, it must be kept in mind that even the most stringent empirical research study does not supply negative proof; it can only provide a probability that, if a treatment produced effects, those effects will have been detected. Those probability calculations are reported in the Summary of Results tables whenever statistical evaluation of results was conducted in a study. But even when the probability of the result is high, extra caution must be used in drawing conclusions because these probability calculations in cerebral palsy research are based on such relatively small numbers of subjects. Large numbers of subjects simply are not available for research because the incidence of cerebral palsy in the general population is low.

    Extra caution must be exercised in regard to the scientific method used to arrive at the levels of evidence; the AACPDM methodology is new and still evolving. While this scientific method for analyzing and weighting studies for bias and error continues to be improved by the Academy, caution should be exercised about drawing conclusions beyond what may be appropriate.

II. REVIEW OF THE EFFECTS OF GASTROSTOMY FEEDING IN YOUNG CHILDREN WITH CEREBRAL PALSY

A. Feeding Problems and Their Consequences

There are a number of potential impediments to normal nutrition in children with cerebral palsy. These children may be unable to eat by mouth due to incoordination of tongue and swallowing muscles, temporomandibular joint contractures, hypoxemia, vomiting and discomfort associated with gastroesophageal reflux, food refusal, and fatigue experienced during feeding (2, 3). The more severe the degree of motor impairment, the greater the oral deficit and gastrointestinal tract dysfunction that leads to inability to ingest or digest sufficient amounts of food.

    Seriously compromised oral feeding has significant consequences (2). After reduced mobility, poor feeding ability is the best single predictor of early death in profoundly disabled individuals with mental retardation (4). Without adequate nutrition in early childhood, it is generally held that potential brain or physical development will not be achieved (5). Malnutrition is associated with diverse complications of health. Decreased muscle strength in the respiratory system reduces the effectiveness of the cough reflex and predisposes to aspiration pneumonia. Vomiting and acid reflux also increase the risk of aspiration. Cold, mottled extremities, frequently seen in malnourished children, are the result of decreased blood circulation. Disturbances in the immune system secondary to malnutrition predispose to infection, particularly in the lungs and urinary tract. Healing of pressure sores is delayed in malnourished children. Malnutrition increases irritability and decreases motivation and energy. Finally, coughing, choking, cyanotic episodes, vomiting, and acid reflux during mealtimes are often associated with feeling sick, which may lead to food refusal.

For these reasons, when conventional treatment (i.e., positioning the child, therapeutic techniques to facilitate lip closure and swallowing, thickened food, and extended feeding time) has failed to resolve severe, chronic feeding disorders, permanent gastrostomy may be considered as a means of by-passing oral-motor and gastrointestinal dysfunctioning. Nasogastric tube feeding, another alternative, is the preferred method for short-term enteral feeding. Its long-term use, however, has several limitations, including nasal discomfort, irritation or penetration of the larynx, recurrent pulmonary aspiration, and blockage or displacement of the tube (6). Moreover, one study of factors affecting survival rate in children with severe neurological disabilities showed that children fed by gastrostomy tube had a statistically significant better survival rate at 10 years than did children fed by nasogastric tube.

B. How Does Gastrostomy Work?

Gastrostomy is a form of enteral feeding that has been used since the late 1800s. Its primary goal is to provide adequate nutrition. A surgical opening is made through the abdominal wall and stomach to insert a feeding tube (4). Today, operative gastrostomy requires a laparotomy with potential surgical and anaesthetic risks, especially in patients with neurological dysfunctions and severe malnutrition. The percutaneous endoscopic gastrostomy (PEG) technique has been increasingly used in disabled children (6). This procedure has been described in the literature and can be performed as a day case, preferably under general anaesthesia (6). Nevertheless, it is recommended only for children who have such a marked degree of oral-motor dysfunction that they (1) require longer than 6 weeks of nasogastric tube feeding; (2) take an inordinately long time to feed; (3) have inadequate weight gain; and (4) have an unsafe swallow (i.e., significant risk of aspiration of food) demonstrated on a contrast videofluoroscopy. Children who have moderate-to-severe gastroesophageal reflux, children with ascites, and children who have had previous abdominal surgery are regarded as unsuitable candidates (6, 7).

Malnutrition and growth failure are no longer accepted as inevitable and irremedial consequences of cerebral palsy. As a result, gastrostomy may play a role in promoting the growth of children with otherwise inadequate dietary intake or malnutrition and in improving their quality of life. What is the documentation of its impact on growth and on quality of life for both the patient and caregiver?

C. Search Results

When the MeSH term "gastrostomy" was added to the search parameters noted earlier, 15 citations were identified. Based on review of the abstracts, nine full-text articles were obtained and examined. Five studies met the inclusion criteria for the review. Four of these studies compared measures of growth made before gastrostomy feeding with those made after a period of gastrostomy feeding. One additional study reported complications, including mortality rates and anecdotal information (8). No study has used a control group.

D. Review of Studies

The five studies are briefly described below and are summarized in Tables 1 and 2. All of these studies compared effects of treatment to no treatment; in other words, effects of feeding via gastrostomy were compared to feeding without gastrostomy (i.e., oral feeding).

In 1986, Shapiro et al. investigated whether growth failure is the result of neurological dysfunction or of nutritional deficiency (9). Changes in weight and height after at least 6 months of feeding by gastrostomy were evaluated. The investigators concluded that nutritional factors appear to have a role in the growth failure of children with cerebral palsy in regard to weight but not in regard to linear growth.

Two years later, Rempel et al. measured weight and height growth in children, half of whom had a gastrostomy during the first 4 years of life and most in the first year (10). Attainment of minimum standards of growth were most frequently seen in the 21 children treated early (before age 2), compared with those treated later (after age 2); only the data for this youngest group are shown in the evidence tables. The authors concluded that gastrostomy feeding can improve nutritional status and even produce an overweight condition. Furthermore, they stated that the high death rate they observed was not related to the gastrostomy surgery but was indicative of the severe morbidity in the children and their significant degree of malnutrition.

In 1990, Sanders et al. investigated the effect of timing of enteral feeding (early, middle, or late start) on reversing nutritional deficit (11). The early group included 14 children whose gastrostomy occurred within 1 year of their central nervous system dysfunction; only their results are included in the evidence tables.

However, the description of all three groups, prior to gastrostomy, demonstrates that the longer a chronic state of malnutrition persists, the greater the morbidity. The early group (those who began gastrostomy feeding within 1 year of the onset of central nervous system dysfunction that restricted feeding) was moderately undernourished for weight but normal for height and weight/height before gastrostomy. The middle group (who began enteral feeding within 8 years of their central nervous system dysfunction) was on the borderline between severely and moderately undernourished for weight, moderately undernourished for height, and moderately undernourished for weight/height. The late group (who had a gastrostomy after 8 years) was quite severely undernourished for weight and for height and had a significant number of chronic secondary conditions, including severe esophagitis and chronic lung disease from repeated pneumonia. The investigators concluded that the earlier adequate nutrition is initiated, the more readily the consequences of malnutrition will be reversed.

A 1992 study analyzed the success of gastrostomy by documenting survival, early and late complications after the procedure, and caregiver satisfaction (8). The authors concluded that noninstitutionalized children with severe cerebral palsy who undergo gastrostomies have a much higher survival rate than adults or severely mentally retarded children undergoing similar procedures.

In 1996, catch-up growth in a series of failure-to-thrive children who had gastrostromy surgery was analyzed according to medical diagnoses and other factors that may affect growth (i.e., age at surgery, ambulatory status, prematurity, or mode of feeding) (4). There was no statistically significant growth in children with scoliosis, chromosomal abnormality, perinatal infection, or sudden trauma, but catch-up growth in children with cerebral palsy was statistically significant in all measures. Only the results of the children with cerebral palsy are reported here. In this study, catch-up growth was found to be more rapid for children older than 2 years.

E. Evidence Tables

Table 3 aggregates all results and demonstrates that treatment outcomes have primarily been investigated in the dimension of impairment. Table 3, Section 1, shows nine measures of impairment; three measures of functional limitation; and one measure in the societal limitation or other context factors dimension. The preponderance of evidence about uniformity of effect is also in the impairment dimension. There is no evidence available about the effects of gastrostomy feeding in the dimensions of pathophysiology or disability/participation.

Table 4 demonstrates that adverse effects have been reported in relation to gastrostomy. Because all of these studies were case series with no control group, neither the rates of these adverse outcomes nor those of the positive outcomes can be compared to those in similar groups of in those studies.

Table 1 Summary of Studies

Section 1. Intervention and subjects.

Study (Ref.)	Treatment	Population sampled	# Total	# CP	Ages
9	Gastrostomy	Severe CP + MR + FTT	19	19	5 mo.–14 yr.
10	Gastrostomy	Severe CP + MR	57	57	3 mo.–18 yr.
	Done < age 2				
11	Enteral feeding	Severe CP	21	21	3 mo.– 15 yr.
	Early		51	51	
			14	14	
8	Gastrostomy	Severe CP	61	61	0–17 yr.
4	Gastrostomy	FTT	75	37	0–6 yr.

CP = cerebral palsy; MR = mental retardation; FTT = failure to thrive.

Section 2. Research methodology

Study (Ref.)	Research design and level of evidence	Duration of Rx	# in Rx group	# in control group
9	Retrospective case series, Level V	6–41 mo.	19	0
10	Retrospective case series, Level V	3 mo.–18 yr.	21	0
11	Prospective case series, Level IV	6 mo.	51	0
	Early treated group		14	0
8	Post Rx descriptive study, Level V	6 yr.	61	0
4	Retrospective case series	18 mo.	37	0

Table 2 Summary of Results

Section 1. Results of gastrostomy compared to no treatment. Outcomes of gastrostomy feeding were compared with outcomes of oral feeding before the gastrostomy.

Study (Ref.)	Outcome	Dim.	Measure	Result	Clin. imp.	Inferential statistics	LOE
9	Weight	I	Wt./length, z score	+	yes	$p < .01$	V
10	Weight	I	<5%ile wt./ht.[a]	+	sml	$p < .01$	V
	Irritability	I	Anecdote	+	yes		V
	Ease of feeding	FL/A	Anecdote	+	yes		V
	Caregiver satisfaction	SL/C	Anecdote	+	yes		V
11[c]	Weight	I	% of ideal wt.[a]	+	yes		IV
	Weight	I	% of wt./ht.[a]	+	sml		IV
	Height	I	% of ideal ht.[a]	+	sml		IV
	Dev. activities		Anecdote	+	yes		V
8	Feeding	FL/A	Estimated time	+	yes		V
4	Weight	FL/A	z score[a]	+		$p = .0001$	V
	Height	I	z score[a]	+		$p = .007$	V
	Height/weight	I	z score[a]	+		$p = .01$	V

[a] National Center for Health Statistics growth charts.
[b] Indices of undernutrition.
[c] Results for early treated group only.
Clin Imp = clinical importance; LOE = Level of evidence; Dim. = Dimension of disablement.

Section 2. Uniformity of results within treated groups.

Study (Ref.)	Dim	Outcome	Measure	+	−	±	LOE
9 ($n = 19$)	I	Weight	Wt./length	84%	16%		V
	I	Weight	Wt./age	84%	16%		V
	I	Length	Length/age	58%	42%		V
10 ($n = 21$)	I	Weight	Wt. for ht.[a]	50%		50%	V
8 ($n = 61$)	FL/A	Abilities/comfort	Phone interview	94%			V
	SL/C	Caregiver satisfact.	Phone interview	93%			V

[a] National Center for Health Statistics growth charts.

Table 3 State of Knowledge About Outcomes of Treatment with Gastrostomy Feeding in Cerebral Palsy

Section 1. Outcomes of treatment compared to no treatment.

The evidence about each outcome is indicated by its level of evidence code (I through V) in the appropriate column showing positive and statistically valid results (+ *); positive (+) or negative (−) results that were not subjected to statistical evaluation; or results that were not different and/or were not statistically significant (± and NS). References to the study that produced the outcome are in parentheses. For example, positive and statistically valid results have been measured for weight growth three times in three different studies (all Level V evidence), and positive results without statistical validity have been measured twice, using different types of measurement, in the same study (both Level IV evidence).

Outcome	+ *	+	−	± or NS
Pathophysiology				
Impairment				
Weight	V(9) V(10) V(4)	IV(11) IV(11)		
Height	V(4) V(4)	IV(11)		
Irritability		V(10)		
Functional limitation/ Activity				
Feeding		V(10) V(8)		
Disability/participation				
Developmental activities		V(11)		
Societal limitation/ Context				
Caregiver satisfaction		V(10)		

Section 2. Uniformity of results within treated groups. Percentages of individuals within studies that demonstrated positive (+), negative (−), or unchanged outcomes (±) with the Level of evidence code for the study which produced the data (i.e., 50% V). References to the study that produced the outcome are in parentheses. For example, two studies (both producing Level V evidence) reported variation in weight growth (using different types of measures) to be 50–84%, 16% weight loss, 50% weight unchanged.

Outcome	+	−	±
Pathophysiology			
Impairment			
Weight	84% V(9)	16% V(9)	
	84% V(9)	16% V(9)	
	50% V(10)		50% V(10)
Functional limitation/Activity			
Abilities/comfort	94% V(8)		
Disability/Participation			
Societal/limitation/Context			
Caregiver satisfaction	93% V(8)		

Table 4 Adverse Effects and Medical Complications

(Ref.)	Type of effect	# of Cases	% of Cases
9 ($n = 19$)	Persistent vomiting	5	Not given
10 ($n = 57$)	Deaths after 1 year	8	23% major com-
	Gastrointestinal bleeding and ulcer-		plications
	ation	5	
	Dehiscence of wound	1	
	Peritonitis and bowel obstruction need-		
	ing reoperation	3	
	Tube migration	2	
	significant postoperative GER requir-		
	ing fundoplication surgery	4	
	Became overweight for height	12	
11 ($n = 51$)	Deaths	7	Not given
	Associated fundoplication surgery for		
	GER	48	
8 ($n = 61$)	Deaths after 2 years	16	32% early com-
	Vomiting, retching, and dumping		plications
	Hiatal hernia	11	
	Unable to bolus feed	7	
	Recurrent reflux and aspiration	1	
	Recurrent reflux aspiration	1	39.3% late com-
	Small bowel obstruction	1	plications
	Recurrent pneumonia/aspiration	4	
	Apnea	1	
	Wound infection	2	
		2	

F. Analyzing the Evidence

1. What Evidence Exists About the Effects of Gastrostomy on Growth Failure (an impairment of structure) and Other Impairments of Structure or Physiological Function in Youngsters with Cerebral Palsy?

Group measures of weight as a function of growth were consistent in showing that gastrostomy feeding promoted weight gain. However, weight gain was not experienced by every child according to two studies that reported the uniformity of effect on weight. These two studies establish a frequency of weight gain to be between 50% and 84% of children studied. Weight decelerated in some children (16%) and was unchanged in others (50%). One of these studies reported that 12 of the children who gained weight became overweight for their height, creating a potential complication for physical management.

Measuring growth as a function of height or, in most cases, recumbent length, also showed improvement on average in two studies. However, these were small gains and a third study reported that only 58% of its subjects increased in length while 42% measured shorter. There may be other factors responsible for failure to document height growth. The tendency of children with severe cerebral palsy to decelerate in rate of linear growth was described as early as 1962 and was attributed, at least in part, to atrophy of the lower extremities or to scoliosis (12). An analysis of factors affecting growth by one of the studies showed that scoliosis was a statistically significant factor in length growth in their sample of children with gastrostomy feeding (4). Obtaining a reliable measurement of length may also contribute to the inconsistent findings, however. Contractures make accurate measurement difficult. Repeated measures of 10 parameters of growth and body composition in a study of a mixed population revealed that recumbent length measurement was extremely unstable (13). Only three measures did prove to be stable: weight, arm muscle, and arm fat stores.

These findings may suggest the presence of subgroups for whom gastrostomy has different effects. Alternatively, it may suggest that each child's caloric needs must be individualized and monitored. In a related study that measured dietary intake and energy expenditure in children with cerebral palsy, an extreme variation in calories needed to maintain ideal weight was found (14). This was also found to be true in one of the case series for children with cerebral palsy fed via gastrostomy; there was a wide variation in the calorie and calcium intake per kilogram needed to produce weight gain in the individuals in the series (11).

Anecdotal evidence suggests that impairment of emotional function was also affected. Children were said to become less irritable and to have "better dispositions."

2. What Evidence Is There About the Effects of Gastrostomy on Pathophysiology, Functional Limitation/Activity, Disability/Participation, and Societal Limitation/Context Factors?

There is no evidence about changes in pathophysiology as a result of feeding via gastrostomy; in other words, changes in cellular or molecular structures or functions have not been investigated. This is also no evidence about changes in the dimension of disability/participation; that is, participation as a family member, the primary societal role of a very young child, has also not been measured.

There is anecdotal evidence about positive effects of gastrostomy feeding in the functional limitation/activity dimension. Eating was easier and faster (a decrease of about 1.5 hours a day). Children engaged in more activities that parents related as demonstrating developmental progress. There is also anecdotal evidence from two studies that caregivers were satisfied with the effects of gastrostomy.

3. What Linkages Exist for Treatment Effects Within and Between These Dimensions of Disablement and in Which Directions?

The evidence is extremely sparse, but it hints at a link between growth (which probably represents better nutrition) and improved well-being and developmental progress.

4. Are There Subgroups for Whom Gastrostomy May Be More or Less Effective?

Uniformity of effect data show that some children's growth improves, some continue to fall behind, and some are unchanged. This suggests that there may be subgroups who respond differently to gastrostomy feeding. Two studies analyzed age as a factor and found that attainment of minimum growth standards appears to occur more frequently in children treated early (10, 11), but other factors have not been identified.

5. What Kinds and Magnitude of Complications Have Been Documented?

For many children in these studies, malnutrition was a serious and potentially life-threatening problem prior to gastrostomy. There were some deaths after children had gastrostomies, but only one occurred in proximity to the surgery (1 month postsurgery). Rempel et al. concluded that the death rate in their case series was indicative of the severe morbidity in the group. In a related study of death rates among children with severe neurological disabilities, the strongest predictor of death was found to be the presence of other significant diseases (15). Comparison of the death rates of three groups in one of these case series would seem to support this; the death rate was distinctly higher in the group of children who had the most pronounced state of malnutrition and most chronic secondary conditions before gastrostomy (11). In contrast, however, another study detected no significant differences between the survivors and non survivors either in the average age at the time of gastrostomy or in the medical procedures or complications that they experienced (8).

The overall rates of major complications in two studies were reported to be 23% (10) and 39.3% (8).

While there is a high incidence of gastroesphogeal reflux (GER) in neurologically impaired children (2), it appears that GER can also be a side effect of gastrostomy feeding. Three studies report or allude to gastrostomy feeding either exacerbating existing GER or causing it (8, 10, 11). However, no study specifically reported the number of cases in which GER developed or became more serious after gastrostomy placement. Despite this lack of data, it is nevertheless being recommended in review articles that children who have moderate-to-severe gastroesophageal reflux be considered unsuitable candidates for gastrostomy placement since GER can cause aspiration pneumonitis and nutrient loss (2).

6. What Is the Strength of the Evidence?

Strength of the evidence depends on several factors: how extensively the population has been sampled reflected in the number of different studies and the overall number of subjects, the consistency of results across the studies, and the robustness of the research methods used. This body of evidence about gastrostomy for very young children with cerebral palsy is very limited in regard to both in the population that has been sampled: only five studies with a total of 152 subjects that had cerebral palsy, not all of whom were infants at the time of gastrostomy placement. The number and types of outcomes that have been measured are few. The credibility of the outcomes is very low (Level V with the exception of one Level IV study). The greatest strength in this body of evidence is the consistency of positive and clinically important group results for weight across the five studies, although this is weakened by the uniformity of results data that show some individuals do not experience improved outcomes.

G. Discussion

The primary goal of gastrostomy feeding is to provide adequate nutrition in children who are failing to thrive and who may, therefore, be at risk for significant morbidity or even death. The evidence tables demonstrate that research to date has successfully identified some possible important outcomes. It appears that gastrostomy feeding improves nutritional status with weight gain in most, but not all, children with cerebral palsy. Elimination of linear growth retardation is less clear. Attainment of minimum growth standards appears to occur more frequently in children treated early (10, 11). However, conclusions about the relationships between nutritional status, growth, morbidity, and developmental potential can only be speculative given the very limited data currently available.

This intervention is associated with a high rate of complications that contributes to the importance of establishing with greater certainty its apparent reversal of malnutrition and its effects. These evidence tables demonstrate that sufficient preliminary research has shown there to be promising positive effects. Gastrostomy feeding is ready for and warrants definitive clinical trials in this population.

Previous research has also been valuable in identifying the need to resolve a critical measurement issue. Before future studies can accurately gauge the effects of nutritional status on growth, reliability of growth measures must be established. Moreover, nutritional guidelines may also need to be redefined for this population since body compositions that are different from typical children have been identified.

Finally, the tables demonstrate a glaring lack of outcomes data across the several dimensions of disablement. Future studies need to incorporate measures across dimensions in order to explore whether reduced impairment (i.e., nutrition, growth, morbidity, and development), if found to be definitively associated with gastrostomy feeding, carries over to improved functional skills or activities, and to increased participation in social roles of daily life. Given that the greatest benefit of gastrostomy feeding may lie in the facilitation of care, future studies also need to document the impact of gastrostomy feeding on the intensity of caregiving that may be required.

III. REVIEW OF THE EFFECTS OF NEURODEVELOPMENTAL THERAPY FOR YOUNG CHILDREN WITH CEREBRAL PALSY

A. How Does Neurodevelopmental Therapy Work?

Neurodevelopmental treatment (NDT), or Bobath therapy, is the approach that has dominated physical, occupational, and speech therapy for children with cerebral palsy for the past 30 years. It was described earlier in Chapter 5, but its mechanism of action will be briefly reviewed again before presenting the evidence.

The proposed mechanism of action of NDT is based on the neuromaturational theory of motor development. The original goal of NDT, as described by Bobath, was to elicit normal patterns of movement through controlled sensorimotor experiences and to prevent the development of contractures and deformities (16). These controlled sensorimotor experiences were assumed to inhibit abnormal reflexes, tone, and movement patterns, and to facilitate more normal movement patterns. According to Bly (17), the theoretical construct and practice of NDT has changed over the years as knowledge of motor control has evolved. NDT techniques now include less emphasis on reflex inhibition and more emphasis on functional activities and active participation of the child. As the same time, other writers continue to define NDT theory and principles using the original concepts (18). Thus, the changing nature of NDT principles, the lack of a consistent and operational definition of NDT in the literature, as well as the variations in how NDT is actually practiced presents a challenge in evaluating outcomes of NDT.

Nevertheless, the goal of most motor therapies in cerebral palsy is to improve motor function and development while preventing the development of contractures and deformities. Improved motor development, in turn, may promote other aspects of child development. Because parental involvement is also stressed in NDT, an additional benefit of increased parenting skills and confidence may be expected. Conversely, the demands it places on parents and family resources may adversely affect family interaction patterns and priorities. Should neurodevelopmental therapy continue to dominate motor therapy in children with cerebral palsy? To what extent does the evidence document its impact on motor and other domains of child development and on quality of life for both the child and family?

B. Search Results

The MeSH terms "neurodevelopmental therapy," "NDT," "physical therapy," and "early intervention" added to "cerebral palsy," "infants," and "young children" produced 32 citations. Based on review of the abstracts, 28 full-text articles were obtained and examined. Reference lists in these studies and review articles as well as researchers knowledgable about this intervention were consulted. Fifty-eight articles were obtained; of that number, 16 potentially relevant studies were identified.

This review included those studies in which the intervention for all the subjects was either: (1) specified as NDT; (2) could be identified as NDT-based (from description of procedures that included inhibition of primitive and pathological reflexes, facilitation of postural reactions, and normalization of muscle tone); or (3) was said to be a mix of NDT with other sensorimotor techniques (a common circumstance in clinical practice). Eight studies of NDT in which the subjects were exclusively infants and very young children and four studies in which the subjects included infants and young children are reported in this review. An early case report about NDT was excluded for lack of measured outcomes (19), and three studies were excluded for the following reasons: treatment approach was too diffuse (i.e., "proprioceptive and neuromuscular facilitation and Bobath approach . . . used extensively in probably more than 50% of the subjects") (20); NDT was confounded with orthopedic surgery (21); and outcomes of CP subjects could not be determined (22).

C. Review of Studies

These 12 studies have used control groups and, in the main, compared NDT to some other intervention; one compared a greater versus lesser intensity of NDT. This was done in deference to the ethical concern of withholding a treatment intervention from a group of children for the formation of a no-treatment control group as well as to investigate whether intensity of therapy makes a difference. The studies are briefly described below and are summarized in Tables 5–6.

The effects of NDT were first investigated in 1973 in a controlled trial that included an external comparison of a group of treated children with an untreated group plus an internal comparison of a third group of children who acted as their own controls (23). Gross motor activities, retention of primary automatic reflexes, and range of motion at the ankle and hip joints were the outcomes of interest. No significant differences were found in measures made after either 6 or 12 months for the treated children. The group findings were generally representative regardless of type of cerebral palsy (diplegia, hemiplegia, or quadriplegia), age (under 6 months of age, 7 to 11 months of age, 12 to 17 months, or 18 months to 6 years of age), or mental ability. Moreover, overall progress was made by children, whether treated or not, as might be expected in a developing child with the passage of time.

Two years later, a study was published that compared an approach based on principles defined by the Bobaths, Rood, and Ayres (termed ''facilitation'') with an approach that emphasized positioning and adaptive hand and self-care skills (termed ''functional'') (24). Children, initially paired by developmental age, type and degree of cerebral palsy, and chronological age, were randomly assigned to one of the two interventions. After 6 weeks of treatment, the children in the facilitation group showed greater gains in all areas of development measured, but only the gross motor gains were statistically significant.

With the neurodevelopmental approach rapidly replacing traditional therapy in the United States, an investigation of an NDT-based therapy versus traditional therapy was undertaken and available for publication in 1976 (25). Infants were randomly assigned to the experimental treatment (positioning and movement to inhibit abnormal and immature reflexes or motor patterns and to facilitate more mature motor development) or the control treatment (passive range of motion and exercises). Measures made at age 2 were compared with measures made at entry to treatment but outcome measures of motor status, social maturation, and home management of parents were not clearly defined. Some children improved and some did not in both groups, but a greater percentage of children in the NDT-based therapy improved on all three measures.

In 1981, a study of the effects of 5 months of NDT-based therapy in severely mentally impaired children with cerebral palsy was published (26). Children, initially matched for age and overall developmental level, were randomly assigned to (1) a direct treatment group that described NDT-based procedures provided by therapists formally trained in Bobath and Rood techniques or (2) a supervised management group. A third group, the control group, received no therapy. Each of the three groups made small and almost identical gains on a developmental score and gross motor age score. No significant difference was found in the appearance of mature developmental reflexes, improvement of gross motor development, or increase of passive joint motion in the children in these three groups.

Immediate effects of NDT were investigated using single subject methodology and reported in 1983 (27). The study was replicated in four very young children. During eight 1-hour sessions over a 5-week period, each infant participated for 25 minutes in NDT therapeutic handling alternating with 25 minutes of simple physical handling during play by a non-therapist. There was not a statistically significant difference in a test of functional position-holding given after each NDT treatment compared with the same test given after each no-treatment play session.

Single subject methodology was also used in a 1985 study to investigate immediate effects of NDT techniques used in a treatment session compared with effects following a free play session (i.e., no-treatment condition) (28). The repeated measures showed improvement in range of motion as measured by ankle dorsiflexion and heel strike during movement to standing following the NDT treatment condition compared to the no treatment conditions.

In 1988, a comparison of the motor, mental, and social outcomes of infants with spastic diplegia who received physical therapy (NDT) versus an infant stimulation control intervention was published (29). The infants were stratified for developmental outcome and randomly allocated to the interventions. The blinded assessment performed at 6 and 12 months showed no motor advantage for the infants in the NDT intervention. Instead, the data favored the infants who received the infant stimulation intervention on the motor quotient measure, and they were more likely to walk as well. There were no significant differences between the groups in the incidence of contractures or the need for bracing or orthopedic surgery. In mental and social outcomes, there also were no significant differences between the groups.

The randomized controlled trial described in the preceding study also yielded additional psychological, behavioral, family, and parenting outcomes data that were published 2 years later (30). Only 1 of 20 measures of infant temperament, maternal–infant interaction, or home environment showed any difference between the groups of infants who had received NDT versus those who had experienced the infant stimulation intervention. There was a statistically significant greater score on maternal responsiveness for mothers of infants in the NDT group.

A replication of design and procedures in the 1983 study was used to investigate effect of NDT on physiological function during dressing (31). Two children were repeatedly assessed over 12 weeks. Observers, blind to the condition being measured, rated specific movements such as shoulder mobility, associated reactions, sitting balance, etc., while the children were engaged in dressing. Function was no different immediately after an NDT treatment than after a play session.

Another 1990 publication of a single subject research design yielded data about the effects of NDT on excessive knee flexion during walking (32). Repeated measures were made during each of five, three-week long phases (A-B-A-BC-A). A was a no treatment phase, B was an NDT treatment phase, and C was an

NDT plus orthosis treatment phase. Trend and level analyses showed improvement during both treatment phases (with greater improvement in the NDT only phase) compared with the no treatment phases.

Whether quantity of therapy has an effect on physiological hand function or quality of movement and on fine motor development was investigated in a randomized controlled trial published in 1991 (33). Power calculations suggest that the study had sufficient power to detect the main effects of NDT. Intensive NDT (45-minute therapy session twice weekly plus 30-minute home program daily) was compared to regularly administered NDT (varied from as little as once a month to as much as once a week plus a 15-minute home program three times a week). Additionally, the combined effect of casting with NDT therapy was studied, but these results are not pertinent to this review. Children were stratified by age (under or over 4 years old) and severity of hand function before random assignment to one of four groups: intensive NDT, regular NDT, intensive NDT + casting, or regular NDT + casting. The results indicated that there were no statistically significant benefits on either outcome from intensive therapy alone. Additional analysis of data suggested that the younger children in the NDT with casting group demonstrated greater improvement. To confirm the possibility of combined effects of NDT with casting in children under 4 years of age, the investigators then conducted the study described next.

Children under age 4 were stratified by age and hand function impairment before random assignment to one of two interventions for 4 months: intensive NDT combined with casting versus OT, which was based on functional activities such as self-help, feeding, and playing (34). A 2-month wash-out period followed, after which the groups crossed over to the opposite intervention. There was blind assessment of measures before and after each intervention period and the wash-out period. Analysis of the outcomes revealed no significant differences between the treatments on any of four measures.

D. Evidence Table

A cursory look at the evidence in Table 7 shows that treatment results have primarily been investigated in the dimension of impairment, that there is only one measure for many of the outcomes, and that most of the results cluster in the column showing no difference between treatment and control conditions. Little is known about the impact of NDT on the child's ability to perform activities, less still about its impact on the family itself and home environment, and nothing about its impact on the youngster's participation in the family. Little is known about the effect of increased amounts of therapy.

Some of the studies attempted to determine other factors that may be responsible for change, or lack of change, when youngsters are exposed to NDT (Table 8). These studies analyzed the relationship between age, intelligence, se-

Table 5 Summary of Studies

Section 1. Intervention and subjects

Study (Ref.)	Rx	Control Rx	Population	# Tot.	Ages
23	NDT	No Rx	Spastic diplegia, hemiplegia, quadriplegia	47	> 6 mo.–6 yr.
24	Facilitation[a]	Functional	Spastic diplegia, hemiplegia, quadriplegia	16	1–5 yr.
25	Neurophysiogic[a]	Traditional	Spastic quadriplegia, hemiplegia; athetosis	22	5–17 mo.
26	NDT[a]	Gr 1 No Rx Gr 2[b]	CP (all types) and severe MR	29	3–22yr.
27	NDT	No Rx (play)	Spastic quadriplegia, hemiplegia, diplegia, hyptonia	4	10–22 mo.
28	NDT	No Rx (play)	Spastic quadriplegia	1	2.5 yr.
29	NDT	6 mo. infant stimulation; 6 mo. NDT	Spastic diplegia	48	12–19 mo.
30	NDT	6 mo. infant stimulation; 6 mo. NDT	Spastic diplegia	48	12–19 mo.
31	NDT	No Rx (play)	Spastic diplegia	2	27, 32 mo.
32	NDT & NDT+ orthotic	No Rx	Spastic diplegia	1	2 yr.
33	1. NDT intensive	1. NDT regular	Spastic hemiplegia or quadriplegia	18[c] ~	18 mo.–8 yr.
34	NDT+ casting	Functional skills OT	Spastic diplegia, hemiplegia and quadriplegia	50	18 mo.–4 yr.

[a] Included neurodevelopmental treatment principles advocated by Bobath, Rood, and Ayres.
[b] Supervised PT management but no direct therapy.
[c] Total $n = 76$ in 4 groups, 2 of which included casting + NDT; the NDT only group data are reported here for those 18 subjects.

Section 2. Research methodology.

Study (Ref.)	Research Design and Level of Evidence	Duration	# in Rx Group	# in Control group
23	RCT (3 groups), Level II			
	External comparison 1	6 mo.	16	31
	External comparison 2	12 mo.	7	10
	Internal comparison	6 mo.	9	9
24	RCT (2 groups), Level II	6 wk.	8	8
25	RCT (2 groups), Level II	7–21 mo.	14	8
26	Concurrent cohort study, Level IV	5 mo.	10	
	Control group 1			9
	Control group 2			10
27	Multiple crossover alternating treatments trial, Level II	5 wk.	4	[a]
28	ABA design, Level III	25 days	1	[a]
29	RCT (2 groups), Level I	12 mo.	25	23
30	RCT (2 groups), Level I	12 mo.	25	22
31	Multiple crossover alternating treatments trial, Level II	12 wk.	2	[a]
32	A-B-A-BC-A trial, Level II	15 wk	1	[a]
33	RCT (2 groups reported), Level I Intensive vs. regular amt. NDT	9 mo.	18	18
34	RCT (2 groups), Level I	10 mo.	50	[a]

[a] Subjects were their own controls.

Table 6 Summary of Results

Section 1. Results of treatment compared to another condition or of greater versus lesser intensity NDT.

Study (Ref.)	Outcome	Dim.	Measure	Result	Clin. imp.	Inferential statistics	LOE
23	Automatic reflexes	I	Rated observation	U	no	NS	II
	ROM (2 movements)	I	Not specified	U	no	NS	II
	Gross motor acts	FL/A	Rated observation	−	no	NS	II
24	Motor age	I	Bayley Motor Sc.	+		$p < .05$	II
	Gross motor age	I	DDST[a], Motor Sc.	+		$p < .05$	II
	Fine motor age	I	DDST, Fine M. Scale	+		NS	II
25	Social age	I	DDST, Social Sc.	+		NS	II
	Language age	I	DDST, Lang. Sc.	+		NS	II
	Physiological function	I	Motor Dev. Eval.	+			II
	Social activities	FL/A	Questionnaire	+			II
	Home management	SL/C	Questionnaire	+			II
26[b]	Dev. reflexes	I	Wilson DR Test	−		NS	II
	Gross motor age	I	Gross Motor Eval.	−		NS	II
	ROM (6 movements)	I	ROM Scale			NS	II
27	Functional positions	FL/A	Rated observations	+		NS	II
28	ROM (dorsiflexion)	I	Biofeedback instrument	+		$p = .002^c$	III
	ROM (heel strike)	I	Biofeedback instrument	+	yes		III
29	Motor age	I	Bayley Motor Sc.	−		$p < .01$	I
	Physiological function	I	Neurological exam	−		$p < .05$	I
	ROM (jt. limitation)	I	Bracing recom.	U		NS	I
	ROM (contractures)	I	Surgery recom.	U		NS	I
	Walking	FL/A	Attained milestone	−	yes	$p = .01$	I
	Mental age	I	Bayley Mental Sc.	−		$p = .3$	I
	Social age	I	Vineland SM Sc.	−		$p = .54$	I

Study	Outcome	Design	Measure	Trend	Clin Imp	Significance	LOE
30	Activity	I	CITQ	−		NS	I
	Rhythmicity	I	CITQ	+		NS	I
	Adaptability	I	CITQ	−		NS	I
	Approach	I	CITQ	U		NS	I
	Threshold	I	CITQ	+		NS	I
	Intensity	I	CITQ	U		NS	I
	Mood	I	CITQ	+		NS	I
	Distractibility	I	CITQ	+		NS	I
	Persistence	I	CITQ	−		NS	I
	Maternal acceptance	SL/C	RMCRC	+		NS	I
	Mater. overprotect.	SL/C	RMCRC	+		NS	I
	Mater. over indulgen.	SL/C	RMCRC	−		NS	I
	Mat. rejection	SL/C	RMCRC	+	no	$p < .04$	I
	Mat. responsiveness	SL/C	HOME	+		NS	I
	Restriction avoidance	SL/C	HOME	+		NS	I
	Envir. organization	SL/C	HOME	+		NS	I
	Play materials	SL/C	HOME	+		NS	I
	Mat. involvement	SL/C	HOME	+		NS	I
	Variety stimulation	SL/C	HOME	+		NS	I
31	Physiological function	I	Rate movements	U		[c]	II
32	ROM (knee flexion)	I	Goniometer and videography	+		[c]	II
33	Fine motor age	I	Peabody FM Scale	−	no	$p = .63$	I
	Physiological hand function	I	QUEST	U	no	$p = .82$	I
34	Fine motor age	I	Peabody FM Scale	U	no	NS	I
	Physiological UE funct	I	QUEST	U	no	NS	I
	Hand activities	FL/A	COPM	U	no	NS	I
	Parent satisfaction	SL/C	Rating scale	U	no	NS	I

[a] Denver Developmental Screening Test.
[b] Results of Rx group compared to aggregated control groups.
[c] Trend and level analysis.
COPM = Canadian Occupational Performance Measure; QUEST = Quality of upper extremity skills scale; U = unchanged; NS = Not statistically significant; LOE = Level of evidence; Clin Imp = Clinical importance; Dim. = Dimension of disablement.

Table 7 State of Knowledge About Outcomes of Treatment with NDT for Youngster with Cerebral Palsy

Section 1. Outcomes of treatment compared with another condition or of greater versus lesser intensity NDT.

The evidence about each outcome is indicated by its level of evidence code (I through V) in the appropriate column showing: positive and statistically valid outcomes (+*), positive (+) or negative (−) results that were not subjected to statistical evaluation, or results that were unchanged, and/or were not statistically significant (U and NS). References to the study that produced the outcome are in parentheses. Outcomes of more intense NDT are shown in italics. For example, only one measure (of five) in one study (of five) detected improved physiological motor responses as a result of NDT. This measure, though Level II evidence, was not subjected to statistical evaluation. Three measures from Level I or II studies, subjected to statistical evaluation, found the group exposed to NDT was not different or less improved than the comparison group not receiving NDT. Two measures (Level I evidence) evaluating the effects of increased intensity of NDT also produced no statistically significant difference.

Outcome	+*	+	−*	U and NS
Pathophysiology				
Impairment				
Physiological motor responses		II(25)	I(29)	II(31) *I(34) I(33)*
Reflexes				II(23) II(26)
Range of motion	III(28) III(28) II(32)			II(23) II(26) I(29) I(29)
Motor age	II(24)		I(29)	
Gross motor age	II(24)			I(26)
Fine motor age				II(24) *I(34) I(33)*
Social age				II(24) I(29)
Mental age				I(29)
Language age				II(24)
Activity				I(30)
Rhythmicity				I(30)
Adaptability				I(30)
Approach				I(30)
Threshold				I(30)
Intensity				I(30)
Mood				I(30)
Distractibility				I(30)
Persistence				I(30)

		Outcome
Functional limitation:		
Activity		
	Gross motor acts	II(23), III(27)
	Walking	I(29)
	Hand activities	II(25)
	Social acts	II(25)
Disability/participation		
Societal limitation/		
Context		
	Home management	I(34)
	M. acceptance	I(30)
	M. overprotection	I(30)
	M. overindulgence	I(30)
	M. rejection	I(30)
	M. responsiveness	I(30)
	M. involvement	I(30)
	M. restrictions	I(30)
	Environment	I(30)
	Play materials	I(30)
	Variety stimulation	I(30)
	Parent satisfaction	I(34)

M. = maternal.

Table 8 Determinants of Change Other than Intervention

Factors subjected to analysis	Statistically significant (Ref.)
Mental development or intelligence	no(23)
	no(33)
	yes(25)
Age	no(25)
	no(26)
	yes(33)
Severity of disability	no(25)
Maternal education level	no(33)
Family income	no(33)
Parental compliance with home program	yes(33)

verity of disability, maternal education, or family income and outcome of exposure to NDT.

E. Analyzing the Evidence Tables

1. What Evidence Is There About the Effects of NDT on Motor Impairment or Impairment in Other Domains of Development?

There are 34 outcomes related to impairment. Of these, 26 results showed no difference between the NDT and control groups; six results favored NDT, two results favored the control condition.

(a) Motor Response.   Benefit of NDT on physiological motor function (including reflex activity) has been measured seven times: benefit was found only once; six measures detected no benefit over the control condition. Specifically, one study found greater improvement in the group that got NDT on an aggregate measure of physiological motor response (25); however, in another study that used a similar aggregate measure, greater improvement was found in the control group (29). The finding that was in favor of NDT was not statistically significant and was produced by a less rigorous study than the one that produced the negative finding for NDT. Two measures each of primitive and mature reflex activity and quality of upper extremity movement, and one measure that combined postural tone, weight shift and bearing, and transitional movement were not statistically significant when scores of the NDT groups were compared with the control groups.

(b) Range of Motion. Three of these seven measures suggest that there may be some immediate effects of NDT on dynamic range of motion. Improved heel strike and ankle dorsiflexion as well as reduction of excessive knee flexion were measured immediately following therapy sessions. Otherwise, the measures detected no difference between the NDT and control groups on joint limitation, contractures, range of hip abduction and ankle dorsiflexion, and on an aggregate measure at several joints.

(c) Motor Development. Normative tests of child development inform about the general degree of impairment in various domains of development through a standardized score, usually a motor, mental, language, or social age (or quotient). There were seven outcomes in which a motor age (gross motor age, fine motor age, or overall motor age) was calculated. Five measures suggest that NDT did not accelerate motor development. In contrast, the two measures that suggest that motor development in the NDT group was accelerated were made in the same group of 12 children.

(d) Other Domains of Child Development and Function. Two measures of social age and one measure each of mental age and language age found no difference between the group that received the NDT and the control group. There were also nine measures of emotional function (i.e., various aspects of infant temperament); none showed results for the NDT group that were significantly different from the control group.

(e) Quantity of Therapy. Two studies evaluated whether more intensive intervention (twice a week plus a home program) compared to a less intensive intervention (once a week or less) would demonstrate greater gains in measures of impairment. (33, 34). Two other studies evaluated outcomes at 6 and again at 12 months to learn whether therapy over a longer period of time would demonstrate greater gains in measures of impairment (23, 29). No beneficial effect of increasing either the intensity of therapy or increasing the period of therapy over time was detected by these studies.

2. What Evidence Is There About the Effects of NDT in Dimensions of Disablement Other than Impairment?

(a) Pathophysiology. There is no evidence regarding changes in cellular or molecular structure or function in individuals as a result of NDT during early childhood.

(b) Functional Limitation/Activity. Unlike the normative tests in the impairment dimension that sample selected activities to yield a comparative developmental domain age or quotient (i.e., motor age or intellectual quotient), this dimension is concerned with quantitative description of the performance of activi-

ties such as walking, dressing, playing, or interacting with other people. Four of the five activities that were measured were concerned with motor performance; one, with social skills. Neither gross nor fine motor activities improved as a result of NDT. In other developmental domains, one study reported that infants displayed more social skills but did not specify what these skills were.

(c) *Disability/Participation.*   Effects of NDT on participation in social roles have also not been investigated.

(d) *Societal Limitation/Context Factors.*   It has been hypothesized that NDT may have indirect benefits for the child by improving the parent–child relationship or by reducing the stress parents experience in caring for a child with atypical motor function. Ten of 12 measures reject this hypothesis. With one exception, measures of mother–child interaction revealed no difference in the outcomes of the mothers whose children received NDT versus mothers whose children did not. Only maternal responsiveness to the child improved as reflected in higher and statistically significant scores for mothers of the NDT group. Four measures detected no difference in the children's environment as a result of children receiving NDT. Parent satisfaction was no higher for parents whose children were in NDT. There was a positive finding for NDT in a questionnaire probing changes in home management; however, this was statistically evaluated.

3.   What Linkages Exist for Treatment Effects Within and Across These Dimensions of Disablement and in Which Directions?

None can be detected for two reasons. Relatively few measures (9 out of 51) detected a treatment effect for NDT. Treatment effects detected were primarily in the impairment dimension (6 of 9); data of effects outside the dimension of impairment are so limited analysis of linkages of effects across dimensions is not possible.

4.   Are There Subgroups for Whom NDT May Be More or Less Effective?

Four of the studies analyzed the relationship between various factors and outcomes of exposure to NDT to identify subgroups of children more or less likely to profit from NDT (see Table 8). Three studies analyzed age as a variable, but it was statistically significant in only one of the studies. The effect of intelligence was analyzed in three studies; it, too, was statistically significant in only one of the studies. One analysis each of severity of disability, maternal education, and family income failed to identify any subgroups. One measure of parental compliance with the home program suggests that only children whose parents follow through with the prescribed treatment are more likely to improve.

5. What Kinds and Magnitude of Complications Have Been Documented?

None.

6. What Is the Strength of the Evidence?

Credibility of the evidence depends on several factors: how extensively the population has been sampled (number of different studies and number of subjects), consistency of results across the studies, and robustness of the research methods used. This body of evidence is relatively limited with regard to the population that has been sampled: 12 studies (two with the same population sample) with a total of 231 different children. On the other hand, it is a fairly robust body of evidence in regard to internal validity: four Level I studies, six Level II studies, and one Level III and IV. Moreover, the outcomes are generally consistent; only 9 of 51 are positive for NDT and these were generally not of clinical importance. Some other determinants of change (age, intelligence, etc.) have also been examined but not consistently found to be factors that could account for the observed outcomes when youngsters have been exposed to NDT.

F. Discussion

The tenets of NDT theory have not been supported by current evidence. There is little evidence that it changes abnormal reflexes, muscle tone, or movement patterns, or that it facilitates either more normal motor development or functional movement activities. More intensive therapy has not conferred a greater benefit. The evidence also has not been able to demonstrate other benefits to children in social-emotional, language, or cognitive domains of development, or in improved parent–child interactions or in better home environments. These conclusions are bolstered by a meta-analysis study of the effectiveness of pediatric therapy, which revealed that NDT effects were detectable with meta-analysis techniques, but that overall treatment effects were small (35).

While these findings are disappointing, this evidence cannot be construed as negative evidence. There are four circumstances that interfere with the ability to detect an intervention effect and make it impossible to draw any definitive conclusions about NDT at this time. These problematic issues are: (1) lack of an operational definition of NDT; (2) lack of known power in the sample sizes to detect effects, had there been effects; (3) the hetergeneous characteristics of the subjects; and (4) lack of valid and reliable outcome measures with which to detect an intervention effect. In addition, we still lack adequate data to indicate whether age, severity of involvement, or other factors influence the effect of NDT.

It is easy to be discouraged by this review. However, given their long-standing commitment to youngsters with cerebral palsy, physical and occupational therapists should view these findings as a call both to more systematic and robust evaluation of the effects of NDT and to the exploration of intervention strategies based on other theoretical models of motor development.

At the same time, the information in this review may allay some anxieties, reduce some conflicts in professional emphasis, and suggest avenues that may prove to be more productive for improving the lives of children with cerebral palsy and their families. These findings may alleviate some of the anxiety that parents, therapists, and other clinicians have felt about children not getting as much NDT therapy as they believed was needed.

These findings may also reduce conflicts between educators and therapists whose interventions derived from different theoretical models (i.e., theories of cognitive and social-emotional development versus the motor theory on which NDT is based). The crux of that professional dilemma has been that NDT, designed to enhance the child's later physical status, may have a secondary deleterious effect upon the child's subsequent intellectual and psychosocial development as a result of the restrictions the therapy may place on the child's preferred movement patterns and resultant sensorimotor experiences (36–38). For example, according to cognitive theory, interaction with the environment is necessary for maximal cognitive development during early childhood. Consequently, youngsters with cerebral palsy who are not encouraged or allowed to use their preferred, albeit abnormal, patterns of movement to position themselves and manipulate objects in the environment may miss out on critical sensorimotor experiences. Likewise, children whose therapeutic experience is focused exclusively on NDT and who are not allowed to use assistive technology to by-pass their motor impairments miss important opportunities for learning and exploring. On the other hand, very young children who use powered devices that allow self-controlled locomotion, electronic communication devices that allow interaction with people, and environmental control devices that activate a variety of objects and toys, can participate in sensorimotor experiences in the normal developmental timetable — and develop a sense of competence and confidence in themselves while they explore their environment and learn.

IV. REVIEW OF THE EFFECTS OF EARLY INTERVENTION WITH PHYSICAL THERAPY FOR INFANTS "AT RISK" FOR CEREBRAL PALSY

A. What Is Early Intervention?

Early intervention programs were first implemented in the 1960s in the United States in its "war on poverty." Their purpose was to alter the cognitive developmental trajectories of *socially* vulnerable children (i.e., to counter the effects of poverty and other frequently coexisting risk factors such as low birth weight, low parental education, and family stress) on cognitive development in children (39, 40). Children born prematurely and with low birth weight are also *biologically* vulnerable. Such infants are disproportionately likely to have major neurodevelopmental deficits, including cerebral palsy. Thus, early intervention has had two meanings. It refers to (1) programs intended to reduce potential cognitive impairment in infants at risk socially and (2) programs intended to reduce potential motor impairment in infants at risk biologically.

For purposes of this review, early intervention is defined as the early initiation of a formal program of physical therapy for infants who are likely to manifest permanent neurological sequelae with motor dysfunction as they develop. This likelihood or risk is calculated on the basis of abnormal birth history (e.g., premature birth, low birth weight, birth asphyxia, low Apgar score at birth) and on various neonatal risk findings after birth (e.g., seizures; abnormal ultrasound scans, computer tomography scans, or EEG tracing during newborn period; abnormal tone or patterns of movement; abnormal persistence of primitive reflexes).

B. Intervention and Timing

Because of the complex developmental nature of cerebral palsy, its diagnosis cannot be made with certainty until motor delay and abnormal motor patterns are well established and other diagnoses ruled out. Except in severe cases, diagnosis of cerebral palsy is often delayed until age 2 or after, when the classic signs of cerebral palsy have become pronounced.

Nevertheless, operating from the neuromaturational premise that the immature nervous system is more adaptable to change and can be more readily influenced than the mature nervous system, it has been thought that intervention begun as early as possible in a child's life will be more beneficial than intervention begun later. Thus, Bobath argued that treatment started before the age of 9 months will give quicker and better results (16). She cited several reasons: the adaptability and plasticity of infantile brain; importance of normal sensorimotor learning; possible mental retardation secondary to sensorimotor deprivation; abnormal postural reflex activity, spasticity and athetosis that grows stronger over time; and opportunity to prevent development of contractures and deformities. Vojta claimed that early intervention may even prevent cerebral palsy. Specifically, he alleged that his method of very early therapy prevents ''uncomplicated'' cerebral palsy (41). By Vojta's definition, ''uncomplicated'' type of cerebral palsy is motor impairment that is not combined with severe mental retardation and/or severe convulsive disorders. On the basis of these assertions or on the basis of neuromaturational theory in general, many therapists and physicians have supported the initiation of therapy as early and as intensively as possible to minimize future handicaps (42). In fact, it has often been presented that early intervention is absolutely essential and that failure to attend therapy sessions and/or administer the recommended home program will compromise the child's future development (43).

Research shows that the predictive validity of early diagnostic signs, while useful, is not perfect. Follow-up studies demonstrate that a greater percentage of high-risk infants do develop cerebral palsy, but many high-risk infants do not. Early differentiation of those infants who will have permanent neurological sequelae from those who will not continues to be difficult.

Clinicians, therefore, face the problem of how to use the information that an infant is at "high risk." One response has been to warn parents about the possibility their infant may have developmental problems, follow the child closely after discharge, and introduce physical therapy only if signs of abnormal muscle tone or motor function develop. Another response is to initiate therapy immediately and discontinue it only after normal motor development has manifested. Today, on the basis of one or more indices of risk factors, even newborns are identified as "at risk" for motor impairment and frequently placed in a physical therapy program.

In addition to potential effect on domains of child development, early physical therapy programs may also offer parental support, foster parent/child relationships, and diminish parental anxiety. Conversely, these programs are demanding both for the infant and for the parent (44). They usually require regular attendance at a clinic for therapy combined with a home program that parents carry out. Many parents are unable to comply fully because it is stressful and time consuming to master and maintain the treatment recommendations (22). Participation in a rigorous intervention program may disrupt family functioning, involve high cost, deflect scarce resources of time, energy, and money exclusively to this enterprise, and even create feelings of guilt in the parents. In addition, from a societal point of view, financial cost associated with early intervention for high-risk infants, some of whom will develop normally without intervention, can be significant.

Is the enthusiasm for early intervention with physical therapy that has prevailed in the past 20 years justified by empirical research? Does early intervention affect motor outcome? Are there other important effects? Do the benefits derived from this early intervention warrant the time and effort expended by parent and child as well as the financial cost?

C. Search Results

The MeSH terms "perinatal risk," "early intervention," "physical therapy," and "developmental outcome" were used with "cerebral palsy," "infants," and "preschool children" to search in Clinical Queries of MEDLINE. Relevant articles were obtained. References in these articles to identify studies missed by electronic searching and knowledgable researchers were consulted. Examination of the article references yielded another six citations for full-text article review. Fourteen full-text articles were obtained and reviewed. Studies were excluded if some of their subjects had already been diagnosed with cerebral palsy at the outset of the study. Ten relevant studies were found.

D. Review of Studies

The ten studies of impact of early intervention with physical therapy on the prevention or minimization of future handicaps are described briefly in the following section and are summarized in Tables 9–10.

The first study, a description of a case series of at-risk infants said to have early signs of cerebral palsy, was highly encouraging (45). In 1966, it was reported that 77% of such children who had had 1 to 4 years of the Bobath method of physical therapy or NDT (clinic sessions plus home program) that began in the first year of life showed almost complete "normalization" of motor function and no longer required treatment. Cerebral palsy was diagnosed in only 23% of the children, and they remained in therapy.

The purpose of a 1980 study was to examine whether early Vojta physical therapy in infants with abnormal reflexes prevented the development of uncomplicated cerebral palsy or, conversely, produced normal motor development, as claimed by Vojta (44). The Vojta method of physical therapy was compared with a control group of children, some of whom got no treatment and some of whom got NDT because their parents were unwilling to accept no treatment at all. There was no difference between the groups in the number of infants who subsequently were found to have normal motor development. On the other hand, no infants with Vojta treatment developed uncomplicated CP compared to four who did in the control group; this was not a statistically significant difference, however.

Another study of Vojta physical therapy appeared the following year. The intent was to compare two forms of motor therapy against each other and to a third control group (41). Children were randomly assigned to participate in a trial of Vojta treatment or a trial of NDT. However, failure to stratify by risk factors of greater severity before randomization resulted in the NDT group being disproportionately and heavily weighted with infants who had risk factors of greater severity (5 out of 6 compared to 5 out of 9 in the Vojta group). This poses a serious threat to the credibility of comparing outcomes of NDT therapy, so the NDT subjects and its data are excluded herein. The control group did not participate in the random allocation; they were exposed to an intervention described only as a "less strictly performed and combined form of physiotherapy." Although 30% more infants in the Vojta-treated grouped turned out to have normal motor development compared to the control group, there was no difference between the groups in the percentage of cases of uncomplicated CP.

A third study of Vojta physical therapy was published in 1983 in which a group of 67 infants at high risk for motor impairment had been treated by the Vojta method (46). The publication reported a case series of 713 children, but only 67 were at high risk for motor impairment and were known to have received this motor intervention. Others received no therapy at all or an alternative therapy; still others had no signs of cerebral coordination disturbance (CCD) or light-to-moderate signs. Thus, only the 67 subjects in the Vojta group and their outcomes are reported herein. Retrospectively, the 713 children were stratified by the severity of CCD signs in the initial examination shown by the medical records, so that outcomes data for the infants most likely to develop cerebral palsy can be examined. Although it is only uncomplicated cerebral palsy that Vojta claims can be prevented, this study did not differentiate complicated versus uncomplicated cerebral palsy. The rate of diagnosis of cerebral palsy was 85% in the 67 children; only 7% of them eventually were found to have normal motor function.

In 1985, 3-month-old graduates from a neonatal intensive care unit who scored as neurologically normal and who scored as neurologically at risk were alternately assigned to a treatment versus a no treatment group, forming four groups to be followed up for a year (47). The developmental quotient of these infants was assessed every 3 months. In neither normal nor at-risk groups did NDT alter the pattern or outcome of overall development.

Five years later, the foregoing subjects were followed up to ascertain whether long-term treatment effects of the early intervention were detectable (43). Of the original 80 children, 49 were available for reassessment. The developmental quotient showed improvement from the 1-year assessment and was similar for both normal and at-risk children. Such improvement, however, appeared to occur naturally and was unaffected by early physical therapy or any subsequent intervention.

A randomized, controlled trial the following year evaluated the impact of early NDT on at-risk infants identified on the basis of low birth weight or adverse birth history (48). The experimental group received physical therapy and a home program carried out by parents for a year; the control group continued in the regular neonatal follow-up of periodic clinic visits. Independent evaluators who were blind to the interventions assessed the children on several developmental and neuromotor measures. Findings failed to provide evidence that early physical therapy as applied in this trial either prevents neuromotor dysfunction or promotes motor development in at-risk infants. Additional analyses of 14 potential determinants of change did not identify effects of treatment in selective groups of experimental children.

Two studies, both published in 1996, tested the hypothesis that the early introduction of physical therapy for children who later developed CP would result in the promotion and acceleration of motor development compared to an approach in which physical therapy is delayed until abnormal neurological signs become apparent.

One of these studies investigated the sensorimotor type of therapy instituted early versus later. The early-start (experimental) group got physical therapy and a home program from age 3 months until their first birthday (49). Delayed-start children began physical therapy sessions only when (and if) they began to demonstrate motor delay. Although cost analyses revealed that the early intervention was almost twice as expensive as the delayed start intervention, annual comprehensive assessments up to age 7 revealed no significant differences in developmental outcomes based on age of start. Anecdotally, one family reported that the involvement of interventionists in the first year, before the family stabilized and got to know their child well, was intrusive rather than helpful.

The other study compared NDT therapy for premature infants, started early versus waiting for abnormal signs to manifest (50). There were no significant differences on a global measure of development, nor on the individual normative subscales at 12 or at 30 months. By 30 months, 45 infants in the early therapy group had developed cerebral palsy compared with 24 in the later therapy group. The subgroup with cerebral palsy in the two groups was further analyzed to determine whether motor development coincident with cerebral palsy had been enhanced by early physical therapy. However, early treatment did not confer a benefit to children with cerebral palsy either in their overall developmental quotient, their locomotor developmental quotient, independent walking, or in development of orthopedic deformities that precipitated surgery.

The final study found that the prevalence of maternal depression was no different for mothers whose premature infants were considered at risk for developing cerebral palsy, compared to mothers of premies not considered at risk, and compared to mothers of healthy full-term infants (51). Of interest to this review of early intervention was the testing of a further hypothesis (i.e., that the rates of depression in mothers whose at risk infants received early physical therapy intervention would be lower than for mothers whose infants were not offered intervention until impaired neurodevelopment manifested). The proportion of mothers who were depressed at 6 weeks, 6 months, and 12 months was higher in the group whose infants were receiving early intervention than in the group whose infants got later intervention. This difference was not statistically significant, however.

E. Evidence Table

A cursory examination of Table 11 shows that most measures have investigated effect of early physical or motor therapy in the dimension of impairment. The

Table 9 Summary of Studies

Section 1. Intervention and subjects.

Study (Ref.)	Rx	Control	Subject sample	#Total	Ages
45	NDT	~	Motor risk Dx	69	<1 yr.
44	Vojta	Mixed: no Rx & NDT	Early signs cerebral coordination disturbance (CCD): Vojta criteria	51	4–7 mo.
41	Vojta	[a]	Early signs CCD: Vojta criteria	18	<6 mo.
46	Vojta		Severe CCD and suspected CP: Vojta criteria	67	<9 mo.
47	NDT	No Rx	VLBW infants from NICU	80	3 mo. CA
43	NDT	No Rx	Same subjects as Goodman study	49	6 yr.
48	NDT	No Rx	LBW infants and/or adverse birth history	134	40 wk. Con. A
49	Early[b] PT	Later[b] PT	Medically fragile NICU infants (IVH or LBW)	65	3 mo.
50	Early[b] PT	Later[b] PT	Analysis 1: Premies with abnormal cranial ultrasound scans	83	36–41 wk.
			Analysis 2: Infants who developed CP	45	
51	Early[b] PT	Later[b] PT	Mothers of infants in early versus late NDT treatment	30	

Section 2. Research Methodology

Study (Ref.)	Research Design and Level of Evidence	Duration	# in Rx Group	# in Control group
45	Retrospective case series without controls, Level V	1–4 yr.	69	0
44	Cohort study with historical control group, Level III	3 yr.	21	30
41	Cohort study with concurrent control group, Level III	4 yr.	10	8
46	Retrospective case series without controls, Level V	1–4 yr.	67	0
47	Treatment outcomes analytic survey, Level II	1 yr.		
	Normal babies (i.e., low NDS)		20	20
	At risk babies (i.e., high NDS)		20	20
43	Treatment outcomes analytic survey, Level III	5 yr.		
	Normal babies (i.e., low NDS)		13	12
	At risk babies (i.e., high NDS)		15	9
48	Randomized controlled trial, Level I	12 mo.	56	59
49	Randomized controlled trial, Level II	7 yr.		
50	Randomized controlled trial, Level I	30 mo.		
	Analysis 1: High-risk infants		42	41
	Analysis 2: Infants that developed CP		23	22
51	Cohort study with concurrent control group, Level II	30 mo.	16	14

[a] "A less strictly performed and combined form of therapy."

[b] Physical therapy started at release from NICU (early) vs. started (later) after Dx of motor delay (later).

LBW or VLBW = low birth weight or very low birth weight; NICU = Neonatal intensive care unit; IVH = Intraventricular hemorrhage; CA = corrected age; Con A = Conceptual age; NDS = Neurodevelopmental scores.

Table 10 Summary of Results

Section 1. Results of treatment compared to another intervention.

Study (Ref.)	Outcome	Dim.	Measure	Result	Clin. Imp.	Inferential Statistics	LOE
44	Uncomplicated CP	I	Rate of uncomplicated CP Dx	+	yes	NS	III
	Normal motor dev.	I	Rate of normal motor Dx	U	no	NS	III
41	Uncomplicated CP	I	Rate of uncomplicated CP Dx	U	no	NS	III
	Normal motor dev.	I	Rate of normal motor Dx	+	yes		III
47[a]	DQ	I	Griffiths MD Scale	U	no	NS	II
43	DQ[a]	I	Griffiths MD Sc. 2	−	no	NS	III
	CP[b]	I	Rate of CP Dx	U	no	NS	III
48	Gross motor activities	FL/A	Wolanski GM Eval	U	no	NS	I
	Physiological motor	I	Milani-Comparetti	U	no	NS	I
	Physiological motor	I	Wilson DR Profile	−	no	NS	I
	DQ	I	Griffiths MD Scale	−	no	NS	I
	Normal motor dev	I	Rate of Dx	−	no	NS	I
	Abnormal motor dev.	I	Rate of Dx	−	no	NS	I
49	Financial cost	SL/C	Cost analysis	−	yes		II
	DQ	I	Battelle Dev. Inv.			NS	II
	IQ	I	Stanford-Binet			NS	II
	Independent beh. age	I	Sc. of Indep. Beh.			NS	II
	Academic ach. age	I	W-J-R			NS	II
	Social age	I	Social Skill Rating			NS	II
	Emotional states	I	CBCL			NS	II
	Stress on child	I	Parent Stress Indx			NS	II

Study	Outcome	Measure	Result[a]	Result[b]	Clin Imp.	p	LOE
50	Analysis 1:						
	DQ	Griffiths MD Scale	I	U	no	p = .7	I
	CP	Limb by Limb. Ass.	I	U	no		I
	Analysis 2:						
	DQ	Griffiths MD Scale	I	–	no	NS	I
	Locomotor dev.	Griffiths Loc subsc	I	–	no	NS	I
	age						
	Independent walking		FL/A	–	no	p = .75	I
	Ortho. deformity	Rate of ortho surg	I	U	no		I
51	Maternal depression	Malaise inventory	I	–	yes	p = .63	II

[a] Results of treated at-risk group compared to untreated at-risk group plus treated and untreated normal groups.
[b] Results of treated at-risk group compared to untreated at-risk group.

DQ = development quotient; AE = Age equivalent; W-J-R = Woodcock Johnson Revised Test of Academic Achievement; CBCL = Child Behavior Checklist; U = unchanged; NS = Not statistically significant; LOE = Level of evidence; Clin Imp. = Clinically important; Dim. = Dimension of disablement.

Section 2. Uniformity of results within treatment groups: rates of normal motor development and development of cerebral palsy.

Study (Ref.)	Cerebral palsy	Normal motor dev.
45 (n = 69)	23%	77%
44 (n = 21)	24%	
46 (n = 67)	85%	7%
50 (n = 42)	55%	

Table 11 State of Knowledge About Outcomes of Early Intervention with Physical Therapy (Outcomes of early treatment compared with no treatment or delayed treatment.)

The evidence about each outcome is indicated by its level of evidence code (I through V) in the appropriate column showing: positive and statistically significant results (+*) or negative (−*), positive (+) or negative (−) results that were not subjected to statistical evaluation, or results that were not different and/or were not statistically significant (U and NS). References to the study that produced the outcome are in parentheses. For example, six measures of developmental quotient made in five studies have found no statistical difference in favor of infants receiving early intervention; these findings represent Level I, II, and III evidence about effect on overall development.

Outcome	+*	+	−*	U or NS
Pathophysiology				
Impairment				
Uncomplicated CP				III(44) III(41)
CP				III(43) I(50)
Abnormal motor dev.				I(48)
Normal motor dev.		III(41)		III(44) I(48)
Locomotor development				I(50)
Physiological motor function				I(48) I(48)
Orthopedic deformity				I(50)
Developmental quotient				II(47) I(48) III(43) II(49) I(50) I(50)
IQ				II(49)
Academic achiev. age				II(49)
Indep. behavior age				II(49)
Social age				II(49)
Emotional states				II(49)
Stress on child				II(49)
Functional limitation/				
Activity				
Gross motor activities				I(48)
Independent walking				I(50)
Disability/participation				
Societal limitation/				
Context				
Financial cost			II(49)	
Maternal depression				II(51)

preponderance of evidence shows no difference as a result of early intervention in this or any dimension.

F. Analyzing the Evidence

1. What Evidence Exists About the Effects of Early Intervention on Domains of Child Development?

The results are remarkably consistent across a variety of measures that have been used. Only one measure supported any benefit of early motor therapy, and it was not evaluated for its statistical validity. The rates of normal motor development or minimal residual motor disability (or conversely, cerebral palsy) were reported in four studies (44–46, 50). When rates of CP, abnormal motor development, or normal motor development were compared with the rates in control groups of children (41, 43, 44, 50), the rates were not lower in groups exposed to early intervention nor were rates of normal motor diagnosis higher. Motor development, as reflected by motor quotients or ages or physiological motor function appeared to be unaffected by early intervention. No effects in other developmental domains were detected.

2. What Evidence Exists for Effects in Other Dimensions of Disablement?

Only two measures have been made in each of two other dimensions.

(a) Pathophysiology. None.

(b) Functional Limitation/Activity. One measure of activities of a gross motor nature found no significant difference for the group with early intervention.

(c) Disability/Participation. None.

(d) Societal Limitation/Context Factors. If early intervention had no direct remedial value for the child as shown by the measures of impairment or activity, did it work to help families cope with the possibility of their infants developing cerebral palsy? One study investigating rates of maternal depression found that the proportion of mothers who were depressed was actually higher in the group receiving early intervention than in the group receiving intervention only after cerebral palsy manifested. However, there was not a statistical difference between these groups of mothers. The only other bit of evidence about families is an anecdote that also suggests early intervention is not necessarily supportive to parents (49). It was reported that the involvement of interventionists in the life, schedule, and home of the family in the first year was felt to be intrusive. Time to get to know their child and stabilize the family was said to be important before ''outsiders'' entered the picture. Finally, in this dimension,

the cost of early intervention was found to be double the cost of intervening after cerebral palsy has been diagnosed; thus, this is a negative outcome.

3. What Linkages Exist for Treatment Effects Within and Between These Dimensions and in Which Directions?

None.

4. Are There Subgroups for Whom Early Intervention is More or Less Effective?

Three studies attempted to identify subgroups of experimental children through statistical analysis of interaction effects (43, 48, 49). Their analyses showed that, regardless of group assignment, long-term developmental outcomes were better for infants who did not have (1) very low birth weight (>750 g); (2) medical complications at birth (especially intraventricular hemorrhage); or (3) low socio-economic status (especially low maternal education).

5. What Kinds and Magnitude of Complications Have Been Reported?

None.

6. What Is the Strength of the Evidence?

Ten studies provide results from a total of 616 children and 30 mothers. Two case series without controls contributed information about rates of cerebral palsy and normal motor development in groups exposed to early intervention (45, 46); however, all other studies employed control groups. The greatest strength of this body of evidence is the consistency of its results. The outcomes are also credible in that 12 of the 25 results are Level I evidence and 10 are Level II evidence. Thus, the body of evidence is relatively definitive; its greatest weakness is the relatively small number of subjects on which it is based.

G. Discussion

The first description, in 1966, of a series of at-risk infants who had received physical therapy in the first year of life raised hope that early intervention would either prevent neuromotor dysfunction or promote more normal motor development. No subsequent study has been able to demonstrate statistical evidence to support that hope for NDT, Votja, or any other form of physical therapy that has been studied. There is relatively strong evidence that very early physical therapy yields neither short-term nor long-term effect on motor development or on other domains of child development. Even children considered to be at risk at one year of age showed improvement over the next five years; such improvement seemed to occur naturally and was unaffected by early physical therapy (43). There is surprising, though quite limited, evidence that early intervention may not necessarily be supportive to families either.

Certainly this evidence challenges any recommendation that early physical therapy for at-risk infants is essential and that failure to attend clinics and/or administer the home program will compromise the child's future development. The cost estimates underscore an economic imperative that is particularly compelling in the absence of measurable clinical difference. The evidence suggests that a "wait and see" approach to treatment is preferable. The skills of physical therapists are needed for the on-going assessment of those children initially identified as high risk and for management of cerebral palsy after its diagnosis.

V. SUMMARY

This chapter has demonstrated that evidence tables constructed on the AACPDM framework can consolidate evidence for specific as well as diffuse types of interventions. Assessment of factors to determine the levels of evidence of a study, as well as the dimensions of disablement represented by the results, tends to be a relatively subjective enterprise. Thus, a review itself is subject to bias. This bias can be partially overcome by adhering to the guidelines set out in the AACPDM methodology for conducting systematic reviews. It can be further overcome by agreement on coding of results and their interpretation by a group of reviewers rather than an individual reviewer. Despite this limitation, however, the concept of systematic reviews of evidence is a useful one and, indeed, is the cornerstone of evidence-based health care.

Use of this particular format for organizing the evidence about interventions can have many additional benefits for the field of developmental disabilities. With such a tool, consensus can be reached about the dimensions for which there is evidence of efficacy in each intervention. Meaningful comparisons between interventions can eventually be made. The dimensions for which adequate information is lacking can be visualized and will invite future research to address the gaps in our knowledge. Use of the model will prompt the research community to include multiple outcome measures in study protocols so that existence of linkage of effects across dimensions can be determined. It will help professionals and clients alike to recognize that recommendations may be seen, not as conflicting, but rather as complementary by showing how different interventions can have effects in different levels. This can help clients make informed decisions about treatment options based on what the treatment offers and how that relates to their own values. It can lead us all to think about intervention differently (i.e., that an individual child may best be served at a particular point by altering the environment rather than attempting to change the child's impairment or by considering whether the disability of social isolation may be caused by depression rather than limited mobility). Finally, it will serve to remind each of us that as individuals in our communities we have the opportunity to reduce further the burden of disability in the dimension of societal limitation by efforts to initiate and support actions to remove all barriers to full participation in society of people with disabilities.

REFERENCES

1. Butler C. AACPDM Methodology for Development of Evidence Tables and Review of Treatment Outcomes Research. Vol. Internet at www.aacpdm.org: American Academy for Cerebral Palsy and Developmental Medicine, 1998. (Last Update: August 1, 1999)
2. Sullivan PB. Gastrointestinal problems in the neurologically impaired child. Baillieres Clin Gastroenterol 1997; 11:529–46.
3. Rogers BT, Arvedson J, Msall M, Demerath RR. Hypoxemia during oral feeding of children with severe cerebral palsy. Dev Med Child Neurol 1993; 35:3–10.
4. Corwin DS, Isaacs JS, Georgeson KE, Bartolucci AA, Cloud HH, Craig CB. Weight and length increases in children after gastrostomy placement. J Am Diet Assoc 1996; 96:874–9.
5. Guesry P. The role of nutrition in brain development. Prev Med 1998; 27:189–94.
6. Eltumi M, Sullivan PB. Nutritional management of the disabled child: the role of percutaneous endoscopic gastrostomy. Dev Med Child Neurol 1997; 39:66–8.
7. McGovern B. Janeway gastrostomy in children with cerebral palsy. J Pediatr Surg 1984; 19:800–2.
8. McGrath SJ, Splaingard ML, Alba HM, Kaufman BH, Glicklick M. Survival and functional outcome of children with severe cerebral palsy following gastrostomy. Arch Phys Med Rehabil 1992; 73:133–7.
9. Shapiro BK, Green P, Krick J, Allen D, Capute AJ. Growth of severely impaired children: neurological versus nutritional factors. Dev Med Child Neurol 1986; 28: 729-33.
10. Rempel GR, Colwell SO, Nelson RP. Growth in children with cerebral palsy fed via gastrostomy [see comments]. Pediatrics 1988; 82:857–62.
11. Sanders KD, Cox K, Cannon R, et al. Growth response to enteral feeding by children with cerebral palsy. J Parenteral Enteral Nutr 1990; 14:23–6.
12. VanGelderen H. Studies in oligophrenia. Acta Paediatr Scand 1962; 51:643–648.
13. Thorne SE, Radford MJ. A comparative longitudinal study of gastrostomy devices in children. West J Nurs Res 1998; 20:145–59, discussion 159–65.
14. Eddy T, Nickolson A, Wheeler E. Energy expenditures and dietary intakes in cerebral palsy. Devel Med Clin Neurol 1965; 7:377-386.
15. Plioplys AV, Kasnicka I, Lewis S, Moller D. Survival rates among children with severe neurologic disabilities. South Med J 1998; 91:161–72.

16. Bobath B. The very early treatment of cerebral palsy. Devel Med Child Neurol 1967; 9:373–390.

17. Bly L. A historical and current view of the basis for NDT. Pediat Phys Ther 1991; 3:131–135.

18. Sant AV. Neurodevelopment treatment and pediatric physical therapy: A commentary. Pediat Phys Ther 1991; 3:137–141.

19. Tyler NB, Kahn N. A home-treatment program for the cerebral-palsied child. Am J Occup Ther 1976; 30:437–40.

20. Goldkamp O. Treatment effectiveness in cerebral palsy. Arch Phys Med Rehabil 1984; 65:232–4.

21. Okawa A, Kajiura I, Hiroshima K. Physical therapeutic and surgical management in spastic diplegia. A Japanese experience. Cini Orthoped 1990; 253:38–44.

22. Mayo N. The effect of physical therapy for children with motor delay and cerebral palsy. Am J of Phys Med and Rehab 1991; 70:258–267.

23. Wright T, Nicholson J. Physiotherapy for the spastic child: An evaluation. Devl Med Child Neurol 1973; 15:146–163.

24. Carlsen PN. Comparison of two occupational therapy approaches for treating the young cerebral-palsied child. Am J Occup Ther 1975; 29:267–72.

25. Scherzer AL, Mike V, Ilson J. Physical therapy as a determinant of change in the cerebral palsied infant. Pediatrics 1976; 58:47–52.

26. Sommerfeld D, Fraser B, Hensinger R, Beresford C. Evaluation of physical therapy service for severely mentally impaired students with cerebral palsy. Phys Ther 1981; 61:338–344.

27. DeGangi GA, Hurley L, Linscheid TR. Toward a methodology of the short-term effects of neurodevelopmental treatment. Am J Occup Ther 1983; 37:479–84.

28. Laskas C, Mullen S, Nelson D, Willson-Broyles M. Enhancement of two motor functions of the lower extremity in a child with spastic quadriplegia. Phys Ther 1985; 65:11–16.

29. Palmer FB, Shapiro BK, Wachtel RC, et al. The effects of physical therapy on cerebral palsy. A controlled trial in infants with spastic diplegia. N Engl J Med 1988; 318:803–8.

30. Palmer FB, Shapiro BK, Allen MC, et al. Infant stimulation curriculum for infants with cerebral palsy: effects on infant temperament, parent-infant interaction, and home environment. Pediatrics 1990; 85:411–5.

31. Lilly L, Powell N. Measuring the effects of neurodevelopmental treatment on the daily living skills of 2 children with cerebral palsy. Am J Occup Ther 1990; 44: 139–145.

32. Embrey D, Yates L, Mott D. Effects of neuro-developmental treatment and orthoses on knee flexion during gait: a single-subject design. Phys Ther 1990; 70:626–637.

33. Law M, Cadman D, Rosenbaum P, Walter S, Russell D, DeMatteo C. Neurodevelopmental therapy and upper-extremity inhibitive casting for children with cerebral palsy [see comments]. Dev Med Child Neurol 1991; 33:379-87.

34. Law M, Russell D, Pollock N, Rosenbaum P, Walter S, King G. A comparison of intensive neurodevelopmental therapy plus casting and a regular occupational therapy program for children with cerebral palsy. Dev Med Child Neurol 1997; 39:664–70.

35. Ottenbacher K, Biocca Z, DeCremer G, Gevelinger M, Jedlovec K, Johnson M. Quantitative Analysis of the Effectiveness of Pediatric Therapy. Phys Ther 1986; 66:1095–1101.

36. Parette H, Hourcade J. Early intervention: A conflict of therapist and educator. Percept Motor Skills 1983; 57:1056–1058.

37. Butler C. High tech tots: Technology for mobility, manipulation, communication, and learning in early childhood. Infants Young Child 1988; 1:66–73.

38. Butler C. Augmentative mobility: Why do it? In: Jaffe K, ed. Pediatric Rehabilitation. Philadelphia: Physical Medicine and Rehabilitation Clinics of North America, 1991.

39. Berlin LJ, Brooks-Gunn J, McCarton C, McCormick MC. The effectiveness of early intervention: examining risk factors and pathways to enhanced development. Prev Med 1998; 27:238–45.

40. Ramey CT, Ramey SL. Prevention of intellectual disabilities: early interventions to improve cognitive development. Prev Med 1998; 27:224–32.

41. d'Avignon M, Noren L, Arman T. Early physiotherapy ad modum Vojta or Bobath in infants with suspected neuromotor disturbance. Neuropediatrics 1981; 12:232–241.

42. Guralnick M, Heiser K, Eaton A, Bennett F, Richardson H, Groom J. Pediatricians' perceptions of the effectiveness of early intervention for at-risk and handicapped children. J Devel Behav Ped 1998; 9:12–18.

43. Rothberg AD, Goodman M, Jacklin LA, Cooper PA. Six-year follow-up of early physiotherapy intervention in very low birth weight infants. Pediatrics 1991; 88:547-52.

44. Brandt S, Lonstrup H, Marner T, Rump K, Selmar P, Schack L. Prevention of cerebral in motor risk infants by treatment ad modum Vojta. Acta Pediatr Scand 1980; 69:283–286.

45. Kong E. Very early treatment of cerebral palsy. Devel Med Child Neurol 1966; 8:198–202.

46. Imamura S, Sakuma K, Takahashi T. Follow-up study of children with cerebral coordination disturbance (CCD, Vojta). Brain Devel 1983; 5:311–314.

47. Goodman M, Rothberg A, Houston-McMillan J, al. et al. Effect of early neurodevelopmental therapy in normal and at-risk survivors of neonatal intensive care. Lancet 1985; 2:1327–1330.

48. Piper M, Kunos V, Willis D, Mazer B, Ramsey M, Silver K. Early physical therapy effects on the high-risk infant: A randomized controlled trial. Pediatrics 1986; 78:216–224.

49. Saylor C, Casto G, Huntington L. Predictors of developmental outcomes for medically fragile early intervention participants. J Ped Psychol 1996; 21:869–887.

50. Weindling A, Hallam P, Gregg J, Klenka H, Rosenbloom L, Hutton J. A randomized controlled trial of early physiotherapy for high-risk infants. Acta Paed 1996; 85:1107–1111.

51. Lambrenos K, Weindlilng A, Calam R, Cox A. The effect of a child's disability on mother's mental health. Arch Dis Child 1996; 74:115–120.

12
Future Perspective on Cerebral Palsy

Alfred L. Scherzer
Joan and Sanford I. Weill Medical College, Cornell University, New York, New York

Charlene Butler
Health and Special Education Consultant, Seattle, Washington

Vidya Bhushan Gupta
Metropolitan Hospital Center, New York Medical College, New York, New York

Margaret J. Barry
Department of Physical Therapy, Youngstown State University, Youngstown, Ohio

Gay L. Girolami
Pathways Center, Glenview, Illinois

Diane Fritts Ryan and Judy M. Gardner
DuPage Easter Seals, Villa Park, Illinois

I. CONSEQUENCES OF CEREBRAL PALSY

Cerebral palsy, as a chronic condition, clearly has significant impact on the individual, the family, and society. As we have seen, it will be a major factor in the growth and development of the child. Psychosocial and emotional maturation will be greatly affected (1). Schooling may present many special difficulties (2, 3). Job training and employment (4) and integration into the adult world will be challenging (5). There will be an increased risk of injuries (6), and associated

331

medical conditions (7). Life expectancy and survival will be inversely related to the extent of functional limitations (8), especially in feeding and mobility (9). Overall, life expectancy for the child with cerebral palsy will be reduced in comparison with the general population, particularly when there are significant associated medical conditions (10–12). In the age range of 15 to 19 years, for example, developmental disabilities are the fifth leading cause of non-traumatic death, with cerebral palsy most often cited (13).

The family is also at risk. The presence of cerebral palsy significantly affects siblings (14), and the mental health of parents (15). There are also special demands associated with providing transportation (16) and dealing with the education and health care systems (17), which present additional burdens.

Society is greatly affected as well. In the United States, 18% of children under 18 years of age (12.6 million) have significant chronic physical, developmental, behavioral, or emotional abnormalities (18). They have 1.5 times more physician visits, 3.5 times more hospital stays, twice the number of school days lost, and are 2.5 times more likely to repeat a grade (19). Additional demands for health and psychological services (20, 21), structural alterations, aids and equipment (22), educational requirements (23), and other community resources (24), have major financial impact. One can only speculate on the potential loss in human contribution from individuals with cerebral palsy who are either unable to fully participate in society, or remain idle (25).

II. THE CHALLENGE TO REDUCE CEREBRAL PALSY

Given the enormous consequences to the child, the family, and society, it behooves us to look for future solutions to reduce cerebral palsy incidence, prevalence, and severity. Prevention would be the approach of choice. However, for the minimum of individuals who are then ultimately involved, means must be found to reduce both the extent and severity of involvement, and to improve function. More efficient and effective educational, health, and community services need to be developed. And, finally, integration into the most appropriate and useful adult lifestyle must be achieved, with full acceptance and equal status within the community. The new millennium offers a fresh perspective from which to view these challenges.

A. Prevention

1. Congenital Cerebral Palsy

Efforts at prevention of congenital cerebral palsy must deal with the following etiological factors discussed previously in Chapter 2: birth asphyxia, prematurity, other perinatal factors, and possible prenatal factors.

(a) *Birth Asphyxia.* The saga of cerebral palsy that started two centuries ago is likely to reach its denouement in this new millennium, when advances in molecular biology will literally take us to the root of this condition. Two centuries ago we identified the phenomenon of cerebral palsy and its two common associations, birth asphyxia and preterm birth. It took us a century to put the horse before the cart. Pioneering discoveries of the National Collaborative Perinatal Project (NCPP) and later work of Nelson and colleagues established that much of the asphyxia seen at term is secondary to an upstream event in the prenatal period, such as maternal infection or fetal malformations (26–28). Developing epidemiological studies are likely to reveal these upstream events, and there is hope that we shall be able to develop strategies to prevent and contain them.

Rapid strides in the last decade have unfolded the cascade from the upstream event to its final destination. We now understand that the neuronal damage in cerebral palsy is mediated by excitatory neurotransmitters such as glutamate, which open the NMDA channels, allowing calcium to enter the cell to disturb mitochondrial function (29, 30). This sets in motion a vicious cycle by further depolarizing the cell membrane and opening more channels, resulting in immediate and programmed cell death, called apoptosis. The more glutamate receptors an area has and the more metabolically active it is, the more vulnerable it will be to asphyxial damage. The basal ganglia and cerebral cortex are the most vulnerable to asphyxia in the term infant. Efforts are now underway to detect this cascade at an earlier point so that it can be nipped in the bud.

New developments in magnetic resonance spectroscopy, near-infrared spectroscopy, and magnetic resonance imaging will enable us to localize and quantify problems in cerebral metabolism following intrapartum hypoxic-ischemic injury (31). In the future, we may be able to monitor changes in cerebral hemodynamics during labor with near-infrared spectroscopy study, thus decreasing our dependence on the much less accurate technique of fetal heart rate monitoring. We may be able to identify hypoxic-ischemic injury early by detecting elevated cerebral lactate concentration. This may allow us to identify infants who could benefit from the new cerebroprotective treatments. These neuronal rescue therapies include drugs that inhibit release of calcium, such as calcium channel blockers, drugs that block glutamate receptors, such as NMDA receptor antagonists, free radical scavengers, nitric oxide synthase inhibitors, and hypothermia (32, 33). The role of carbon dioxide and glucose is being elucidated so that we can manage newborns better.

While there have been many recent innovative developments in the very early identification of hypoxemia/ischemia (34), the technology at present is extremely expensive, still highly complex, and may not be readily available. There is a need for more clinically accessible procedures that can lead to earlier and more widespread use and appropriate intervention.

(b) Prematurity. Another revolutionary achievement of medicine has been the survival of tiny infants, with increasing numbers now born at less than 28 weeks of gestation, often weighing 750 g or less. This has brought in its wake a higher prevalence of disabling conditions, such as cerebral palsy. This millennium holds the promise of saving even tinier newborns and the challenge of saving them without disabling conditions. The preterm brain has its unique pattern of vulnerability to injury. Whereas in the full-term infant the basal ganglia are more prone to hypoxic-ischemic injury, the periventricular white matter bears the brunt of insult in the preterm infant because of the vulnerability of oligodendrocyte precursors to free radicals and inflammatory cytokines (35). Death of oligodentrocytes leads to failure of myelination. It is hoped that we will be able to stop this cascade by preventing oligodendrocyte death through scavenging free radicals, and promoting myelination and axonal growth by providing trophic factors, such as basic fibroblast growth factor and IGF-1 (36). Understanding the molecular basis of cell death and treatments targeted to prevent cell death may finally lead to a decrease in the prevalence of cerebral palsy that has eluded us so far, despite all the advances in obstetrics and neonatal care.

The preterm birth rate in the United States is increasing, and low-birth-weight births (<2500 g) are at the highest level reported since 1973 (37). This is a major factor in the U.S. ranking of 24th in infant mortality among other developed countries (38). Multivariate causality relates to social and economic conditions, and issues of maternal health and nutrition (39). However, many unanswered questions remain concerning the actual mechanisms involved, and there is need to better understand the etiology of adverse pregnancy outcomes along the entire birth weight spectrum (40). Definitive studies are essential to identify and deal with all possible variables, while renewed efforts are made to clearly reduce preventable causes such as maternal use of tobacco, alcohol, and drugs. Certainly, a future hope would be for some form of manipulation affecting the events at the cellular level, and possibly even genetic engineering to mothers at risk.

(c) Other Perinatal Factors. Although there is generally a well-established routine for management of hyperbilirubinemia, possible maternal infection with chlamydia and other pathogens must be identified and treated appropriately (34). Another therapeutic challenge is recently identified maternal clotting disorders that may lead to strokes and cerebral palsy (Leiden mutation) and disorders related to autoimmunity and hypercoaguability (41).

(d) Prenatal Factors. Factors associated with maternal general health and appropriate treatment of remedial conditions, such as thyroid abnormalities and infection, must be addressed vigorously. Likewise, maternal exposure to tobacco, alcohol, drugs, toxins, and radiation needs to be targeted through aggres-

sive public health education and further studies of environmental hazards should be performed.

2. Acquired Cerebral Palsy

Preventive efforts require early identification and treatment of childhood infections and vascular abnormalities that can involve the central nervous system. Trauma also remains a major factor, especially where childhood supervision is limited, and is an increasing peril in areas of the world where landmines are prevalent (42). The international community must be sensitized to the devastating effects of residual land mines causing traumatic brain injury as well as limb deficits where there are the least resources to provide needed care.

3. Genetic Cerebral Palsy

Special populations at risk (43, 44) must be made aware of susceptibility and provided appropriate education and counseling. At the same time, additional studies need to continue case finding and probing definitive genetic etiology.

B. REDUCTION OF EXTENT AND SEVERITY

1. Definition of Cerebral Palsy

Several issues surround the current nosology of cerebral palsy, including lack of a precise and universally agreed definition, difficulty of case ascertainment due to the uncertain time of onset, and changing signs and symptoms during its early evolution. Cerebral palsy is different from other medical conditions in that it is defined as a disability, an abnormality of motor function. However, the degree of motor function that qualifies as cerebral palsy is not standardized. Is clumsiness cerebral palsy? Does abnormal tone, posture, and reflexes, in the absence of significant functional deficit, constitute cerebral palsy?

Cerebral palsy is defined as an injury to the immature brain, but there is no clear consensus on a time frame for delineating congenital and acquired categories. In the United States and Sweden, for example, etiology that occurs beyond the neonatal period is considered acquired, whereas in Australia this designation is used only with events beyond 5 years. Should postneonatal cases in which a definite etiology is identifiable be included as congenital or acquired? Should motor dysfunction due to identifiable chromosomal and genetic conditions be called cerebral palsy? Perhaps a consensus may never be reached on these issues and we may move to a noncategorical definition based entirely upon functional limitations. This latter approach is gaining ground for programmatic and administrative reasons (45).

In this volume, we have attempted to clarify the definition of cerebral palsy as a static encephalopathy with primary motor characteristics. Moreover, it is *developmental* in nature, and must be viewed in relation to changes in the growing infant. The current classification does not sufficiently reflect the dynamic and changing nature of the condition, especially in the young child. A more up-to-date classification is needed to help emphasize the duality of this static condition that has, at the same time, dynamic, changing features. Nevertheless, "cerebral palsy" is not a wastebasket term to be used indiscriminately for any child with possible delays or retardation. These concepts are essential for all health practitioners to understand as a basis for appropriate referral and treatment.

2. Early Diagnostic Referral

We have seen that an orderly, systematic approach to early diagnosis can be achieved with a high degree of specificity; that functional levels and change over time can be predictably measured with a large variety of screening instruments. The procedures, techniques, and many tools are therefore available now. Unfortunately, the extent of very early referral continues to be limited for infants with developmental delay (46), although well accepted for those with a clear diagnosis (47). Renewed efforts must be made to acquaint health professionals with the techniques and value of early diagnosis so that appropriate referral can be made for both management and treatment, even if there are not sufficient criteria for a specific label.

3. Management

Assistance to families with daily care and management of the infant with cerebral palsy is a cornerstone in early intervention. This is an area with few relevant studies and needs more data regarding parental communication, cross-cultural variables, and specific techniques for dealing with both the child and the environment.

4. Therapy

(a) Treatment Outcomes Research. As indicated in Chapter 11, the available levels of evidence provided by published research studies do not presently substantiate specific long-term benefits of either neurodevelopmental therapy (NDT), or early intervention for any method of physical therapy for infants who are eventually diagnosed with cerebral palsy. This does not mean that these approaches are ineffective, nor does it mean that these studies supply negative proof. On the contrary, the evidence tables and reviews of treatment outcomes in Chapter 11 demonstrate that for all three interventions reviewed there is a paucity of adequate studies from which we may learn about the efficacy of inter-

ventions. This is in fact true for all interventions in cerebral palsy—and, indeed, for almost all interventions in health care because it is in an interim period. Health care is in the process of leaving behind a paradigm that is exclusively based on the compelling logic of current understanding about the mechanism of action of interventions in human biology. It is entering a paradigm that requires empirical evidence in addition to this compelling logic of biology and theory. Health care is just beginning to build this empirical base.

The AACPDM methodology for systematic reviews is already pointing out gaps in research that need to be filled by future research, particularly the lack of any data outside the dimension of impairment. There is an immediate need for research protocols to include multiple measures across dimensions of disablement. Also, the internal validity of the majority of current studies is wanting. Thus, there is an urgent need for more studies, especially those that produce stronger levels of evidence.

Conducting definitive research studies in cerebral palsy is more difficult than in other areas of health care, but these problems will be overcome as the requirement for empirical evidence grows. One of the thorny issues is how to conduct treatment evaluation in chronic, sometimes severe, and often complex disabilities present from early childhood. Group research that has a long tradition in medicine is not well suited to the study of such disabilities. There are, however, other approaches that do lend themselves to treatment evaluation in low-incidence, highly heterogeneous populations, notably, single subject research (or within subjects methods).

The group and single subjects approaches are differentiated by the type of variation each method measures. Group research is limited to a measure of the variation of results at a group level. Single subject research measures the variation of results for an individual. But when multiple individuals are studied, single subject research can also measure the consistency of variation for the group and produce a group result.

Single subject research offers an alternative to group research and is the method of choice in two situations. One of these situations is the study of interventions in populations so heterogeneous in nature that any summative statements of groups as a whole might be terribly misleading. Another situation is the study of low-density populations in which it is not feasible to muster even the smallest of group sizes that would be acceptable for a reasonable group study. Both of these situations exist in the study of interventions for individuals with cerebral palsy.

In treatment evaluation, single subject strategies can prove to be as powerful and persuasive as group strategies. While most of the same factors can threaten the credibility of findings from a group or single subject study, the group methods usually seek to control for those threats by distributing potentially confounding factors evenly among the various groups. The uneven (albeit unknown and unintentional) distribution of these factors in one group provides one of the most common threats to validity (called biased subject selection) in group studies. Single subject methods obviate this particular threat to internal validity because, with no groups, there is no potential for unknown bias in one of the groups. In addition, single subject methods allow for the direct observation and analysis of other threats. Thus, single subject methods can produce strong credibility (internal validity) that the observed changes can be attributed to the intervention, or conversely, that the intervention was not efficacious (not able to bring about the desired result).

In single subject methods, the same person is exposed to both the treatment and the control condition(s), thus acting as his or her own control. Attributing the measured difference to the intervention depends on comparing stability of outcomes measured repeatedly during each condition, and on shifts in the obtained differences being consistently coincident with the shifts between the treatment and control conditions.

Most researchers in developmental disabilities are currently unfamiliar with single subjects methods. As they begin to appreciate and embrace this research methodology along with group methodology, however, there will be increased opportunity to produce definitive research.

(b)   Evolving Therapy Approaches.   Therapeutic theory, methods, and clinical application will naturally continue to evolve as therapists look for models that more closely mirror the CNS acquisition of motor control. The dynamic systems approach, which emphasizes environmental interaction for function, has become prominent in recent years. Rather than being a new and separate therapy modality, it strongly supports a trend of all therapy interventions to become more successful at achieving and maintaining *function*. It may also become an important factor in how all therapy procedures evolve. Further research and appropriate evidence-based studies will be needed to substantiate its relevance and effectiveness.

In whatever direction research may guide the therapy process in the future, it is clear that there will always be a need for sound clinical judgment in selecting treatment alternatives. Moreover, therapy should not be considered a way of life in itself, but a means to help improve function and, thereby, quality of life. Interventions must fit into a family's daily routine, not consume them. And the word "compliance" should be taken out of our vocabulary. There should be no adverse judgments about a family's acceptance or rejection of our recommendations.

5.   Other Treatment Modalities

Botulinum A toxin, intrathecal baclofen, and selective dorsal rhizotomy have all gained widespread acceptance in recent years, each with strong adherents and varied approaches to clinical use. Unfortunately, there are very few conclusive data about any of these treatments that support their effects on individual functional change or long-term benefit. Moreover, there is no uniformity or standardization of protocols in using these modalities either individually or in combination. Appropriate studies are urgently needed to enable a more rational approach to these current practices, and to achieve professionally agreed-upon standards of uniform criteria and clinical application.

It should also be noted that new treatment modalities have come into clinical practice in the past largely through trial and error, or as an extension from other established uses. The new theoretical insights of the central nervous system at the molecular level now offer possibilities for planned prospective studies in the future that are unparalleled. These should include such approaches as genetic engineering, changes in neurotransmitters, and alteration of brain tissue, among others.

6. Technology

Cerebral palsy is more appropriately regarded as a developmental disorder than a musculoskeletal condition. For some years, there has been a growing recognition in child development fields that physical and psychological development are interrelated and that early experiences influence all subsequent behavior. When development along any line (motor, cognitive, social, emotional) is restricted, delayed, or distorted, the other lines of development are adversely affected as well. Motor skills that develop rapidly during the first 3 years of life are the primary vehicle for learning and socialization. They foster a sense of competence and independence. Through their motor interactions, infants and toddlers learn about things and people in their world, and also discover they can cause things to happen. They become active initiators and participants rather than passive recipients of experience.

Infants and toddlers with cerebral palsy often lack the necessary movements for locomotion, manipulation, and speech that make it possible for them to engage and act on their environment. Thus, learning opportunities are hindered. Equally important, their inability to influence the environment, that is, to affect or alter it through their own actions, leads to a condition of learned helplessness in which children give up trying to control their own world (48). Repeated failure in exploring and mastering situations leads to a self-perception of incompetence and a passive resignation that extinguishes further attempts (49). A sense of helplessness (or a sense of incompetence) is well established by four years of age (50, 51).

With the assistance of technology, even very young children with cerebral palsy can experience more success in directly controlling their environment, thereby reducing or avoiding secondary social-emotional and intellectual disabilities (52). Increasingly, opportunities for using technology have become available to the birth to 3 population. Computer applications, powered mobility, augmentative communication devices, environmental control systems, and battery-powered toys have been successfully demonstrated in research settings. Infants as young as 3 months have interacted with computers, 18-month-old children have driven powered mobility devices skillfully and safely, and 2-year old children have talked via speech synthesizers. For severely involved children, use of these assistive technologies depends on first learning to use switches and/or scanning techniques on which they may always have to rely for control of all their mobility, communication, independent learning, and environmental interaction. Children who are competent users of these technologies by the time they enter school have a greater potential for achieving success in mainstream education, and for participating in other normal social roles in their families and communities.

Assistive technologies in the use of adaptive, supportive, and mobility equipment will be greatly enhanced in the future as the demand for appropriate hardware and software for this young population grows. Families will increasingly understand that use of these technologies will not demotivate youngsters to strive to walk, talk, and manipulate things with their hands, but instead offer a means by which motor disabilities can be by-passed. Appropriate timing for their use is not after children have failed to achieve normal movement through extensive casting, bracing, surgery, and therapy, but when a particular motor skill or activity appears in normal development. If, for example, there is no efficient ambulation shortly after the age of one year, a developmental approach to management would substitute as an alternative means of mobility using assistive technology. The aim would be to promote overall development rather than merely improve the musculoskeletal disorder, although the latter cannot be ignored. Planned, total integration in the anticipation of and use of all assistive devices for a given child requires priority consideration, and must be built into the overall intervention program as it develops (53, 54).

7. Effective Use of Services

Community health, education, and social services for the child with cerebral palsy vary widely in accessibility and ease of use. On the one hand, many similar treatment facilities may exist in a given area, creating confusion about what would be most appropriate. On the other hand, the lack of facilities in some localities requires extensive travel to obtain services. Moreover, often both practitioners and parents are not knowledgeable about available resources, and it is not unusual for families to be endlessly confused about where to obtain help. Health facilities, schools, and social agencies need to provide information to professionals about available services in a more centralized way, which must then be communicated more effectively to families. And, in turn, education of parents must focus on providing a clear understanding of how to become better involved in the health, education, and social systems with which they will have to deal.

Habilitation of the very young child implies the use of a wide variety of services over a long period of time. Costs of health care, transportation, and the financial implications of lost work time to utilize services are all important factors that bear on family interaction and ultimate benefit to the child. The burden of organizing and paying for needed services can be staggering for families, especially those at the low end of the economic scale. The current managed care health system in the United States is not designed to deal effectively and efficiently with the need for coordinated, multispecialty care required by the infant with cerebral palsy. Dealing with this system has added to the demands placed upon the families of children who increasingly benefit from the new technological advances that enable very early diagnosis and referral. This paradoxical situation requires strong advocacy as legislation and administrative changes continue to be made in the evolving health care system.

8.   Integration into the Community

Ultimate success of the early diagnosis and treatment process will depend on how well the child with cerebral palsy can be integrated into the adult community. There are many existing gaps and inconsistencies in education and training that need to be addressed, and a much more organized transition process to adulthood must become an integral part of the education process. A goal of full and equal employment remains more a hope than an achievement, while societal acceptance with total participation is a dream that will continue to require continuous and vigorous efforts at attitude change. A new millennium could provide the impetus to jump-start efforts to achieve these goals, providing we are motivated to make them a high priority.

III.   CEREBRAL PALSY IN THE DEVELOPING WORLD

The United States and the western industrial nations have had the resources and technological capability to develop what is considered to be the "standard" of treatment in this field. This is the case even though we continue to lack adequate scientific validity of our own methods, as we have seen. At any rate, we have until recently applied our procedures as best we can, primarily within our own societies and cultures.

We can now begin to see some extension in the application of our technology beyond our own borders, for a new revolutionary component is upon us. In spite of ever-present infectious diseases and malnutrition, increasing numbers of children are now surviving with greater frequency. According to United Nations estimates (55), and international surveys (56), some two thirds of the world's 500 million handicapped children live in Third World nations.

A number of official agencies such as UNICEF, WHO, individual governments, and nongovernmental organizations are now actively involved in working with these areas on the problems of children with handicaps. Confusion, overlapping, and duplication of efforts continue to be a mark in some of these activities, largely due to the numbers of agencies and programs involved, as well as problems in communication and information exchange between them.

More important, the direct application of our purely Western technology and methods is obviously impractical economically, and clearly inappropriate culturally. Both WHO and UNICEF recognized the need to overcome these obstacles several years ago and helped initiate the Community-Based Rehabilitation (CBR) movement (57). In a large number of Third World countries, projects begun at the grass roots level in the 1980s (often initiated locally) have continued to flourish (58). Technical personnel train local individuals in rudimentary early identification of handicaps, simple methods of treatment, and use of local materials for needed equipment (59–61). This type of activity will surely be in greater demand as we can anticipate increasing survival of children with handicaps in these areas and little likelihood of improved resources in the foreseeable future.

Of major concern is the continued presence of land mines. The resultant brain and limb trauma to untold numbers of children is a major factor in the incidence of acquired cerebral palsy. Although some additional rehabilitation services are being made available, the demands are staggering, while resources and even recognition of the problem remain less than acceptable (62).

Therefore, the time has come for us to increasingly use our expertise to assist in this effort. We need to have a firmer grasp on the relevance of our own therapy and treatment methods through the kinds of studies we have previously indicated. We must then have the skill and wisdom to adapt them to cultures elsewhere, such as the Third World, where there is need for a simple, economically feasible, and practical approach (63). Any system of therapy and treatment that evolves will have little relevance unless it takes into account the social and cultural context of a disability rather than simply the diagnosis alone. An opportunity and an obligation is now before us to bring this kind of world perspective into our treatment efforts.

REFERENCES

1. Darrow D, Stephens S. Interferences in psychosocial development of seriously health-impaired and physically disabled children. Educational implications. Acta Paedopsychiatr 1992; 55:41–44.
2. Hall CD, Porter P. School intervention for the neuromuscularly handicapped child. J Pediatr 1983; 102:210-214.

3. Ross G, Lipper EG, Auld PA. Educational status and school-related abilities of very low birth weight premature children. Pediatrics 1991; 88:1125–1134.
4. O'Grady RS, Nishimura DM, Kohn JG, Bruvold WH. Vocational predictions compared with vocational status of 60 young adults with cerebral palsy. Dev Med Child Neurol 1985; 27:775–784.
5. Fiorentino L, Datta D, Gentle S, Hall DM, Harpin V, Phippis D, Walker A. Transition from school to adult life for physically disabled young people. Arch Dis Child 1988; 79:306–311.
6. Dunne RG, Asher KN, Rivara FP. Injuries in young people with developmental disabilities. Comparative investigation from the 1988 National Health Survey. Ment Retard 1993; 31:83–88.
7. Cathels BA, Reddihough DS. The health care of young adults with cerebral palsy. Med J Aust 1993; 159:444–446.
8. Hutton JL, Cooke T, Pharoah PO. Life expectancy in children with cerebral palsy. Br Med J 1994; 309:431–435.
9. Strauss P, Shavelle R. Life expectancy of adults with cerebral palsy. Dev Med Child Neurol 1998; 40:369–375.
10. Chrichton JU, Mackinnon M, White CP. Life expectancy of persons with cerebral palsy. Dev Med Child Neurol 1995; 37:567–576.
11. Plioplys AV, Kasnicka I, Lewis S, Moller D. Survival rates among children with severe neurologic disabilities. South Med J 1998; 91:161–172.
12. Strauss D, Cable W, Shavelle R. Causes of excess mortality in cerebral palsy. Dev Med Child Neurol 1999; 41:580–585.
13. Boyle CA, Decoufle P, Holmgreen P. Contribution of developmental disabilities to childhood mortality in the United States: a multiple cause of death analysis. Paediatr Perinat Epidemiol 1994; 18:411–422.
14. Dallas E, Stevenson J, McGurk H. Cerebral palsied children's interaction with siblings II. Interactional structure. J Child Psychol Psychiatry 1993; 34:649–671.
15. Lambrenos K, Weindling AM, Calam R, Cox AD. The effect of a child's disability on mother's mental health. Arch Dis Child 1996; 74:115–120.
16. Paley K, Walker JL, Cromwell F, Enlow C. Transportation of children with special seating needs. South Med J 1993; 86:1339–1341.
17. Sloper P, Turner S. Service needs of families of children with severe physical disability. Child Care Health Dev 1992; 18:259–282.
18. Newacheck PW, Strickland B, Shonkoff JP, Perrin JM, McPherson M, McManus M, Lauver C, Fox H, Arango P. An epidemiologic profile of children with special health care needs. Pediatrics 1998; 102:117–123.
19. Boyle CA, Decoufle P, Yeargin-Allsopp M. Prevalence and health impact of developmental disabilities in United States children. Pediatrics 1994; 93:399–403.
20. Ireys HT, Anderson GF, Shaffer TJ, Neff JM. Expenditures for care of children with chronic illnesses enrolled in the Washington State Medicaid Program, fiscal year 1993. Pediatrics 1997; 100:197–204.
21. Rodman J, Weill K, Driscoll M, Fenton T, Alpert H, Salem-Schatz S, Palfrey JS. A nation-wide survey of financing health related services for special education students. J School Health 1999; 69:133–139.
22. Hull R, Prouse P, Sherratt C, Brennan D, Townsend J, Frank A. Capital costs of supporting young disabled people at home. Health Trends 1994; 26:80–85.

23. Parrish TB, Chambers JG. Financing special education. Future Child 1996; 6:121–138.

24. Prouse P, Ross-Smith K, Brill M, Singh M, Brennan P, Frank A. Community support for young physically handicapped people. Health Trends 1991; 23:105–109.

25. Ireys HT, Salkever DS, Kolodner KB, Bijur PE. Schooling, employment, and idleness in young adults with serious physical health conditions: effects of age, disability status, and parental education. J Adolesc Health 1996; 19:25–33.

26. Nelson KB, Ellenberg J. Antecedents of cerebral palsy, multivariate analysis of risk. N Engl J Med 1986; 315:81-86.

27. Nelson KB, Grethers JK. Potentially asphyxiating conditions and spastic cerebral palsy in infants of normal birth weight. Am J Obset Gynecol 1998; 179:507–513.

28. Susser M, Hauser WA, Kiely JL, Paneth N, and Stein Z. Quantitative estimates of prenatal and perinatal risk factors for perinatal mortality, cerebral palsy, mental retardation and epilepsy. In: Prenatal and Perinatal Factors Associated with Brain Disorders, John M. Freeman, ed. Washington, D.C.: US Department of Health and Human Services, 1985.

29. Choi DW, Rothman SM. The role of glutamate neurotoxicity in hypoxic-ischemic neuronal death. Ann Rev Neurosci 1990; 13:171–182.

30. Frandsen A, Schousboe A. Mobilization of dantrolene-sensitive intracellular calcium pools involved in the cytotoxicity induced by quisqualate and N-methyl -D-aspartate but not by 2-amino-3-(3-hydroxy-5-methylisoxazol-4-yl)propionate and kainate in cultured cerebral cortical neurons. Proc Natl Acad Sci USA 1992; 89:2590–2594.

31. Wyatt JS. Magnetic resonance spectroscopy and near-infrared spectroscopy in the assessment of asphyxiated term infant. Ment Retard and Develop Disabilities Res Rev. 1997; 3:42–48.

32. Clemens JA, Panetta JA. Neuroprotection by antioxidants in models of global and focal ischemia. Ann NY Acad Sci 1994; 738:250–256.

33. Xue D, Huang Z-G, Smith KE et al. Immediate or delayed mild hypothermia prevents focal cerebral infarction. Brain Res 1992; 587:66–72.

34. Nelson K. Changing horizons in understanding pathophysiology: prevention and treatment of infant brain injury. Fifty-Third Annual Meeting of the American Academy for Cerebral Palsy and Developmental Medicine, Washington, D.C., Sept 15–18, 1999.

35. Selmaj K, Raine CS, Farooq et al. Cytokine cytotoxicity against oligoodendrocytes: apoptosis induced by lymphotoxin. J Immunol 1991; 147:1522–1529.

36. Mattson MP, Cheng B, Smith-Swintosky VL. Mechanisms of neurotrophic factor protection against calcium- and free radical-mediated excitotoxic injury: Implications for treating neurodegenerative disorders. Exp Neurol 1993; 124:89–95.

37. Ventura SJ, Martin JA, Curtin SC, Mathews TJ. Births: final data for 1997. Nat Vital Stat Rep 1999; 47:1–96.

38. Guyer B, Hoyert DL, Martin JA, Ventura SJ, MacDorman MF, Strobino DM. Annual summary of vital stastics 1998. Pediatrics 1999; 104:1229–1246.

39. Meis PJ, Goldenberg RL, Mercer BM, Iams JD, Moawad AIT, Miodovnik M, Menard MK, Caritis SN, Thurnau GR, Bottoms SF, Das A, Roberts JM, McNellis D. The preterm prediction study: risk factors for indicated preterm births. Maternal-

fetal medicine units. Network of NICHHD. Am J Obstet Gynecol 1998; 178:562–567.

40. Lang JM, Lieberman E, Cohen A. A comparison of risk factors for preterm labor and term small-for-gestational-age birth. Epidemiology 1996; 7:369–376.

41. Harum KH, Hoon AH, Casella JF. Factor-V Leiden: a risk factor for cerebral palsy. Dev Med Child Neurol 1999; 41:781–785.

42. Forjuoh SN, Zwi AB. Violence against children and adolescents. International perspectives. Pediatr Clin North Am 1998; 45:415–426.

43. Sinha G, Corry P, Subesinghe D, Wild J, Levene MI. Prevalence and type of cerebral palsy in a British ethnic community: the role of consanguinity. Dev Med Child Neurol 1997; 39:259–262.

44. Mitchell S, Bundy S. Symmetry of neurological signs in Pakistani patients with probable inherited spastic cerebral palsy. Clin Genet 1997; 51:7–14.

45. Kuroda MM and Durkin M. The categorical and non- categorical approaches to identifying children with cerebral palsy: results from the National Health Interview Survey. Dev Med Child Neurol 1999; 41(suppl)8.

46. Reddihough DS, Tinworth S, Moore TG, Ibsen E. Early intervention: professional views and referral practices of Australian paediatricians. J. Paediatr Child Health 1996; 32:246–250.

47. Liptak GS. The role of the pediatrician in caring for children with developmental disabilities: overview. Pediatr Ann 1995; 24:232–237.

48. Rosenbloom L. Consequences of impaired movement: A hypothesis and review. In: Holt KS, ed. Movement and Child Development. Philadelphia: Lippincott, 1975: 159–162.

49. Lewis M, Goldberg S. Perceptual-cognitive development in infancy: A generalized expectancy model as a function of the mother-infant interaction. Merrill-Palmer Q 1969; 15:81–100.

50. Harter S. Effectance motivation revisited: Toward a developmental model. Hum Devel 1978; 21:34–64.

51. Safford P, Arbitman D. Developmental Intervention with Young Physically Handicapped Children. Springfield, IL: Charles C Thomas, 1975.

52. Kohn M. Symptoms and Underachievement in Childhood: A Longitudinal Perspective. New York: Wiley, 1977.

53. Butler C. High tech tots: Technology for mobility, manipulation, communication, and learning in early childhood. Infants Young Child 1988; 1:66–73.

54. Nisbet P. Integrating assistive technologies: current practices and future possibilities. Med Eng Phys 1996; 18:193–202.

55. Hammerman S, Irwin M. Community based rehabilitation: essence of the new strategy in childhood rerhabilitation. UNICEF/RI One in Ten 1981; 1:1.

56. Renker K. World statistics on disabled persons. Int J Rehabil Res 1982; 5:167–177.

57. Helander E, Mendis P, Nelson G. Training Disabled People in the Community – A Manual on Community Based Rehabilitation for Developing Countries. Geneva: WHO, 1983.

58. Finnstam J, Grimby G, Nelson G, Rashid S. Evaluation of community based rehabilitation in Punjab, Pakistan I: Use of the WHO Manual, 'Training disabled people in the community.' Int Disabil Stud 1988; 10:54 58.

59. Hardoff D, Chigier E. Developing community based services for youth with disabilities. Pediatrician 1991; 18:157–162.
60. Rao PH, Venkatesan, Svepuri VG. Community based rehabilitation services for people with disabilities: an experimental study. Int J Rehabil Res 1993; 16:245–250.
61. Parver CP, Levin B. Community-based rehabilitation programs in five countries. Caring 1997; 16:26–28, 30, 32-34.
62. Kakar F, Bassani F, Romer CJ, Gunn SW. The consequences of land mines on public health. Prehospital Disaster Med 1996; 11:2–10.
63. Werner D. Disabled Village Children—A guide for Community Health Workers, Rehabilitation Workers, and Families. Palo Alto: Hesperian Foundation, 1987.

Index

Abnormal infant neurologic development, 51–52
 consequences of, 96–101
  discordant neurologic maturation, 96
  motor patterns of behavior and deprivation, 99–100
  oral development deficits, 100–101
  sensory deficit and function, 98–99
  specific motor abnormality; posture and movement, 100
  tone abnormality, 96–97
 developmental milestones, 52
 general movements, 51
 motor abnormality, 52
 prediction of, 52–55
 tone, 52
American Academy for Cerebral Palsy:
 becomes AACPDM, 12
 establishment, 10
 founders, 10

American Academy for Cerebral Palsy and Developmental Medicine:
 classification of levels of evidence, 275–277
 treatment outcomes framework, 272–273
Apgar score, and prediction of developmental abnormality, 32, 52–53
Appraisal of treatment outcomes literature, problems in, 271–272
Assessment and treatment planning, case study, 229–266
 assessment, 229–238
  assessment work sheet, 232
  written assessment, 232–234
 charting progress, 259
 initial treatment plan, 238–259
  treatment planning worksheet, 251, 254
  treatment strategies, 254, 259
Assessment models of disability:
 National Center for Medical Rehabilitation Research, 130, 142, 271, 273
 World Health Organization ICIDH-2, 130, 142, 271, 273

About the Editor

ALFRED L. SCHERZER is Clinical Professor Emeritus of Pediatrics at Cornell University—Joan and Sanford I. Weill Medical College, New York, N.Y., and Clinical Professor of Preventative Medicine, State University of New York at Stony Brook. He is Director of the Child Habilitation Center and is also in Private Consultation Practice specializing in Developmental Pediatrics. The author or coauthor of over 70 publications, he is an Emeritus Fellow of the American Academy of Pediatrics and a past president of the American Academy for Cerebral Palsy and Developmental Medicine, among numerous other professional affiliations. Professor Scherzer received his medical degree from Columbia University and also holds degrees in public health, sociology, and education.